The Little Black Book of Geriatrics

Series Editor: Daniel K

FOURTH EDITION

Karen Gershman, MD, CMD, CAQ Geriatrics
Associate Professor of Community and
Family Medicine
Dartmouth Medical School
Faculty, Maine–Dartmouth Family Practice
Residency Program,
Director of Geriatric Fellowship
Augusta, Maine

JONES AND BARTLETT PUBLISHERS
Sudbury, Massachusetts
BOSTON TORONTO LONDON SINGAPORE

World Headquarters
Jones and Bartlett Publishers
40 Tall Pine Drive
Sudbury, MA 01776
978-443-5000
info@jbpub.com
www.jbpub.com

Jones and Bartlett Publishers Canada
6339 Ormindale Way
Mississauga, ON L5V 1J2
CANADA

Jones and Bartlett Publishers International
Barb House, Barb Mews
London W6 7PA
UK

Jones and Bartlett's books and products are available through most bookstores and online booksellers. To contact Jones and Bartlett Publishers directly, call 800-832-0034, fax 978-443-8000, or visit our website at www.jbpub.com.

Substantial discounts on bulk quantities of Jones and Bartlett's publications are available to corporations, professional associations, and other qualified organizations. For details and specific discount information, contact the special sales department at Jones and Bartlett via the above contact information, or send an email to specialsales@jbpub.com.

Copyright © 2009 by Jones and Bartlett Publishers, LLC

All rights reserved. No part of the material protected by this copyright may be reproduced or utilized in any form, electronic or mechanical, including photocopying, recording, or by any information storage and retrieval system, without written permission from the copyright owner.

Library of Congress Cataloging-in-Publication Data
Gershman, Karen
The little black book of geriatrics / Karen Gershman. — 4th ed.
p. ; cm. — (Jones and Bartlett little black book series)
Includes bibliographical references and index.
ISBN-13: 978-0-7637-5771-7
ISBN-10: 0-7637-5771-3
1. Geriatrics—Handbooks, manuals, etc. I. Title. II. Series: Little black book series.
[DNLM: 1. Geriatrics—Handbooks. WT 39 G381L 2009]
RC952.55.G485 2009
618.97—dc22
6048 2008013659

Production Credits
Executive Publisher: Christopher Davis
Senior Acquisitions Editor: Nancy Anastasi Duffy
Production Director: Amy Rose
Associate Editor: Kathy Richardson
Associate Production Editor: Mike Boblitt
Associate Marketing Manager: Ilana Goddess
Manufacturing Buyer: Therese Connell
Composition: ATLIS Graphics
Cover Design: Anne Spencer
Cover Images: © Photos.com
Printing and Binding: Malloy, Inc.
Cover Printing: Malloy, Inc.

Printed in the United States of America
12 11 10 09 10 9 8 7 6 5 4 3 2

Dedication

To Melaine Gershman-Tewksbury, MD, who in kindling hope in her patients has given off a great light.

To my parents, Professor Elaine S. Gershman and Professor Melvin Gershman, who thought I should be a physician, and whose excellent examples as teachers inspired me to be both.

K.G.

Contents

Preface to the First Edition

In college, I had the habit of reading good literature in the bathtub, late at night, sometimes until 2 or 3 in the morning. As my eyelids and hands went limp, lulled by the warm water and slumber, the book would inevitably tumble. Now, most of my treasured library is a bit waterlogged, the pages bunched and wrinkled after hanging to dry.

I could attribute my novels' misadventures to my father, a professor of microbiology. It was he who insisted that the dreaded sciences: organic chemistry, comparative physiology, physics, be tackled early in the evening. "Save the humanities for later." My precious humanities were like dessert. They accompanied the reward of a tepid tub after an arduous day of classes.

In Herman Hesse's *The Glass Bead Game,* the main character of the book, the aged and esteemed master of the glass bead game, has taken on a young apprentice. The student is unfocused, inexperienced, and restless, yet the sage sees potential in him. So he sets about enticing his pupil down the difficult road of erudition. First he must create a bond with the youth. He will gain his trust by joining the student where the student is most comfortable and unthreatened. Thus, the tutor chooses an exhilarating walk in the early morning cold.

They come to a pond. The apprentice impulsively dives into its icy depths and begins swimming its length, preferring the physical challenge, one that he knows he can master and escape for a time the embarrassment of ignorance he's apt to feel with his tutor in the cognitive realm. Left on the shore, the scholar gazes at his pupil, hoping that this is the place where they shall meet, where the bond will be created. Without pondering his own physical limitations, he plunges into the rough chill of the waters and drowns.

I still see myself in that silly bathtub, the water gone cold, blubbering over the death of a fictitious teacher, and sharing with his pupil the remorse of a missed opportunity, the loss of a mentor.

Hesse's novel left me with a lasting admiration for the teacher who reaches more than halfway to capture the imagination of a novice and crosses the chasm, whether it be generational, cultural, class, or gender, to work together in shaping a discipline.

As I learn who my students are, it is each student's story that becomes the study, myself the pupil. Their uniqueness changes the nuance of the didactic, the approach to the patient. Family practice residents have contributed to the writing of this book, enriching its repertoire.

Its earliest form was a collaborative effort among doctors and nurses. Its aim was to emphasize the geriatric patient's independence and individuality. Multiple disciplines in concert with medicine are needed to achieve this, hence the "team management" sections of this book.

Dan Onion asked me to develop the next in a series of books based on the format he used in his book, *The Little Black Book of Primary Care*. Having learned a great deal from Dan's scientific approach to medicine, one which supplied references for current controversies, I could see the utility of such a geriatric manual. Dennis McCullough, a mentor since our first meeting at the Chapel Hill Family Practice Fellowship, has provided wise pearls of family practice experience. During the last legs of the book's production, I was diagnosed with breast cancer. Dennis' support and detailed review of the page proofs allowed for the book's timely completion.

One day this summer while sitting alongside my own pond, recuperating from chemotherapy, I was visited by a resident who had come to invoke a resurgence of my bone marrow. It was her notion that an exhilarating swim would do the trick. My fears of deep water made me an unwilling student and encumbered her cure. Eventually, she coached me across the pond and back, keeping me afloat as my colleagues have done these past months.

I hope you, the reader, whether primary care provider, student, or resident, will find what we've put together useful, knowing all along that your patients will be most helped by what you bring of yourself to the patient encounter.

K.G.

Addendum

From the Second Edition:

Since the publication of the first edition, the author has recovered from breast cancer and lost a mentor who she capriciously thought would live to be 100, her father. As with our parents, we are grateful to our patients for their enduring lessons.

Our patients, well into their 80s, foster an apprenticeship, continuing to parent generations younger than themselves, preparing us to do the same. We decided to dedicate the second edition to our respective children: Jackie, Abu, and Kate. They will always be our children no matter how old we get.

This book includes new topics such as hypothermia, liver failure, executive function testing of dementias, and family phases of adaption to chronic illness. There are expanded areas as well, e.g., hospice management. Wherever possible we have used tables and decision trees to facilitate acquisition of disease entities.

Karen Gershman and Dennis M. McCullough

Special thanks to Dennis M. McCullough whose help in the first two editions have made this third edition possible.

Medical Abbreviations

<	Less than
<<	Much less than
>	More than
>>	Much more than
A_2	Aortic (first) component of S_2
AA	Alcoholics Anonymous
AAA	Abdominal Aortic Aneurysm
AADLs	Advanced activities of daily living
AAML	Age-associated memory loss
abd	Abdomen/abdominal
ABGs	Arterial blood gases
ABW	Actual body weight
abx	Antibiotics
ac	Before meals
ACE	Angiotensin-converting enzyme
ACTH	Adrenocorticotropic hormone
AD	Alzheimer's dementia
ADA	American Diabetic Diet
ADLs	Activities of daily living
Æ	Leads to
AFB	Acid-fast bacillus
Afib	Atrial fibrillation
Aflut	Atrial flutter
AGS	American Geriatrics Society
ALS	Amyotrophic lateral sclerosis
ALT	SGPT; alanine aminotransferase
ANA	Antinuclear antibody
ANP	Atrial natriuretic peptide
antibx	Antibiotics
ARB	Angiotensin receptor blocker
ARDS	Adult respiratory distress syndrome
AS	Aortic stenosis
ASA	Aspirin
ASCVD	Arteriosclerotic cardiovascular disease
ASHD	Asteriosclerotic heart disease
AST	SGOT; aspartate transferase
ASVD	Atherio sclerotic vascular disease
asx	Asymptomatic
ATP	Adenosine triphosphate
AV	Arteriovenous; or atrial-ventricular
AZT	zidovudine
Ba	Barium
BBB	Bundle branch block
bcp's	Birth control pills
BE	Barium enema
bid	Twice a day
BiPAP	Bi-positive airway pressure

bm	Bowel movement
BMD	Bone mineral densitometry
BMI	Body Mass Index
BNP	Brain natriuretic peptide
BP	Blood pressure
BPH	Benign Prostatic Hypertrophy
bpm	Beats per minute
BS	Blood sugar
BUN	Blood urea nitrogen
bx	Biopsy
Ca	Calcium
CABG	Coronary artery bypass graft
CAD	Coronary artery disease
CAGE	Alcohol screening test
cal	Calories
CBC	Complete blood count
CCU	Critical care unit
CEA	Carcinoembryonic antigen
cGMP	Cyclic GMP
CHD	Congenital heart disease
CHF	Congestive heart failure
CHO	Carbohydrate
CIWA	Scale for assessing alcohol withdrawal
cm	Centimeter
CML	Chronic myelocytic leukemia
cmplc	Complications
CMV	Cytomegalovirus
CN	Cranial nerve
CNS	Central Nervous System
COMT	Catechol O-methyl-transferase
COPD	Chronic obstructive lung disease
COX	Cyclooxygenase
CPAP	Continuous positive airway pressure
CPK	Creatine phosphokinase
CPR	Cardiopulmonary resuscitation
Cr	Creatinine
CRF	Chronic renal failure
CRP	C reactive protein
crs	Course
CSF	Cerebrospinal fluid
CT	Computed tomography
CV	Cardiovascular
CVA	Cerebrovasular accident
CVP	Central venous pressure
CXR	Chest X-ray
d	Day/s
DAT	Dementia, Alzheimer's type
dB	Decibel
DEXA	Dual-energy X-ray absorptiometry
DI	Diabetes insipidus
dias	Diastolic
DIC	Disseminated intravascular coagulation
diff	Differential
dig	Digoxin
DJD	Degenerative Joint disease
dL	Deciliter
DLBD	Diffuse Lewy Body disease
DM	Diabetes Mellitus
DMARD	Disease-modifying antirheumatic drug

DNA Deoxyribonucleic acid
DNR Do not resuscitate
DRE Digital rectal exam
DSM Diagnostic and Statistical Manual
DTRs Deep tendon reflexes
DVT Deep venous thrombosis
dx Diagnosis

ECT Electroconvulsive therapy
EEG Electroencephalogram
EF Ejection fraction
EKG Electrocardiogram
EORA Elderly-onset RA
Epidem Epidemiology
EPS Electrophysiologic studies; extrapyramidal side effects
ERCP Endoscopic retrograde cholangiopancreatography
ESR Erythrocyte sedimentation rate
ETOH Ethanol
ETT Exercise tolerance test

F Female; or Fahrenheit
f/u Follow up
FA Fatty acid
FBG Fasting blood glucose
FBS Fasting blood sugar
FDA Food and Drug Administration
Fe Iron
FEV_1 Forced expiratory vital capacity in 1 second
FFA Free fatty acids
FFP Fresh frozen plasma
FICSIT Frailty and Injuries: Cooperative Studies of Intervention Techniques
FSH Follicle-stimulating hormone
FTA Fluorescent treponemal antibody
fx Fracture

GABA γ-aminobutyric acid
GDS Geriatric Depression Scale
GE Gastroesophageal
GERD Gastroesophageal reflux disease
GFR Glomerular filtration rate
GHRH Growth hormone-releasing hormone
gi Gastrointestinal
gm Gram
GnRH Gonadotropin-releasing hormone
GTT Glucose tolerance test
gu Genitourinary

h/o History of
HCl Hydrochloric acid
HCM Health Care Maintenance
hct Hematocrit
HCTZ Hydrochlorothiazide
HDL High-density lipoprotein
hep Hepatitis
HF Heart Failure
hgb Hemoglobin
HHNC Hyperosmolar hyperglycemic nonketotic coma
hL Nanoliter(s)

HLA Human leukocyte antigens
HMG-COA Hydroxy-methylglutaryl-coenzyme A
HN High nitrogen
hr hour(s)
hs At bedtime
HT Hypertension
hx History
Hz Hertz

IADLs Instrumental activities of daily living
IBD Inflammatory bowel disease
IBW Ideal body weight
ICD Implantable cardioverter-defibrillator
ICU Intensive care unit
IgA Immunoglobulin A
IgG Immunoglobulin G
IgM Immunoglobulin M
IHSS Idiopathic hypertrophic subaortic stenosis
IL Interleukin
im Intramuscular
IMA Inferior mesenteric artery
IMI Inferior myocardial infarction
incr Increased
INH Isoniazid
IPG Impedance plethysmography
IU International units
iv Intravenous
IVP Intravenous pyelogram

JVD Jugular venous distension
JVP Jugular venous pressure/pulse

K Potassium
kcal Kilocalorie
kg Kilogram

L Liter; or left
LA Left atrium
lb Pound
LBBB Left bundle branch block
LBP Lower back pain
LDH Lactate dehydrogenase
LDL Low-density lipoproteins
LFTs Liver function tests
LH Luteinizing hormone
LMWH Low molecular weight heparin
LOC Loss of consciousness
LP Lumbar puncture
LR Lactated Ringer's
LS Lumbosacral
LV Left ventricle
LVEF Left ventricular ejection fraction
LVH Left ventricular hypertrophy

M Male
m Meter(s)
m Micron(s)
M/F Male/Female
MAC *Micobacterium avium* complex
MAO Monoamine oxidase
MAP Mean arterial pressure

MAT	Multifocal atrial tachycardia
MB	Isoform 2 of CPK, mainly found in heart
mcg	Microgram
MCI	Mild Cognitive Impairment
MCV	Mean corpuscular volume
MDI	Metered-dose inhaler
meds	Medications
mets	Metastases
Mg	Magnesium
mg	Milligram
mgm	Microgram(s)
MI	Myocardial infarction; or mitral insufficiency
MIC	Minimum inhibitory concentration
min	Minute(s)
mL	Milliliter
MMA	Methylmalonic acid
M:MS	Methadone:Morphine sulfate
MMSE	Mini-Mental State Exam
mo	Month
MOM	Milk of Magnesia
mOsm	Milliosmole(s)
MPTP	1-methyl-4-phenyl-1,2,3,6-tetrahydropyridine
MRA	Magnetic resonance angiography
MRFIT	Multiple risk factor intervention trial
MRI	Magnetic resonance imaging
MS	Multiple sclerosis; or mitral stenosis
n	Nanogram(s)
NA	Narcotics Anonymous
neg	Negative
NG	Nasogastric
NH	Nursing home
NIDDM	Non-insulin-dependent diabetes mellitus
nl	Normal
nm	Nanometer(s)
NMDA	N-methyl-D-aspartate
NMS	Neuroleptic Malignant Syndrome
NNT	Number needed to treat
NPH	Normal-pressure hydrocephalus
npo	Nothing by mouth
NS	Normal saline
NSAID	Nonsteroidal anti-inflammatory drug
NSR	Normal sinus rhythm
NYHA	New York Heart Association
O_2	Oxygen
OA	Osteoarthritis
OBRA	Omnibus Budget Reconciliation Act
OCD	Obsessive Compulsive Disorder
OGIT	Oral glucose tolerance test
OT	Occupational therapy
OTC	Over the counter
P	Pulse
Pap	Papanicolaou
PAP	Pulmonary artery pressure

PAT	Paroxysmal atrial tachycardia
patho-phys	Pathophysiology
Pb	Lead
pc	After meals
PCI	Percutaneous coronary intervention
PCN VK	Penicillin
PCP	Pneumocystis carinii pneumonia
PCWP	Pulmonary capillary wedge pressure
PE	Pulmonary embolism; or Physical examination
periumb	Periumbilical
PET	Positron emission tomography
PFTs	Pulmonary function tests
PGE	Prostaglandin E
pH	acidity
PMI	Point of maximal impulse of heart
PMN	Polymorphonuclear neutrophils
PMNLs	Polymorphonuclear leukocytes
PMR	Polymyalgia rheumatica
pn	Pain
PND	Paroxysmal nocturnal dyspnea
po	By mouth
POAG	Primary open angle glaucoma
pos	Positive
ppd	Pack per day
PPD	Tuberculin skin test
PPI	Proton pump inhibitor
pr	Per rectum
prep	Preparation
prn	As needed
PSA	Prostate-specific antigen
PT	Prothrombin time; physical therapy
pt(s)	Patient(s)
PTCA	Percutaneous Transluminal Coronary Angioplasty
PTH	Parathormone
PTSD	Post-traumatic stress disorder
PTT	Partial thomboplastin time
PTU	Propylthiouracil
PUD	Peptic ulcer disease
PVC	Premature ventricular tachycardia
PVD	Peripheral vascular disease
PVR	Postvoid residual
px	Prognosis
q	Every
qd	Daily
qid	4 times a day
qod	Every other day
QRS	QRS wave form on EKG
r/o	Rule out
RA	Rheumatoid arthritis
RAAS	Renin-angiotensin-aldosterone system
RBBB	Right bundle branch block
rbc	Red blood cell
re	About

rehab	Rehabilitation
REM	Rapid eye movement
Rh	Rhesus factor
RLQ	Right lower quadrant
RNA	Ribonucleic acid
ROM	Range of motion
RPR	Rapid plasma reagin
RR	Respiratory rate
RSD	Reflex sympathetic dystrophy
RSV	Respiratory syncytial virus
rv	Review
RV	Right ventricle
rx	Treatment
s/p	Status post
S_1	First heart sound
S_2	Second heart sound
S_3	Third heart sound, gallop
S_4	Fourth heart sound, gallop
SAD	Seasonal affective disorder
sc	Subcutaneous
se	Side effects
sens	Sensitivity
SGOT	Serum Glutamic Oxaloacetic Transaminase
SHEP	Systolic Hypertention European Project
si	Sign(s)
SIADH	Syndrome of inappropriate ADH
sl	Sublingual
SLE	Systemic lupus erythematosis
SNP	Supranuclear palsy
soln	Solution
specif	Specificity
SPECT	Single-photon emission computed tomography
SPEP	Serum protein electrophoresis
SS	Sickle cell disease
SSRI	Selective serotonin reuptake inhibitor
SSS	Sick sinus syndrome
ST	ST segment of EKG
SVT	Supraventricular tachycardia
sx	Symptom(s)
sys	Systolic
T°	Fever/temperature
tab	Tablet
TAH	Total abdominal hysterectomy
Tbc	Tuberculosis
TCA	Tricyclic antidepressant
TEE	Transesophageal echocardiogram
TFA	Trans fatty acid
TFV	Tenofovir
TG	Triglycerides
TIA	Transient ischemic attack
TIBC	Total iron-binding capacity
tid	Three times a day
Tm/S	Trimethoprim/sulfa
TMP	Trimethorprim
TNF	Tumor necrosis factor
TNG	Nitroglycerine
TPA	Tissue plasminogen activator

TPN Total parenteral nutrition
TSH Thyroid-stimulating hormone
tsp Teaspoon
TTP Thrombotic thrombocytopenic purpura
TURP Transurethral resection of prostate

U Units
U.S. United States
UA Urinalysis
UGI Upper gastrointestinal
UPEP Urine Protein Electrophloresis
URI Upper respiratory illness
US Ultrasound
UTI Urinary tract infection
UV Ultraviolet

VDR Venereal Disease Research Lab
ves Vessel
Vfib Ventricular fibrillation
vit Vitamin
VRE Vancomycin-resistant Enterococci
vs Versus

w With
w/o Without
w/u Work up
wbc White blood cells; or White blood count
wgt Weight
wk Weeks(s)
WPW Wolff-Parkinson-White syndrome

YORA Young-onset RA
yr Year(s)

Zn Zinc

Journal Abbreviations

Acta Neurol Scand	Acta Neurologica Scandinavica
Acta Psychiatr Scand	Acta Psychiatrica Scandinavica
Adv Studies Med	Advanced Studies in Medicine
Adv Wound Care	Advances in Wound Care
Age Aging	Age and Aging
Am Coll Phys J Club	American College of Physicians Journal Club
Am Coll Psychiatrists	American College of Psychiatrists
Am Fam Phys	American Family Physician
Am Hrt J	American Heart Journal
Am J Cardiol	American Journal of Cardiology
Am J Clin Nutr	American Journal of Nutrition
Am J Clin Oncol	American Journal of Clinical Oncology
Am J Epidem	American Journal of Epidemiology
Am J Gastroenterol	American Journal of Gastroenterology
Am J Ger Cardiol	American Journal of Geriatric Cardiology
Am J Ger Psychiatry	American Journal of Geriatric Psychiatry
Am J Hlth Sys Pharm	American Journal of Health-System Pharmacy
Am J Hosp Palliat Care	American Journal of Hospice and Palliative Care
Am J Hosp Pharm	American Journal of Hospital Pharmacy
Am J Kidney Dis	American Journal of Kidney Diseases

Am J Med	American Journal of Medicine
Am J Med Sci	American Journal of Medical Science
Am J Neuroradiol	American Journal of Neuroradiology
Am J Nurs	American Journal of Nursing
Am J Obgyn	American Journal of Obstetrics and Gynecology
Am J Occup Ther	American Journal of Occupational Therapy
Am J Phys Med Rehabil	American Journal of Physical Medicine and Rehabilitation
Am J Psych	American Journal of Psychiatry
Am J Pub Hlth	American Journal of Public Health
Am J Resp Care Med	American Journal of Respiratory Care Medicine
Am J Surg	American Journal of Surgery
Am Pain Soc Bull	American Journal of Pain Society Bulletin
Am Psych Association	American Journal of Psychiatric Association
Am Rheum Dis	American Journal of Rheumotologic Diseases
Am Rv Respir Dis	American Review of Respiratory Disease
Anesthesiology	Anesthesiology
Ann EM	Annals of Emergency Medicine
Ann IM	Annals of Internal Medicine
Ann Long-Term Care	Annals of Long-Term Care
Ann Neurol	Annals of Neurology
Ann Oncol	Annals of Oncology
Ann Pharmacother	The Annals of Pharmacotherapy
Ann Rheum Dis	Annals of Rheumatic Diseases
Ann Rv Public Health	Annual Review of Public Health
Ann Surg	Annals of Surgery
Ann Vasc Surg	Annals of Vascular Surgery

Abbreviation	Journal
Arch Derm	Archives of Dermatology
Arch Fam Med	Archives of Family Medicine
Arch Gen Psychiatry	Archives of General Psychiatry
Arch IM	Archives of Internal Medicine
Arch Neurol	Archives of Neurology
Arch Ophthalm	Archives of Ophthalmology
Arch Phys Med Rehab	Archives of Physical Medicine and Rehabilitation
Arch Sex Behav	Archives of Sexual Behavior
Arch Surg	Archives of Surgery
Arthritis Rheum	Arthritis and Rheumatism
Aust N Z J Surg	Australian and New Zealand Journal of Surgery
Basic Res Cardiol	Basic Research in Cardiology
Biol Psych	Biological Psychiatry
Blood	Blood
BMJ	British Medical Journal
Bone Miner	Bone and Mineral
Br J Cancer	British Journal of Cancer
Br J Clin Pract	British Journal of Clinical Practice
Br J Psych	British Journal of Psychiatry
Brit J Rheum	British Journal of Rheumatology
Br J Surg	British Journal of Surgery
Br J Urology Int	British Journal of Urology
Bull Rheum Dis	Bulletin of Rheumatic Diseases
CA	A Cancer Journal for Clinicians
Can CME	Canadian CME
Can J Ophthalm	Canadian Journal of Ophthalmology
Can J Psychiatry	Canadian Journal of Psychiatry
Can Med Assoc J	Canadian Medical Association Journal
Cancer J	Cancer Journal
Cancer Nurs	Cancer Nursing

Cardiol Clin	Cardiology Clinics
Cancer Pract	Cancer Practice
Cardiovasc Surg	Cardiovascular Surgery
Cell	Cell
Chest	Chest
Circ	Circulation
Clin Diabetes	Clinical Diabetes
Clin Endocrinol	Clinical Endocrinology (Oxford)
Clin Gastroenter	Clinics in Gastroenterology
Clin Ger	Clinical Geriatrics
Clin Ger Med	Clinics in Geriatric Medicine
Clin Gerontol	Clinical Gerontology
Clin Infect Dis	Clinical Infectious Diseases
Clin Obgyn	Clinical Obstetrics and Gynecology
Clin Orthop	Clinical Orthopedics and Related Research
Clin Pharmacol Ther	Clinical Pharmacology and Therapeutics
Clin Pract Guidelines	Clinical Practice Guidelines
Clin Symp	Clinical Symposia
Clin Ther	Clinical Therapeutics
CNS Drugs	Central Nervous System Drugs
Conn Med	Connecticut Medicine
Consult Pharm	Consultant Pharmacist
Convuls Ther	Convulsive Therapy
Crit Care Clin	Critical Care Clinics
Curr Clin Top Infect Dis	Current Clinical Topics in Infectious Disease
Curr Concepts Cerebro Dis	Current Concepts of Cerebrovascular Disease
Curr Med Res Opin	Current Medical Research and Opinion
Curr Opin Neurol	Current Opinion in Neurology
Curr Opin Clin Nutr Metab Care	Current Opinion in Clinical Nutrition and Metabolic Care
Curr Probl Cancer	Current Problems in Cancer
Curr Probl Cardiol	Current Problems in Cardiology

Decubitus	Decubitus
Depress Anxiety	Depression and Anxiety
DHHS Publc	Department of Health and Human Services Publication
Diab Care	Diabetes Care
Diabetes	Diabetes
Diabetes Med	Diabetes Medicine
Diabetes Metab Rev	Diabetes/Metabolism Reviews
Dis Mo	Disease-a-Month
Dis Nerv Syst Clin Neurobiol	Diseases of the Nervous System and Clinical Neurobiology
Drugs	Drugs
Drugs Aging	Drugs and Aging
Ear Hear	Ear and Hearing
Emerg Med Clin N Am	Emergency Medical Clinics of North America
Eur Hrt J	European Heart Journal
Eur J Cancer	European Journal of Cancer
Eur J Neurol	European Journal Neurology
Eur J Surg Oncol	European Journal of Surgical Oncology
Eur Respir J	European Respiratory Journal
Exp Aging Res	Experimental Aging Research
Fortschr Neurol Psychiatrie	Fortschritte der Neurologie-Psychiatrie
Gastroenterol Clin N Am	Gastroenterology Clinics of North America
Gastroenterol Int	Gastroenterology International
Gastrointest Endosc Clin N Am	Gastrointestinal Endoscopy Clinics of North America
GE	Gastroenterology
Ger Clin	Geriatric Clinics
Ger Clin N Am	Geriatric Clinics of North America

Ger Med Today	Geriatric Medicine Today
Ger Nurs	Geriatric Nursing
Gerontol Clin	Gerontologia Clinica
Ger Rv Syllabus	Geriatric Review Syllabus
Geriatrics	Geriatrics
Gerontol	Gerontologist
GFT	Geriatrics at Your Fingertips
GRS	Geriatric Review Syllabus
Gut	Gut
Hlth Serv Res	Health Services Research
Heart	Heart
Heart Lung	Heart and Lung
Horm Metab Res	Hormone and Metabolic Research
Hosp Pract	Hospital Practice
HT	Hypertension
Inf Contr Hosp Epidem	Infection Control and Hospital Epidemiology
Int J Addict	International Journal of Addiction
Int J Aging Hum Dev	International Journal of Aging and Human Development
Int J Cardiol	International Journal of Cardiology
Int J Epidem	International Journal of Epidemiology
Int J Geriatr Psychiatry	International Journal of Geriatric Psychiatry
Int J Integrative Med	International Journal of Integrative Medicine
Int J Psychiatr Med	International Journal of Psychiatry in Medicine
Intern Med	Internal Medicine
JAMDA	Journal of the American Medical Directors Association
J Acoustic Soc Am	Journal of the Acoustical Society of America

J Acquir Immune Defic Syndr	Journal of Acquired Immune Deficiency Syndromes
J Affect Disord	Journal of Affective Disorders
J Allergy Clin Immunol	Journal of Allergy and Clinical Immunology
J Am Acad Derm	Journal of the American Academy of Dermatology
J Am Board Fam Pract	Journal of the American Board of Family Practice
J Am Coll Cardiol	Journal of the American College of Cardiology
J Am Diet Assoc	Journal of the American Dietetic Association
J Am Ger Soc	Journal of the American Geriatric Society
Jama	Journal of the American Medical Association
Jamda	Journal of the American Medical Directors Association
J Am Optom Assoc	Journal of the American Optometric Association
J Am Soc Nephrology	Journal of the American Society of Nephrology
J Anxiety Disord	Journal of Anxiety Disorders
J Bone Joint Surg Am	Journal of Bone and Joint Surgery (American)
J Bone Joint Surg Br	Journal of Bone and Joint Surgery (British)
J Bone Miner Res	Journal of Bone and Mineral Research
J Clin Invest	Journal of Clinical Investigation
J Chronic Dis	Journal of Chronic Disease
J Clin Endocrinol Metab	Journal of Clinical Endocrinology and Metabolism
J Clin Epidem	Journal of Clinical Epidemiology
J Clin Oncol	Journal of Clinical Oncology
J Clin Psychiatry	Journal of Clinical Psychiatry

J Clin Psychopharmacol	Journal of Clinical Psychopharmacology
J Comm Hlth	Journal of Community Health
J Consult Clin Psychol	Journal of Consultant Clinical Psychology
J ECT	Journal of Electroconvulsant Therapy
J Emerg Med	Journal of Emergency Medicine
J Endourol	Journal of Endourology
J Fam Pract	Journal of Family Practice
J Fla Med Assoc	Journal of the Florida Medical Association
J Gen Intern Med	Journal of General Internal Medicine
J Ger Psych Neurol	Journal of Geriatric Psychiatry and Neurology
J Gerontol	Journal of Gerontology
J Gerontol A Biol Sci Med Sci	Journal of Gerontology Acta Biological Science and Science
J Gerontol Med Sci	Journal of Gerontology Series A Biological Sciences and Medical Sciences
J Gerontol Nurs	Journal of Gerontological Nursing
J Hosp Infect	Journal of Hospital Infection
J Hypertens	Journal of Hypertension
J Hypertens Suppl	Journal of Hypertension Supplement
J Intern Med	Journal of Internal Medicine
J Midwife Women Hlth	Journal of Midwifery and Women's Health
J Natl Cancer Inst	Journal of the National Cancer Institute
J Neurol	Journal of Neurology
J Neurol Sci	Journal of the Neurological Sciences
J Neurol Neurosurg Psychiatry	Journal of Neurology, Neurosurgery & Psychiatry

J Neurosurg	Journal of Neurosurgery
J Neuropsych Clin Neurosci	Journal of Neuropsychiatry and Clinical Neuroscience
J Obgyn	Journal of Obstetrics and Gynecology
J Oral Maxillofac Surg	Journal of Oral Maxillofacial Surgery
J Psych	Journal of Psychiatry
J Psych Pract	Journal of Psychiatric Practice
J Psychol Nurs	Journal of Psychological Nursing
J Rheum	Journal of Rheumatology
J Thorac Cardiovasc Surg	Journal of Thoracic and Cardiovascular Surgery
J Trauma	Journal of Trauma—Injury, Infection and Critical Care
J Urol	Journal of Urology
Lancet	Lancet
Leuk Lymphoma	Leukemia & Lymphoma
Leukemia	Leukemia
Life Sci	Life Sciences
Maturitas	Maturitas
Mayo Clin Proc	Mayo Clinic Proceedings
Md State Med Assoc J	Maryland State Medical Association Journal
Mech Age Dev	Mechanisms of Aging and Development
Med Care	Medical Care
Med Clin N Am	Medical Clinics of North America
Med Lett	The Medical Letter on Drugs and Therapeutics
Med Lett Drugs Ther	Medical Letter of Drugs and Therapeutics
Millbank Q	Millbank Quarterly
Minn Med	Minnesota Medicine

Mod Concepts Cardiovasc Dis	Modern Concepts of Cardiovascular Disease
N Am Med	North American Medicine Clinics
Natl Ctr Hlth Stat	National Center for Health Statistics
Nature	Nature
Nejm	New England Journal of Medicine
Nephrol Dial Transplant	Nephrology Dialysis Transplantation
Neurol Clin	Neurologic Clinics
Neurol Res	Neurological Research
Neurol	Neurology
Neuropsychopharm	Neuropharmacology
Neuroscience	Neuroscience
Nurs Home Med	Nursing Home Medicine
Nurs Home Pract	Nursing Home Practice
Nutr	Nutrition
Nutr Rev	Nutrition Review
Obgyn	Obstetrics and Gynecology
Oncology	Oncology
Ophthalm	Ophthalmology
Osteoporos Int	Osteoporosis International
Pain	Pain
Palliatr Med	Palliative Care Medicine
Ped Derm	Pediatric Dermatology
Pharmacotherapy	Pharmacotherapy
Phys Ther	Physical Therapy
Post Grad Med J	Postgraduate Medicine Journal
Prim Care	Primary Care
Prog Clin Biol Res	Progress in Clinical and Biological Research
Psychiatr Clin N Am	Psychiatric Clinics of North America
Psychotherapy and Psychosomatics	Psychother Psychosom

Radiol Clin N Am	Radiologic Clinics of North America
Schizophr Bull	Schizophrenia Bulletin
Sci Am	Scientific American
Sci Am Med	Scientific American Medicine
Science	Science
Semin Oncol	Seminars in Oncology
Semin Spine Surg	Seminars in Spine Surgery
Sleep Med Rv	Sleep Medicine Review
South Med J	Southern Medical Journal
Spine	Spine
Stroke	Stroke
Surg Clin N Am	Surgical Clinics of North America
Surgery	Surgery
Surv Ophthalmol	Survey of Ophthalmology
Treat GuideL Med Lett	Treatment Guidelines from the Medical Letter
Urol Clin N Am	Urologic Clinics of North America

Acknowledgments

Several primary care providers and medical students have contributed to the writing of various sections of this book. They include:

Maine–Dartmouth Family Practice Residency = MDFPR

Contributor	Section
Benjamin Brown, MD, MDFPR, Sabahat Iqbal, MD, MDFPR	Diabetes Mellitus; MI
Diana Berger, MD, Hanover, NH	Gout
Laura Chapman, Hanover, NH	Meningitis
Sandy Colt, GNP, Maine General Medical Center	UTIs/Constipation
Ahmed Aldilaimi, MD, MDFPR	Atrial fibrilation
Rod Forrey, PA, MDFPR	NMS
Alicia Forster, MD, MDFPR	Prostate Cancer
James Glazer, MD, MDFPR	Osteomyelitis; Hypothermia
Rick Hobbs, MD, MDFPR	Hospice & Palliative Care
Kristin Burdick, MD, MDFPR	Syncope
Janis B. Petzel, MD, Augusta, ME	Depression; Anxiety
Jonathan Kilroy, DO, MDFPR	Thrombolytics
Nate Harmon, MDFPR	Parkinson's
Cory Ingram, MD, MDFPR	HTN
Kathryn Wistar, MD, MDFPR	ETOH Abuse
Chi Jokonya, MD, MDFPR	HIV
Catherine Neilsen, MD, MDFPR	Elderly Abuse
Daniel K. Onion, MD, MDFPR	Cardiology
Rebecca Reeves, Albany, NY	Endocarditis
Cheryl Seymour, MD, MDFPR	CHF
Shannon Tome-Kenney, Biddeford, ME	Skin Infections
Stephanie Waecker, DO, MDFPR	Ovarian Cancer
Richard Wallingford, III, MD, MDFPR	TB

Delvina Saraqini, MD, MDFPR, Chris Lutrzykowski, MD, MDFPR	Adhesive Capsulitis
Danielle Saad, DO	Dementia
Sanjaya Soori, MD, MDFPR, Musgrave, Katje, DO, MDFPR	COPD
Gail Rowell, DO, Biddeford, ME	Osteoarthritis
Gayle Smith, DO, MDFPR	Urinary Incontinence
Ferdinand Saran, MD, MDFPR	Tube Feeding
Tonya Campus, MD, MDFPR, Rachael Blake, UMass Med	Geriatric Obesity

Special thanks to Michele Lazerow for editing the fourth edition with grace and aplomb. We would also like to thank Davene Fitch for her help with additions of new tables and Kathleen Keene.

Notice

We have made every attempt to summarize accurately and concisely a multitude of references. However, the reader is reminded that times and medical knowledge change, transcription or understanding error is always possible, and crucial details are omitted whenever such a comprehensive distillation as this is attempted in limited space. And the primary purpose of this compilation is to cite literature on various sides of controversial issues; knowing where "truth" lies is usually difficult. We cannot, therefore, guarantee that every bit of information is absolutely accurate or complete. The reader should affirm that cited recommendations are reasonable still, by reading the original articles and checking other sources, including local consultants as well as recent literature, before applying them.

Drugs and medical devices are discussed that may have limited availability controlled by the Food and Drug Administration (FDA) for use only in research study or clinical trial. The drug information presented has been derived from reference sources, recently published data, and pharmaceutical tests. Research, clinical practice, and government regulations often change the accepted standard in this field. When consideration is being given to use of any drug in the clinical setting, the clinician or reader is responsible for determining FDA status of the drug, reading the package insert, and prescribing information for the most up-to-date recommendations on dose, precautions, and contraindications and determining the appropriate usage for the product. This is especially important in the case of drugs that are new or seldom used.

Chapter 1

Common Geriatric Problems

1.1 Dysfunction in the Elderly

Cause: Loss of physical, mental, social function, excessive family burden (Gerontol 1980;20:649)

Epidem: In 1985, 20% of elderly were disabled; by 2060, 30% will be disabled (J Gerontol 1992;47:S253), although there have been improvements in life style and risk factors decreasing old age disability over the past decade (Jama 2003:289:3137,3164): among individuals 65 yr and older: > 20% have difficulty walking a half mile; > 30% have difficulty doing heavy housework; 50% have difficulty pulling or pushing large objects, such as furniture. 30% community elders live alone: M/F ratio = 1:3; the remainder live in family settings: 54% w spouse, 13% w children, 3% w non-relatives (DHHS Publc 1990; PF3029912900 d996).

NH spending 48% Medicaid, 12% Medicare, and 38% private spending (GRS 2004, 5th ed., p101).

Sx: Loss of self-care/independent living skills; social, psychological, emotional isolation.

Si: Inability to read 20/40; inability to hear and answer short, whispered question such as "What is your name?"; urinary incontinence; weight below acceptable range for height; inability to recall 3 objects after 1 min; often sad or depressed; can't get out of bed, make own meals, do own shopping; trouble with stairs, bathtubs, rugs, lighting; doesn't know where to call in emergency or if ill (Ann IM 1990;112:699); inability to touch back of head with both hands, touch back of waist, or contralateral hip; inability to sit and touch toe of shoe; no grip strength (J Fam Pract 1993;17:429).

ADLs: Katz functional assessment (Gerontol 1970;10:20) records loss of independence in 6 skills (in the order in which they are lost: bathing, dressing, toileting, transferring, continence, feeding); usually they are regained in the reverse order; assess actual capacity, not reported performance (Nejm 1990; 322:1207); Mahoney and Barthel ADL scale has more specific questions (Md State Med Assoc J 1965;14:61); speed and pain in performing ADLs in arthritis pts (J Chronic Dis 1978;31:557); use of rehabilitation for ADLs (Arch Phys Med Rehab 1988; 69:337); falls and incontinence associated w lower and upper extremity impairment (Jama 1995;273:1348).

Instrumental activities of daily living (IADLs): more complex activities like shopping, seeking transportation, preparing food, climbing stairs, managing finances, housework, telephone, meds, and job (Fillenbaum IADLs - Jags 1985;33:698); mnemonic: SHAFT: shopping, housework, accounting, food preparation, transportation (Mayo Clin Proc 1995;70:891).

Other IADL scales: home assessment (Clin Ger Med 1991;7:677); nutrition (Am Fam Phys 1993;48:1395); driving (Clin Ger Med 1993;9:349): states where standard vision tests required for driver license renewal have fewer fatalities, whereas states requiring cognitive function test show no difference in fatalities (Jama 1995;274:1026); identify older pts at risk for functional decline after acute medical illness and hospitalization w scoring system based on Mini Mental State Exam (MMSE), IADLs, and age (Jags 1996;44:251); IADLs helpful in community-dwelling elderly.

Crs: For every 5 adults with 5-6 limitations in ADLs, 1 pt may be expected to improve in all ADLs in 2 yr (Milbank Q 1990;68:445);

pts who have trouble performing IADLs have 12 × the baseline probability of developing dementia (Jags 1992;40:1129).

Cmplc: NH placement; Medicaid eligibility for NH admission requires a medical or behavioral dx, plus 2 impaired ADLs; caregiver burnout: 70% of primary caregivers are middle-aged, married women; 30% are elderly themselves (Gerontol 1987;27:616); prevalence of depression among caregivers is 30%-50% (J Gerontol 1990;45:P181); measures of function strong predictors of 90-d and 2-yr mortality (Jama 1998;279:1163).

Lab: CBC, TSH, routine blood chemistries.

Team Management: Annual geriatric evaluation (Nejm 1995; 333:184); rehab; change medical regimen so as not to inhibit function; solicit community services; be vigilant about underlying depression; PT, OT evaluation and instruction (Jama 1997; 278:1321).

1.2 Falls in the Elderly (see also falls under HCM)

Ann IM 1994;121:442; Nejm 1994;331:821; 1990;322:1441; Rubenstein LZ, UCLA intensive geriatric review course, 1996; Am Fam Phys 2000;61:2163; Jags 2001;49:664; 1995;43:1146

Cause:

Intrinsic:

- Visual: cataracts, acuity loss, glare, dark adaptation (Jags 1991;39:1194; Nejm 1991;324:1326).
- Vestibular: previous ear infection, ear surgery, aminoglycosides, quinidine, furosemide (Lasix).
- Proprioceptive: peripheral neuropathy, cervical degeneration; one-third of elderly have abnormal position sense (Jama 1988;259:1190).

- CNS: stroke, Parkinson's, NPH, dementias (or Alzheimer's Disease—end stage).
- Cognitive: dementia, delirium.
- Musculoskeletal: deconditioning, lower extremity weakness, eg, severe arthritis (Nejm 1988;319:1701; Jags 2002;50:671); leg weakness imparts 5 × the risk of fall compared with balance or gait problem, which imparts only 3 × the risk of fall, vs balance most important factor (Age Aging 1999;28:513); knee extension (quads) and ankle plantar flexion (gastrocnemius and soleus) strength contribute to gait velocity and step length (Jama 1995;273:1341); foot problems like thick nails, calluses, bunions, toe deformities, ill-fitting shoes (Jags 1988;36:266).
- Drugs (> 4 meds a risk factor) especially long-acting benzodiazepines, psychoactive drugs (Jags 1999;47:30), tricyclics (Nejm 1998;339:875).

NH Falls (Ann IM 1994;121:442; Jags 2000;48:652):

20% are cardiovascular, eg, hypotension—drug-induced, postprandial, postural or bradycardia (J Gerontol 1991;46:M114); 5% due to acute illness such as pneumonia, febrile illness, UTI, CHF (Am J Med 1986;80:429); only 3% falls from overwhelming intrinsic event, eg, syncope, seizure, stroke, psychoactive drugs (Nejm 1992;327:168).

Extrinsic:

- Environmental hazards > 50% , eg, cords, furniture, small objects, optical patterns on escalators, stairs, floors (Clin Ger Med 1985;1:555); majority occur with mild-moderate activity, eg, walking, stepping up, stepping down, changing position; 70% at home, 10% on stairs (descending > ascending) (Age Aging 1979;8:251).

NH: (Paradoxically) restraints (Ann IM 1992;116:369; Jags 1999;47:1202); higher fall rate during shift changes and when staffing ratios inadequate (Jags 1987;35:503).

Epidem: Accidents 5th leading cause of death in elderly; falls constitute two-thirds of accidental deaths; two-thirds of falls are preventable; 33% of elderly (> 65) living in the community fall each year; females > males, whites > blacks (Nejm 1994;330:1555); active elderly at greater risk than frail elderly for injury (Jags 1991;39:46).

Over 50% of all NH pts fall during their stay (Jags 1995;45:1257) because of greater frailty, but rate may be high because better reporting (Jags 1988;36:266).

Pathophys: Fracture risk from falls increased in elderly because of decreased capability for energy absorption in tissue and impaired protective responses such as reaction time, muscle strength, level of alertness, cognition (J Gerontol 1991;46:M164).

Falls from standing height provide sufficient energy to fracture hip (Nejm 1991;332:1326; Jama 1994;271:128); more likely to fracture a wrist than a hip when falling forward bracing a fall; falling backward more hazardous because of risk of breaking hip (Jags 1993;41:1226).

In old age the strategy for maintaining balance after a slip changes from weight shifting at hip when younger to rapid forward stepping when older (Rubenstein LZ, 1996).

Sx: H/o hypotensive sx posturally, postprandially, on micturition; may have h/o PAT, SSS, AS, hemiplegia, neuropathy, seizures, anemia, hypothyroidism, poor nutritional status, ETOH abuse, intercurrent illness (UTI, pneumonia, CHF); or use of antihypertensives, antidepressants, sedatives, hypoglycemics, phenothiazines, or carbamazepine.

Si: Evaluate environment: stairs, floors (slippery from urine, high-polish linoleum, thick-pile rugs), low-lying furniture, pets, shower, lighting, stairway handrails, toilet grab bars, footwear, slippers.

1.3 Tinetti Gait/Balance Assessment

Balance: Upon immediate standing (if abnormal, consider myopathy, arthritis, Parkinson's, postural hypotension, deconditioning, hip disease, hemiparesis).

With eyes closed and feet together (if abnormal, consider multisensory deficit or diminished proprioception).

If unstable with sternal nudge or turning 360° (consider Parkinson's, NPH, CNS disease, back problems, cervical spondylosis); especially important to determine prior to beginning exercise classes.

While sitting (if abnormal, consider impaired vision, proximal myopathy, ataxia).

When turning neck (if abnormal, consider cervical arthritis or spondylosis, vertebrobasilar insufficiency).

When reaching up, bending down, standing on one leg are screening tests for higher-functioning individuals in the community; if unable to perform, at risk for falls at home (Jags 1986; 34:119).

6% of F > 65, 38% > 85; 63% NH residents have gait abnormality (Jags 1996;44:434); timed 8-foot walk and other lower extremity function tests predict mobility-related ADL disability in 4 yr (Nejm 1995;332:556); NH pt's self-selected gait speed and perception of physical disability are predictive of functional loss (Jags 1995;43:93); comfortable walking speed better predictor than treadmill test of cardiac status in pts w CHF; changes w normal aging: broader-based, smaller steps, diminished arm swing, stooped posture, slower turning.

Step Height (See Table 1.1):

- Frontal lobe gait: seen in vascular dementia, most common gait abnormality: wide-based, slightly flexed, small shuffling steps, hesitant steps, can't initiate step: "glued to floor" (Nejm 1990;322:1441).

Table 1.1 Tinetti Gait Assessment

Gait Abnormality	Type of Gait	Description	Etiology	Dx/Rx
Step height/length	Spastic	Wide-based, slightly flexed, small shuffling steps, hesitant steps, can't initiate step, "glued to floor"	Vascular dementia	Trochanteric pads decrease hip fx
		Circumduction, scrape foot along floor, hand-arm spasticity	Stroke	Surgery
		Bilateral circumduction, sometimes increase urinary frequency and urgency	Spinal stenosis	Surgery
	NPH	Short steps, decreased velocity of stride length and associated shoulder movements, increased sway, poor balance, difficulty turning		Shunt
	Parkinson's	Lacks arm swing, turn en bloc (moves whole body when turns), hesitation, gets stuck while walking especially in open spaces like doorways, festination		Front-wheeled walker
	Steppage	W foot slap	Seen in distal motor neuropathies	Foot orthotics
Path deviation	Vestibular	Broad-based foot stamping, pt looks at feet	Sensory ataxia	Pos Romberg/ position/ vibration sensitivity at ankle
		Unsteady on one side and then the other	Peripheral neuropathy	
	Weakness	Slow unsteady swagger, use furniture to grab onto when walking	Deconditioning	Atrophy, 2/5 strength

continues

COMMON GERIATRIC PROBLEMS

Table 1.1 continued

Gait Abnormality	Type of Gait	Description	Etiology	Dx/Rx
Postural sway				
	Cerebellar	Wide-based, irregular, unsteady, veering, truncal titubation	MS	
	Waddling	Broad based	Seen with severe arthritis, myositis, PMR	
	Antalgic	Seen with arthritis of hip when cane held incorrectly on same side Throwing trunk out over affected hip, resulting in stress on hip and low back		Analgesics, hip replacement
Hysterical				
		Hemiparesis without circumduction, hemiparetic arm normal during walking, good strength lying down but ataxia when walking, staggering a long time to get to opposite wall, tightrope walking, pt drags person assisting them down to the ground		Reassurance

- Spastic gait: seen in stroke w circumduction, scrape foot along floor, hand-arm spasticity; also seen w cervical stenosis and myopathy w bilateral circumduction, sometimes increased urinary frequency and urgency (Jags 1996;44:A).
- Parkinsonian gait: lacks arm swing, turns en bloc (moves whole body when turns), hesitation, gets stuck while walking ("freezing"), especially in open spaces like doorways, festination (involuntary increase in speed of walking in attempt to catch up with displaced center of gravity forward), 4th most common gait abnormality.
- NPH: short steps, decreased velocity of stride length and associated shoulder movements, increased sway, poor balance, difficulty turning; overlap between NPH and vascular etiologies, eg, hydrocephalus from stroke may account for similar gait abnormalities (Jags 1996;44:434).
- Steppage gait w foot slap: seen in distal motor neuropathies.

Path Deviation: Observe from behind, one foot at a time in relation to midline; abnormal path deviation in:

- Vestibular gait, seen with sensory ataxia, 2nd most common gait abnormality, broad-based, foot stamping, pt looks at feet; and peripheral neuropathy gait, 3rd most common, unsteady on one side and then the other, Romberg (pt unable to maintain balance w eyes closed).
- Muscle weakness, slow unsteady swagger, grabs onto furniture when walking.

Postural Sway: Observe from behind for truncal side-to-side motion; seen in:

- Cerebellar gait, 5th most common gait disturbance, wide-based, irregular, unsteady, veering, truncal titubation (shimmying of thorax with respect to the rest of the body).
- Antalgic gait, seen with arthritis of hip when cane held incorrectly on same side, throwing trunk out over affected hip resulting in stress on hip and low back (Ger Med Today 1985;4:47; Jags 1996;44:434).

- Waddling gait, broad-based, seen with severe arthritis, myositis, PMR.
- Hysterical gait: hemiparesis w/o circumduction, hemiparetic arm normal during walking, good strength lying down but ataxia when walking, staggering, takes a long time to get to opposite wall, gait resembles attempts at tightrope walking, pt drags person assisting them down to the ground, not known to occur in pts > 70 yr (Jags 1996;44:434).

Cmplc: Clustering of falls associated with high 6-mo mortality (Age Aging 1977;6:201), 6% fracture some bone, of these one-fourth fx hip (Jags 1995;43:1146); 2% of injurious falls are fatal, of those 13% die from pulmonary embolus; white men 85 yr and older have highest rate of deaths attributable to falls, exceeding 180/100,000 population (Ann Rv Pub Hlth 1992;13:489); 5% serious soft tissue injury (Nejm 1988;319:1701).

Prolonged lies while waiting for help (< 10% of falls); if > 1 hr may cause dehydration, pressure sores, rhabdomyolysis, pneumonia (Jama 1993;268:65).

25% of fallers subsequently avoid ADLs, IADLs, and AADLs for fear of falling again (J Gerontol 1994;49:M140; Nejm 1988;319:1701).

NH Admissions (Am J Pub Hlth 1992;82:395; Nejm 1997;337:1279):

Increased use of health care services (Med Care 1992; 30:587); approximately 50% of pts that are hospitalized for falls may end up in NHs (Emerg Med Clin N Am 1990;8:309)

Lab: Routine w/u: CBC w differential, UA, routine blood chemistries, stool guaiacs, TSH, vit B_{12}, Folate, and ESR (r/o PMR), EKG, CXR, and/or CT as hx indicates.

Noninvasive: No need for Holter monitor; prevalence of ventricular arrhythmia is 82% in both fallers and non-fallers; no sx reported with these arrhythmias (Jags 1989;37:430).

Rx:

Prevention: Programs reduce falls by one-third (Nejm 1994;331:821; Jama 1997;278:557)

- Assessing falls in elderly (Jags 1993;41:309,315,479): Medicare allowable charges for the evaluation of falls: CBC, EKG, MRI, neurologic, orthopedic, PT consultation, safety and functional evaluation of pt's home (Jama 1996;276:59); w questionnaire assess those at risk of immobility because of fear of falling (J Gerontol Med Sci 1995;45:239); pt education sheet (Am Fam Phys 1997;56:1815).
- Minimizing number of meds and using lowest possible doses.
- Vit D reduces falls (Jama 2004;274:291; Jags 2005;53:1881).
- Exercise programs: (Nejm 1994;330:1769) to increase muscle strength and flexibility (FICSIT trials - Jama 1995;273:1341; Jags 1996;44:513), in > 80 yr old (BMJ 1997;315:1065; Age Aging 1999;28:513; Jags 2002;50:1119,1121). Interventions for fear of falling (Jags 2007;55:603).
- Resistance training: to improve weakness, which may be more of a limiting factor than endurance (Jags 1994;42:937).
- Flexibility programs: to increase range of motion for tight hip flexors common in thoracic kyphosis, tightness in hip abductors and adductors.
- Balance and gait training: especially getting in and out of chairs, turning around; NH standard PT is of moderate benefit (Jama 1994;271:519); perturbation training (pushes in different directions to stimulate postural responses) more useful in community setting.
- Endurance training: to help compensate for extra energy cost gait dysfunctions impose; using crutches requires 60% more energy than nl walking; 3-wk bed rest decreases VO_2 max by 27%.
- Tai Chi: cardiorespiratory function better among older Tai Chi practitioners (Jags 1995;43:1222); Tai Chi decreases falls (Jags 1996;44:489,498; 2007;55:1185; Phys Ther 1999;77:371);

decreases fear of falling (Jags 2005;53:1168) vs studies need to be more uniform in choice of subject to conclude there is a positive effect of Tai Chi (Jags 2002;50:756).

- Assistive aids: 23% of noninstitutionalized elderly use assistive aids; of those who use assistive aids, 49% use a cane (70% use incorrectly), 24% use a walker, 12% use a wheelchair (Natl Ctr Hlth Stat 1992;217:1).
- Trochanteric pads: decrease hip fractures (Jama 1994;271:128; Nejm 2000;343:1562), facilitate compliance w gradual implementation; pts are more likely to wear them if the trochanteric pads are worn only at pt-specified limited time periods (Jags 1993;41:338).
- Yaktrax Walker (Jags 2005;53:943)
- Neck collars for vertebral insufficiency (Rubenstein LZ, 1996).
- Proper shoes: high-heel shoes decrease balance in elderly women (Jags 1996;44:434).
- Chairs and toilet seats should have arm rests and increased seat height.
- Obstacle-free, glare-free, adequately lit environment.
- Avoid physical and pharmacologic restraints (Jama 1991; 265:468; Ann IM 1992;116:369), fewer serious injuries in hospital without bedrails (Jags 1999;47:529); alternatives: special areas for walking, lower beds, floor pads, alarm systems (Am Fam Phys 1992;45:763), surveillance by staff; avoid sleep meds w potential for falls: instead tape player w headphones w tapes of favorite music, talking books and family messages (Neufeld R, Phoenix, AZ, 1997); encourage sitting instead of wandering w table containing diversionary activity, eg, meal, playing cards (Ann of Long-Term Care 1999;7:17); hospital alternatives: use of family visitors, professional sitters, lower beds, "functional" ICUs.

1.4 Geriatric Pharmacology

Family practice review course, Seattle, WA, March 95; Mayo Clin Proc 1995;70:685; Jama 2003;289:1107

Underused Drugs: β-blockers s/p MI (Jama 1999;282:113; 1998;280:623; 1997;277:115; Lancet 1999;353:955; Nejm 1998;339:489).

Overused Chronically Administered Drugs: TNG patches and paste, isosorbide dinitrate, sleeping meds, antipsychotics for dementia, antidepressants, digoxin, diuretics, antihypertensives, antiepileptics, laxatives and vitamins, NSAIDs, H_2 blockers and sucralfate (Nurs Home Med 1995;3:254); 5-28% of all acute medical hospital admissions of geriatric pts are due to adverse drug reactions (Ger Rv Syllabus, 5th ed, 2002); most common—drug-drug interactions—causing side effects leading to hospitalization are diuretics, benzodiazepines, ACE inhibitors causing hyperkalemia (Jags 1996;44:944; Ann IM 1995;123:195), hypoglycemia on glyburide, digoxin toxicity (Jama 2003;289:1652); (see Table 1.2).

Table 1.2 Most Commonly Prescribed Medication on the Beers Criteria

Medication	Number of Patients	Reason to Avoid in Elderly	Severity Rating
Diphenhydramine	76	May cause confusion and sedation; should not be used as a hypnotic	High
Naproxen	75	Potential for gi bleed, renal failure, high blood pressure, and heart failure	High
Propoxyphene	63	Offers few analgesic advantages over acetaminophen, yet has the adverse effects of other narcotic drugs	High
Amitriptylline	31	Anticholinergic and sedative effects	High
Clonidine	29	Orthostatic hypotension, CNS adverse effects	Low
Promethazine	28	Poorly tolerated in elderly, due to anticholinergic adverse effects, sedation, and weakness	High
Cyclobenzaprine	28	Potent anticholinergic effects	High
Ketorolac	24	High incidence of adverse gi effects	High
Oral estrogen	23	Potentially carcinogenic, lacks cardio-protective effects in older women	Low
Hydroxyzine	21	Potent anticholinergic effects	High
Ferrous sulfate > 325 mg/day	18	Increases incidence of constipation, but no increase in amount absorbed	Low
Oxybutynin	17	Poorly tolerated in elderly, due to anti-cholinergic adverse effects, sedation, and weakness	High
Methocarbamol	17		High
Indomethacin	15	Most CNS adverse effects of all the NSAIDs	High
Nitrofurantoin	14	Potential renal failure	High
Piroxicam	11	Potential for gi bleed, renal failure, high blood pressure, and heart failure	High
Digoxin > 0.125 mg/d	10	Decreased renal clearance may lead to increased risk of toxic effects	Low
Lorazepam > 3 mg/d	9	Highly anticholinergic, questionable effectiveness	High

continues

Table 1.2 continued

Medication	Number of Patients	Reason to Avoid in Elderly	Severity Rating
Hyoscyamine	9	Increased sensitivity seen in elderly patients, smaller doses are desired	High
Meperidine	6	Oral dosing not effective, potential for CNS adverse effects, safer alternatives	High

Adapted from Table 1, *Arch Inter Med.* 2003;163:2719-20.

Pharmacokinetics:

Absorption: Absorption of ciprofloxacin decreased by concomitant administration of antacids or sucralfate (Pharmacotherapy 1996;16:314); omeprazole inhibits cyanocobalamin absorption.

Distribution: Pts taking interacting meds or with low albumin states such as renal failure and malnutrition may show evidence of toxicity despite normal serum levels, e.g., nystagmus w phenytoin; warfarin displaced and therefore potentiated by allopurinol, metronidazole (Flagyl), Tm/S (Bactrim); phenytoin (Dilantin) potentiated by INH, benzodiazepines, phenothiazines; increase in plasma B_1-acid glycoprotein leads to increased protein binding of alkaline drugs, thereby decreasing amount of free active drug, eg, lidocaine and propranolol.

Adipose tissue proportion increases with aging from 18% to 36% (men) and from 36% to 48% (women); total body water decreases by 15% from ages 20 to 80 yr; therefore, increase in volume of distribution of lipophilic drugs resulting in longer time to reach steady state and longer time to be eliminated from the body eg, diazepam, flurazepam, trazadone, haloperiodol; and decrease in volume of distribution of hydrophilic drugs, resulting in higher initial blood levels, eg, digoxin, aminoglycosides, penicillins (Mayo Clin Proc 2003;78:1564).

Excretion: Decrease in renal blood flow 1%/yr after age 50, GFR decreased by 35% between 3rd and 10th decades of life.

Creatinine Clearance:

$$\text{Creat Cl} = [(140 - \text{age}) \times \text{ideal body weight in kg/serum creatinine} \times 72] \ (\times\ 0.85 \text{ if woman})$$

If < 30, cut the drug dose by half; digoxin toxicity not always recognized in the elderly, so imperative to base dose on creatinine clearance (Jags 1996;44:54); can either lengthen drug interval or decrease dose (Drugs 1994;48:380):

$$\text{Drug interval} = (\text{nl Creat Cl/pt's Creat Cl}) \times \text{nl interval}$$

$$\text{Drug dose} = (\text{pt's Creat Cl/nl Creat Cl}) \times \text{nl dose}$$

Measured creatinine clearance may be better than estimated in higher-functioning elderly (Jags 1993;41:716); drug levels should be drawn just prior to scheduled dose after 3-5 half-lives of dosing; aminoglycosides may have same efficacy w once daily dosage (Clin Infect Dis 2000;30:433); half-life determines interval and loading dose while Vd determines dose (Mayo Clin Proc 2003;78:1564).

Metabolism: Drugs requiring phase 1 (oxidation, reduction, hydrolysis), eg, diazepam (Valium), lidocaine, isosorbide, are affected by decreased enzymatic activity of P-450 with aging (Med Lett 1999;41:59); phase 2 (conjugation), eg, oxazepam (Serax), lorazepam (Ativan), metabolism is not affected by aging (Figure 1.1.) (Med Lett 1996;38:75).

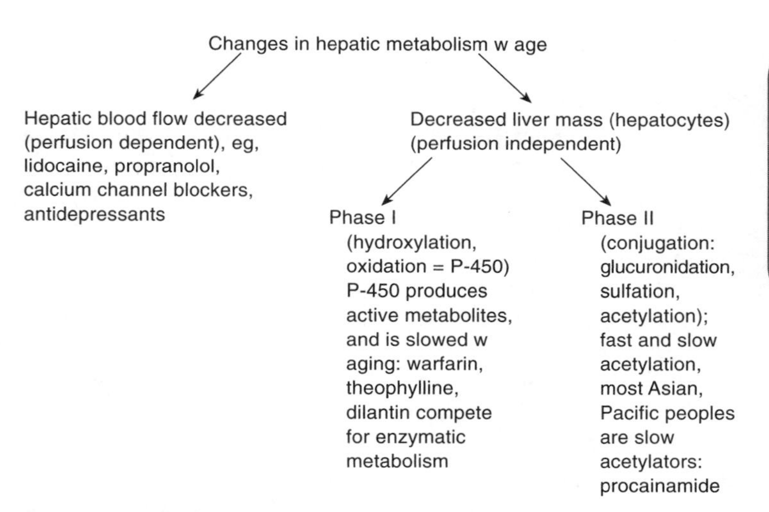

Figure 1.1 Changes in Hepatic Metabolism with Age

More adverse drug interactions when renally excreted drugs used simultaneously, eg, digoxin not cleared when given with quinidine or verapamil; lithium not cleared when given with NSAIDs or thiazides. Types of renal-drug interactions: (1) allergic is not dose-related and takes weeks to resolve, eg, methicillin, ACE inhibitors, NSAIDs, trimethoprim, cimetidine; (2) hemodynamic is dose-related and takes days to resolve, eg, anti-inflammatory drugs, ACE inhibitors; (3) toxic is dose-related and takes weeks to resolve, eg, gentamicin, phenacetin, lithium; (4) pseudo azotemia is dose-related and takes days to resolve, eg, trimethoprim, cimetidine (Am J Kidney Dis 1996;27:162).

Drug-drug interactions (Ger Rv Syllabus 1999-2001, 4th ed., p 33) and conditions necessary for notable drug-drug interactions: 1) drug > 80% bound to albumin, 2) narrow therapeutic index, 3) small Vd (Mayo Clin Proc 2003;78:1564).

Common drug interactions:

- Tricyclic antidepressants and type I antiarrhythmics have potentially fatal interactions.
- Warfarin interacts with many drugs, eg, inhibits metabolism of sulfonylureas leading to hypoglycemia (Mayo Clin Proc 2003;78:1564).
- Erythromycin may raise levels of theophylline and digoxin.
- Iv contrast is contraindicated for pts who have taken metformin.
- Quinidine raises serum levels of digoxin.
- Selegiline taken with some antidepressants can cause severe delirium.
- Statins may interact with other lipid-lowering drugs (eg, gemfibrozil, niacin) to cause rhabdomyolysis.
- Sucralfate interferes with absorption of quinolones.

Pharmacodynamics: Decreased receptor response: norepinephrine and dopamine concentration decreased so decreased effect of adrenergic medications, eg, α-adrenergic agonists, α-adrenergic blockers, increased sensitivity to dopamine blockers eg, metoclopramide.

Increased receptor response: MAO activity increased; increased effect of opiates, eg, morphine, and increased effect of benzodiazepines, eg, diazepam; clonazepam 0.5 mg hs and increase by 0.5 mg q 1-2 wk (drug half-life 48 hr) and assess pt's gait.

Pain: (Management of Cancer Pain, US Department of Health and Human Services Agency of Health Care Policy and Research; Storey P, Primer of Palliative Care, Academy of Hospice Physicians; Pain, in Kemp C, terminal illness, JB Lippincott, 1995:112)

Nonacetylated salicylates less gi se (Treat GuideL Med Lett 2007;5:23)

Midrin, sumatriptan safer for migraines than for ergots.

Acetaminophen < 4 gm/d can cause hepatotoxicity in the elderly (Ger Rv Syllabus 1999-2001, p255)

Post-herpetic neuralgia: nortriptyline or desipramine 10-25 mg increased slowly to maximum of 75 mg qd as tolerated (Jags 2007;55:1176); gabapentin (Neurontin) start at 100 mg q hs, up to 100-600 mg tid; SSRIs less effective than tricyclics; lidocaine topical patch (Am Fam Phys 2005;71:806); Herpes Zoster vaccine (Ann IM 2006;145:317,386).

Serotonin and norepinephrine dampen peripheral pain signals (Neuroscience 2000;100:861).

Neuropathic pain: tricyclic anti-depressants, or venalfaxine which has fewer side effects, or lidocaine patch for peripheral neuropathic pain, or gabapentin (Adv Studies Med 2004;4:88) or baclofen. Gabapentin for fibromyalgia (Arthritis Rheum 2007; 56:1336). Acupuncture for LBP (BMJ 2006;332:680,696).

Opioids for severe pain (Med Lett Drugs Ther 1993;35:1): morphine sulfate for cancer or postop pain; liquid morphine sulfate, start with10 mg q 4 hr with rescue dose (5-15% of the total 24-hr dose q 1 hr prn); slow-release morphine q 12 hr must be accompanied by immediate-release morphine for breakthrough pain (10% of 24-hr slow-release dose (sl, po, or pr); drowsiness occurs within first few hr of therapy, onset unlikely after this period; tolerance requires wks to mo of continuous administration, and may not develop in some pts; respiratory depression unlikely to develop if none present in 2-3 d, monitor sleep respiratory rate, if does not fall below 12 breaths/min when dose increased, will not develop respiratory depression; physical or psychological dependence does not occur early in its administration; bisphosphonates good adjuvant analgesic for bone pain; pts get equally confused after the administration of epidural or general anesthesia (Jama 1995;274:44).

Avoid propoxyphene and meperidine in the elderly (accumulation of active metabolites of meperidine leads to myoclonus, delirium).

When switching between opiates, calculate equianalgesic dose; decrease by 25% for severe pain and 50% for moderate pain to allow for incomplete cross tolerance (see Table 1.3).

Table 1.3 Opioid Conversion Chart

Medication	Single Dose Equivalent Parenteral	Oral	Daily Dose Equivalent Parenteral	Oral	Using Starting Dose Parenteral	Oral
Morphine	10 mg	30 mg	12 mg (2 mg q4hr)	30 mg (5 mg q4hr)	2 mg q4hr	5 mg q4hr
Morphine SR	NA	NA	NA	30 mg (15 mg q12hr)	NA	15 mg q12hr MS Contin Kaian 20 q24hr Avinza 30 q4
Oxycodon	NA	20 mg	NA	30-40 mg (5 mg q3-4hr)	NA	5 mg q4hr
Oxycodon SR	NA	20-30 mg	NA	20 mg (10 mg q12hr)	NA	10 mg q12hr
Methadone	1.5 mg			2 to 1 up to 20:1 for MS1000 <50 mg M:MS=1:2 10-100 M:MS=1:3		

				101-300 M:MS=1:5 301-600 M:MS=1:10 601-800 M:MS=1:12 801-1000 M:MS=1:15 > 1000 mg M:MS=1:20		
Hydromorphone	1.5 mg	7.5 mg	1 mg q12hr	2 mg q3-4hr	1 mg q4hr	2 mg q4hr
Hydrocodone	NA	30 mg	NA	20 mg 5-10 mg q6hr	NA	5 mg q6hr
Codeine with acetaminophen	NA	200 mg	NA	15 mg q4-6hr (NR)	NA	15 mg q4hr
Tramodol	NA	150-300 mg	NA	25-50 mg q4-6hr (NR)	NA	50 mg q8hr
Fentanyl	NA	NA	25 mcg/hr patch 300 mcg/hr patch equiv to 1035-1124 mg/24 MS P.O.		25 mcg/hr patch	

Adapted from Advanced Studies in Medicine 2004;4:(2):88-99
NA = not applicable; NR = not recommended

Management of Opioid-Induced Constipation (Nejm 1996;335:1124):

Prevention: Docusate sodium 100 mg po bid and senna po 1-2 tabs hs; bisacodyl suppository prn; add sorbitol 70%, 15-30 mL bid (less expensive than lactulose); if no bm × 4 days, enema; need to disimpact manually or with enemas if pt is impacted, prior to starting laxatives (Ger Rv Syllabus, 5th ed, 2002, p110).

Alternative Pain Therapies: Topical therapy: add capsaicin cream 0.25%-0.75%, lower potency for first 2 wk, then switch to higher potency; may tolerate better if applied w lidocaine ointment 2.5%-5.0% for first few d of rx; may interfere w substance P (Life Sci 1979;25:1273), reduces tenderness and pain with only adverse effect of localized transient burning (J Rheum 1992;19:604; Ann IM 1994;121:133); consider neural blockade after all else fails.

Herbs:

- Potentially dangerous herbs include charparral, comfreyn (liver toxicity; Ephadra, (HT); Lobela (acts like nicotine); Yohimbine (weakness); Ginkgo biloba (increases bleeding time) (Arch IM 1998;158:2000)
- May use Chamomile, Echinacea, Ginger for nausea, and Saw Palmetto for BPH (Arch Fam Med 1998;7:523)

Vitamins:

- 1-6 gm vit C reduces cold sx by 21% and shortens course by 1 d
- Vit E boosts immune system response in elderly (Jama 1997;277:1380)
- Folic acid for vascular dementia prevention (Arch of Neurol 1998;55:1449)
- Zinc improved cell-mediated response especially for chronic infection (Jags 1998;46:19).

Alternatives to Oral Estrogen:

- Phytoestrogens (Obgyn 1996;87:897) in high-soy diet of Japanese women associated w infrequent hot flashes and other menopausal sx (Lancet 1992;339:1233); ½ cup soybeans = 200 mg isoflavone/d (~0.3 mg conjugated steroidal estrogen), 100 mg/d isoflavin reduces menopausal sx, LDL cholesterol (Obgyn 2002;99:389).
- One gm estrogen cream qd hs 3 × wk for friable mucosa (Am J Med Sci 1197;14:262), may still have to use progesterone to avoid hyperplasia (Jama 2004;291:1701).

1.5 Urinary Tract Colonization/Infection

Jags 1996;44:927,1235,4120; Clin Ger Med 1990;6:1; Ann IM 1990;150:1389; 1995;122:749

Cause: *Escherichia coli* predominant pathogen (50%) in elderly; instrumentation and institutionalization lead to *Proteus mirabilis*, *Klebsiella*, *Enterobacter*, *Serratia*, and *Pseudomonas aeruginosa;* 25% of elderly with urinary catheters have *Enterococci* in urine; coagulase-neg *Staphylococci* in ambulatory elderly; resistant organisms, eg, *Citrobacter freundii*, *Providencia stuartii*.

Epidem: F/M = 2:1; UTIs cause 30%-50% of all bacteremia and septicemia; catheter bacteriuria increases by 3%-10%/d; bacteriuria increased in NH (33%) secondary to immobility, DM, fecal/urinary incontinence, deteriorating mental status.

Pathophys: Attachment of bacteria to epithelial cells of the bladder is promoted by the changing hormonal status of the elderly pt, BPH, prostatic or renal stone formation, a decrease in bacteriostatic prostatic secretions, increased vaginal pH, decreased lactobacillus, anatomic weakening of pelvic floor; MS, DM, CVA, Alzheimer's cause impaired bladder emptying, bacterial colonization; fecal incontinence causes retrograde colonization.

Sx: Dysuria, fever, urinary urgency, frequency, hematuria, suprapubic discomfort are UTI-specific sx; nonspecific sx of UTI much more frequent, eg, change in mental status, change in functional capacity, acute-onset incontinence, decreased appetite, weakness, falls, hypotension, abdominal pain, nausea and vomiting, increased blood sugar in diabetics; must have specific or nonspecific sx before beginning treatment.

Si: Foul-smelling urine more indicative of dehydration than UTI (Nurs Home Med 1997;5:101).

Crs:

Uncomplicated: Infrequent UTIs (separated by at least 2-3 mo) occurring in a functionally independent, community-based elder with no h/o gu complications and improving within 24-48 hr of beginning therapy.

Complicated: Hospitalized pt or recurrent UTIs (separated by 4 wk), recent instrumentation or gu complications; relapsing infection (separated by 2 wk; bacterial persistence) less common, r/o stones, chronic prostatitis (pos UA after prostatic massage), pyelonephritis, and fistulas.

Cmplc: Sepsis, chronic pyelonephritis, incontinence.

Lab: Clean-catch UA: combined pos reading for nitrates, leukocyte esterase highly predictive of a UTI; whether to culture if UA pos debatable; replace catheter to obtain fresh specimen.

X-Ray: Bladder US for PVR; renal US if suspect chronic pyelonephritis, obstruction.

Rx: Rx of asx bacteriuria not shown to decrease morbidity or mortality (Nejm 2002;347:1576).

Preventive:

Indwelling Catheter When:

1. Retention unmanageable surgically
2. Risk of wound infection from incontinence high

3. Terminally ill pt w pain on movement w change of clothes
4. Pt preference when not responding to other incontinence therapy
5. Bacteriuria 48 hr after short-term catheter: rx as sx UTI

Cranberry Juice: unsweetened 8 oz tid or cranberry extract tabs 1 (300-400 mg) bid (Am Fam Phys 2004;70:22175), 2 gm vit C; separating pts w indwelling catheters in NH in different rooms reduces risk of UTI (J Hosp Infect 1997;36:147).

Suppress recurrent infections (> 3/yr) or w h/o urosepsis: Tm/S (1 tab qd in M and ½ tab in F) and continue as long as UA neg; may use nitrofurantoin in this setting, as well; intravaginal estrogen decreases pH, reducing colonization w Gram-neg bacilli (Nejm 1993;329:753) vs recommendation against suppression (Ger Rv Syllabus, 5th ed, 2002, p310).

Chronic Catheter Care: Change monthly because leakage typical secondary to encrusted debris 16-18 french w 5-10 ml balloon; do not irrigate routinely (J Clin Epidem 1989;42:835).

Therapeutic: Treat symptomatic bacteriuria × 7-10 d in F, 14 d in M; rx nonspecific sxs at their first occurrence; if they do not respond to rx, sx may not be indicative of UTI; rx asymptomatic bacteriuria in pts with h/o short-term catheters, urinary manipulation and instrumentation (Arch IM 1990;150:1389). Consider covering MRSA, enterococcus, pseudomonas in chronically catheterized pts w urosepsis (Jama 2006;7:388).

Uncomplicated: Tm/S or amoxicillin; if resistance is suspected or drug allergy exists, use a quinolone (ciprofloxacin or levofloxacin 250-500 mg qd); replace catheter. In vitro resistance to sulfa drugs not always clinically relevant (Arch IM 2006;166:635).

Complicated:

- In stable outpatient or NH pt, start with a quinolone and change to narrower-spectrum drug once sensitivities have returned; ×14 d for T° > 101 for upper UTI; replace catheter.

- Unstable: In NH pt, ampicillin and ceftriaxone im q 12-24 hr, remove and replace catheters; in hospitalized pt, ampicillin and gentamicin iv, vancomycin and gentamicin iv, fluoroquinolones and ampicillin iv, 3rd generation cephalosporin or aztreonam iv (Nurs Home Med 1997;5:100); chronic bacterial prostatitis: Tm/S or quinolone × 4 wk; linezolid (Zyvox) po bid × 10 d for VRE or MRSA, vancomycin for MRSA.
- 0.5 mg Estriol hs × 2 wk, then 2/wk × 8 mo decreases recurrent UTI without risk to endometrium (Nurs Home Med 1998;6:77).
- Yeast usually represents colonization, unless in acute care setting (Jags 1998;46:849).

1.6 Constipation

Mayo Clin Proc 1996;71:81; Jags 1993;41:1130; 1994;42:701; Geriatrics 1989;44:53

Cause:

Primary Causes: Slowed colonic transit; pelvic floor dysfunction (Jags 2000;48:1142); decrease in large-bowel motility due to decreased fiber, decreased fluid, immobility, laxative abuse.

Secondary Causes:

- Neurologic: CNS central lesions, Parkinson's, CVA, dementia
- Obstructive (more common): Colonic-anorectal disorders (diverticula, irritable bowel, megacolon, hemorrhoids, strictures, polyps, colorectal cancer)
- Metabolic: Constipation can be 1st sign of DM, hypothyroid, hypercalcemia, heavy metal intoxication, hyper/hypoparathyroidism, hypokalemia
- Drugs: Iron, anticholinergics, Ca channel blockers (verapamil), antipsychotics, diuretics, narcotics, anti-Parkinsonian medications

Epidem: Most common digestive complaint, subjective nature of the complaint makes accurate determination of the prevalence of true constipation difficult; 10% for those > 75 (Gerontol Clin 1972;14:56); 30%-50% of elders use laxatives regularly.

Pathophys:

Definitions:

Functional constipation, for at least 12 wks not necessarily consecutive: straining > 25% of time or hard stools > 25% of time or feeling of incomplete evacuation > 25% of time or < 3 bms/wk; or sense of anorectal obstruction in > 25% of bms; or manual aid to facilitate > 25% of bms; or hard or lumpy stools > 25% bms; loose stool should not be present—no sx of irritable bowel syndrome.

Rectal outlet delay (prolonged defecation secondary to anorectal dysfunction): anal blockage and prolonged defecation or manual disimpaction needed (Gastroenterol Int 1991;4:99).

Frail/institutionalized pts w increased total gut transit time develop colonic dilatation due to decrease in intraluminal pressures; increased gut transit time also caused by a disruption in coordinated segmental motion of the colonic circular smooth muscle, impaired rectal sensation and tone; also rectal dyschezia or increased rectal tone (irritable bowel syndrome); weakening of abdominal muscles and decreased external and internal anal sphincter tone.

Sx: Change in usual bowel frequency (< 3 bms/wk); straining with evacuation and prolonged defecation (10 min or more for completion of bm); sense of incomplete defecation; fecal soiling and/or fecal incontinence; abdominal distension and discomfort; need for manual disimpaction.

Si: Diminished bowel sounds; lax abdominal musculature; masses in sigmoid, transverse, and descending colon; decreased rectal tone; decreased perianal sensation and anal reflex; presence of hard stool in rectal vault (empty vault common and does not preclude a high impaction); soft stool impacted in rectal vault may indicate rectal dysfunction; masses, hemorrhoids, fissures, oozing stool (overflow diarrhea); distended abdomen; nausea/vomiting; hard stool in rectum or colon; chronic or semi-acute dehydration with tenting of skin.

Crs: May be chronic or acute; r/o irritable bowel syndrome (usually associated with a long h/o of bowel disorders; "gas problems;" abdominal pain relieved by defecation and alternation between constipation and diarrhea); colorectal cancer w obstruction, anal fissure, rectal ischemia, and anorectal tumor may be associated w rectal pain on defecation.

Cmplc: Cardiovascular (angina, MI, arrhythmias); megacolon (volvulus of sigmoid, cecal rupture); rectal prolapse; fecal incontinence (UTIs and sepsis, decubitus ulcers); hemorrhoids; laxative abuse.

Lab: Fasting glucose, TSH (r/o hypothyroidism), calcium, potassium, BUN, creatinine, guaiac stool, urine specific gravity, heavy metal screen

X-Ray: Flat plate of abdomen to r/o impaction; barium studies not recommended due to barium retention; colonoscopy, if colonic cancer is suspected (anemia, family hx or guaiac-pos stools) (Mayo Clin Proc 1996;71:81).

Rx:

Preventive: Increase fluid intake to 1200-2000 mL/d; then increase fiber intake (dietary fiber or OTC supplements, eg, methylcellulose (Citruce), psyllium (Metamucil)—must take at least 1200 mL fluid/d, if using fiber supplementation; begin regular exercise program; adjust toileting schedule to coincide with natural urge to defecate; consider morning coffee or tea; avoid meds that lead to constipation; avoid routine use of stimulant laxatives.

Therapeutic: Initiate preventive regime, as above; increase fiber (Citrucel) 1 tsp up to tid, except if pt is bedridden, has < 1000 mL fluid intake/d or has a h/o megacolon or volvulus.

For slow transit, use laxatives in increasing order of strength as follows: sorbitol 15-30 mL qd to tid; (Jamda 2005;6:532) MOM 15-30 mL qd or bid (contraindicated in moderate renal insufficiency); senna 1-2 tabs qhs 3 ×/wk or qd hs (for maintenance); bisacodyl 10 mg supplement up to 3 ×/wk; for rectal dyschezia: glycerin supplement 3 ×/wk or up to qd; tap water enema, 500 mL, as needed; mineral oil enema, 100-250 mL, qd.

For fecal impaction: digital disimpaction, followed by oil retention enemas and subsequent tap water enemas qd until clear; follow with cathartics to cleanse colon; senna 30 mg up to tid and sorbitol 30 mL up to tid; if large fecal load still present (but without obstruction), give 1-2 L polyethylene glycol (GoLYTELY, MiraLax).

When abdominal x-ray is clear of impaction, begin maintenance bowel regime as above; stool softeners, eg, docusate sodium (Colace), only when straining is to be avoided (post-MI, angina, hemorrhoids, post-surgery); always avoid use of highly irritant laxatives.

Team Management: Nursing staff, family assist pt to upright commode when urge to defecate occurs; osteopathic maneuvers, eg, sacral rocking (gentle pressure on sacrum w inspiration while pt prone).

1.7 Malnutrition

Nurs Home Med 1994;2:206; Geriatrics 1990;45:7; Rueben D, Nutritional problems and assessment, UCLA intensive geriatric review course, 1/19/96; Jags 1995;43:415; 2002;50:1996; Ger Rv Syllabus, 3rd ed, 1996, 145.

Cause:

- Inadequate intake, inadequate dentition, poverty and inadequate range of food groups, malabsorption, nutrient-drug interactions, chronic disease, or acute insult; taste decreased secondary to decreased olfaction w age (J Gerontol 1986;41:460).

- Dehydration: reduced access to fluids, decreased thirst perception, reduced response to serum osmolality, decreased ability to concentrate urine following fluid deprivation.

Epidem: Malnutrition occurs in 37%-40% of community elderly, 35%-65% of hospitalized elderly, 19%-58% of institutionalized elderly (Nurs Home Med 1994;2:206).

Sx: Nutritional hx from the pt or caregiver regarding eating preferences, restrictions, and allergies; use of mineral/vit supplements and nonprescription meds; taste change, chewing, swallowing problems, nausea/vomiting/diarrhea.

Si: DENTAL Screening Survey (Jags 1996;44:980):

- Dry mouth
- Eating difficulty
- No recent dental care
- Tooth or mouth pain
- Alteration or change in food selection
- Lesions, sores or lumps in the mouth

Changes seen in nutritional deficiencies may be mistaken for changes occurring with aging on screening exam (brittle hair and nails, sunken eyes, pale sclerae, prominence of the bony skeleton, especially the extremities and chest); may also see cracked lips, sores around the mouth, poor dentition, magenta tongue, muscle wasting, peripheral edema, blunted mental status.

Height and weight most reliable of the anthropomorphic measurements; assess ability to self-feed; when intake is difficult to assess or is obviously poor, obtain a 24-72 hr calorie count (in NH 2 wk after admission, allowing the pt to settle into environment).

Meds That Interfere w Vits:

- Trimethoprim and phenytoin interfere w folate
- Cholestyramine, mineral oil, and neomycin interfere w vit A absorption, causing night blindness

- Hydralazine is a vit B_6 antagonist; INH increases vit B_6 urinary excretion

Lab:

BMI wt(kg)/ht(m2) < 18.5 = malnutrition; 25-50% < RDA

Assess the severity of wgt loss by determining the ratio of the pt's ABW to IBW; for M calculated at 106 lbs for the first 5 feet and 6 lbs for each inch above 5 feet; for F it is 100 lbs for the first 5 feet and 5 lbs for each inch above 5 feet.

Knee height measurements, arm span, or summation of body part measurements may be used to accurately assess height in pts who are unable to stand erect (Gottschlich M, Matavese L, Shronts EP, eds, Nutrition Support Dietetics Core Curriculum, 2nd ed, Silver Spring, MD, American Society of Parenteral and Enteral Nutrition, 1993:44); take into account ethnic variation and compare to other family members. ABW is affected by hydration status, and therefore dehydration should be r/o before other causes of wgt loss are investigated. Significant wgt loss: 2% in 1 wk or 5% in 1 mo; 7.5% in 3 mo; 10% decrease in wgt from the UBW in 6 mo.

Crs: B vitamins and vit C become deficient over wk to mo while fat-soluble vits (A, D, E, K) take longer because of enterohepatic circulation; obesity about the waist and abdomen increases free fatty-acids in the portal system leading to increased lipid production and CAD.

Cmplc: Pressure sore formation, compromised immune function, increased rate of infection, longer recuperation periods, and consequent loss of independence.

Rx:

Prevention: Rx oral hygiene problems with medicated chewing gum chlorhexidine, xylitol (Jags 2002;50:1348).

Older pts trying to gain wgt require 30-35 kcal/kg IBW; check lytes prior to aggressive nutritional support; if tube feeding indicated, start at 20 kcal/kg IBW and slowly advance to 30-35 kcal/kg IBW; energy needs for pts whose wgt is < 76% of IBW should be calculated using ABW, not IBW, which could result in an overestimate of caloric requirements, extreme fluid, and electrolyte shifts.

Estimate protein needs using albumin levels; albumin has half-life of 21 d, reflects previous protein expenditure due to a number of causes, eg, liver disease, infection, nephrotic syndrome, post-op status, inadequate intake and malabsorption; dehydration may falsely elevate albumin; albumin levels of 3.1-3.5 gm/dL indicate mild depletion; 2.6-3.1 gm/dL moderate depletion; and < 2.6 gm/dL severe depletion; low albumin a predictor of mortality, as well (Jama 1994;272:1036); single best predictor of death in malnourished NH pt is cholesterol below 150 mg/dL (Jags 1996;44:37).

Protein RDA 1.0gm/kgbody wt/d: NH pts require 1 gm/kg IBW/d of protein; this increases to 1.2 gm/kg IBW in presence of infection or pressure sores and to 1.5 gm/kg IBW w overwhelming infection and after major surgery. Protein provides 20% of the energy from regular diet, therefore 1800-cal diet furnishes 90 gm of protein. Most dietary supplements provide 10 gm of protein/can (240 mL). Protein food sources expensive for elderly in poverty.

Restrictive Diets: 3 gm Na, ADA diet not likely to improve the status of CHF or DM in old-age, more likely to cause protein-energy malnutrition.

Poor Wound Healing: Consider vit C 500 mg/d and zinc sulfate 220-mg tid (Ann IM 1988;109:890).

Treatment:

Dehydration: Fluid requirements of 1500 mL/d; can consider sc fluid infusion for dehydration (Jags 2000;48:795); clysis (subcutaneous hydration or hypodermoclysis) as good as iv rehydration (Jags 2003;51:155); useful in NH.

Hypernatremia: Require 30-mL free water/kg body weight or replace 25%-30% of deficit/d: Free water deficit = 0.6 × IBW × (1-140/measured serum Na) (Nejm 1977;297:1444).

Vitamin Supplementation: Low-dose multivitamin enhances lymphocyte proliferation, IL-2 production, decreases infection risk in elderly; selenium decreases risk: prostate, lung, colon CA. Vit E risk: HD in women, prostatic CA in men, CA in smokers. Vit A risk: stomach CA. Vits C, E, carotenoids, Zn, Omega 3 FA's slow progression of macular degeneration (Ann IM 2006;145:364).

With Aging Skin: Vit D synthesis from sunlight decreased, therefore supplement those at risk for osteoporosis (especially important in institutionalized elderly); vit K also helps w bone metabolism.

Vit B_6: Helps maintain glucose tolerance, cognitive function; enhances aging immune system, but decreases the effectiveness of L-dopa in treatment of Parkinson's.

Vit B_{12}: Protects against high homocysteine levels associated w stroke; neither vit B_{12} nor folic acid absorbed well in atrophic gastritis; screen for vit B_{12} deficiency (Jags 1995;43:1290); oral B_{12} (1000-2000 gm/d) effective in absence of intrinsic factor.

Increased Consumption of Leafy Vegetables: Rich in retinoids, decreases risk of age-related macular degeneration (Jama 1994;272:1413).

Antioxidant Vits C, E, and β-Carotene: may reduce risk of cancer, cataracts, and heart disease (Nutr Rev 1994;52:S15) vs β-carotenes not shown to help (Nejm 1996;334:1145,1150).

Fiber: Psyllium-containing products also lower cholesterol when given w meals; phytate (cereals, legumes, vegetables) can impair Ca and Zn absorption.

Use Herbs and Spices for Hot Foods: To compensate for loss of sense of smell and taste, avoid excessive use of salt and sugar.

1.8 Geriatric Obesity

Clin Ger Med 2005;21:684,694,758,777

Cause: American dietary habits and sedentary life style

Epidem: 60-69 yr, 42.5% women and 38.1% men, BMI 30+; 70-79 yr, 20% to 28% in men from 1994-2000 and 25% to 31% in women from 1994-2000, BMI weight (kg/height m^2)

Pathophys: Pro-inflammatory state causes erosion of muscle mass leading to sarcopenia. Muscle mass starts to decrease at 30s to 40s and intra-abdominal fat increases with age.

Sx: Sob, joint pain, gait disturbance, sleep disturbance, chest pain

Si: Negative effects on get up and go test, walking speed, chair stand and reach test; BMI > 30; waist circumference > 35 inches in female and > 40 inches in men may be better predictor of mortality than BMI (Arch IM 2001;161:1194)

Skin tags/acanthosis nigricans indicating possible hyperinsulinemia; leg edema secondary to pannus pressure on lymphatics; rash in intertriginous areas; malnutrition can cause muscle wasting, weakness, edema, neuropathy, and angular cheilosis.

Crs: Gait disturbance exacerbated by sedentary lifestyle and functional decline, BMI > 35, greater chance for becoming homebound risk 75% higher

Cmplc: Osteoarthritis knees, diabetes, HT, ASCVD, metabolic syndrome. In men, increase risk for colorectal and prostate cancer. In women, higher risk for gall bladder, endometrial, cervical, ovarian, and breast cancers, renal disease, and functional impairments including immobility, pain, and incontinence (Jags 2001;49: 398), Parkinsons (Am Acad Neurology 2006;67), AD (Arch IM 2003;163:1524), cerebral atrophy. Risk of temporal atrophy increased 13% to 16% per 1.0 kg/m^2, increase in BMI ($p < 0.05$) 24-yr study not causal data (Neurology 2004; 63).

Depression: 25% to 30%. Strong societal bias and discrimination against individuals who are obese extends to healthcare professionals, including nurses and professionals specializing in obesity. Individuals who are obese frequently experience societal mistreatment because of their obesity, and stigmatizing experience may lead to poor image and psychological function. Need for staff education, sensitivity training, and interventions to facilitate an atmosphere of caring.

OSA: 10% to 15% older adults, apnea/hypopnea index doubles every 10 yr, but report of symptoms decreases over age 65, not clear if this is due to decreased reporting. OSA associated with HT, CAD, CHF; atrial fibrillation increase mortality and cognitive function (sustained attention, visuospatial learning and motor performance). Treatment with CPAP may improve all these problems and improve quality of life.

Skin: candidiasis in skin folds, pressure ulcers, venous stasis dermatitis and stasis ulcers, cellulitis, surgical wound dehiscence. Risk for thromboembolism impaired mobility. R/o insulinoma, Cushing's syndrome.

X-ray: Diagnostic tests may be difficult to obtain because of equipment or transport limitations.

Lab: Blood glucose, uric acid, BUN/creatinine, AST/ALT/Alk phos, total and direct bilirubin (hepatic steatosis and gallbladder disease), fasting lipid panel, TSH urinalysis, 2-hr postprandial insulin level in some patients, screen for specific conditions based on presentation of symptoms/index of suspicion.

Rx:

Prevention: Consider stopping meds associated with weight gain. 89% of people who are counseled by their primary care physician actively try to lose weight and are 3 times more likely to try to lose weight.

Prevention of ulcers: Repositioning q2 hr with repositioning of skin folds, use of hair dryer or cooler air to dry area between skin folds.

Prevention of staff injuries in nursing homes: Multifactor interventions that combine training with mechanical and other assistive patient-handling equipment are more successful in preventing injuries (Spine 2001;26:1739).

Therapeutic:

- NIH Clinical Guidelines, and Treatment of Overweight and Obesity in Adults (Circ 2004;109:3244)
  - Diet: increase daily intake of fruits, vegetables, whole grains, and fish and reduction of total fat intake within the limits of estimated caloric need; minimize restrictions.
  - Nutritional treatment; low fat, low carbohydrate, low glycemic, low calorie diet for weight loss recommended but also found to have low adherence by patients and not as effective as Mediterranean diet (Lancet 2004;364:897).
  - Appropriate calories/d Harris Benedict formula 25-30 kcal/kg/d overestimates calorie needs. Instead, estimated calorie requirement for obese patients is IBW + 25% or 120% IBW.
  - Protein requirement increase in elderly to 1 g/kg/d; in healthy adults to 1.25; in patients with acute illness or pressure ulcers to 1.5 g/kg/d; and in severe conditions to 2 g/kg/d.
- Active lifestyle, resistance strength training, and aerobic activities increase strength and muscle mass, decreases risk for death; stretching exercises for flexibility; 10% weight loss in 6 mo 1-2 lbs/wk, then maintain; appointments w/ physician 2-4 wk first month then once a month first 6 months.
  - Exercise causes weight and abdominal circumference reduction, weight maintenance, preservation of lean body mass

and bone during weight loss, and helps prevent functional decline.

- Tx contraindicated in pt with terminal illness, osteoporosis, and cholelithiasis may become worse with weight loss; intentional weight loss benefits older people, unintentional associated with increased mortality; patients are 3 times more likely to attempt weight loss when it is recommended in an office visit.

Pharmacotherapy:

Orlistat: Inhibit pancreatic lipases (Diabetes Care 204;27:115); side effects: flatulence, nephrolitiasis; interacts with warfarin; expensive

Sibutramine: Serotonin, dopamine, and norepinephrine reuptake inhibitor decrease appetite; increase pulse; increase blood pressure; contraindicated in CAD, glaucoma, sz, many complications in elderly

Bile acid-resins improve glycemic control and ameliorate obesity and fatty liver in diabetics (Diabetes 2007;56:239)

- Surgery: BMI > 40 or > 30 with comorbidities; gastric bypass surgery age 50-65, rarely performed > 65

Team Management: Physician, dietician, psychologist, nurse, and nurse practitioner

Bariatric unit in nursing home: physician, PT, OT, nurse, risk manager, safety specialist, ergonomist, CNAs, administrator Educational information (NIH Publication No 00-4084; Clin Ger Med 2005;21:698; Curr Opin Nutr Metab Care 2004;7:3)

Safety

Bariatric unit nursing home: Special equipment/clothing for high weight and width of patients, including wide chairs, expandable beds that can be lowered and tilted, pressure reduction, noncompressible mattress, wide bed pans and toilet, heavy duty lifts, wide walkers, wide wheelchairs, appropriately sized gowns and incontinence briefs, wide blood pressure cuffs and scales (Clin Ger Med 2005;21:771)

Providing appropriate nursing home care to residents who are obese requires environmental modifications, specialized equipment, and staff training. Nursing home bariatric units' nurses must be aware of common postoperative complications (Mayo Clin Proc 2004;79:1158).

1.9 Vision

Cataracts

UCLA intensive geriatric review course, 1/96; Ger Rv Syllabus, 3rd ed, 1996, p138, Treat GuideL Med Lett 2007;5:1.

Cause: Sun exposure, age, trauma, uveitis, retinitis pigmentosa, intraocular malignancies, DM, hypoparathyroidism, hypothyroidism, steroids (topical, as well as systemic), congenital, environmental/UV radiation, smoking, diets low in antioxidants.

Epidem: 18% of those age 65-74 yr and 46% age > 75 yr; leading cause of reversible blindness in the U.S.; second leading cause of overall blindness in the U.S.; cataract extraction is the most frequently performed surgical intervention on the Medicare population.

Pathophys: Water-insoluble proteins increase w age, leading to brown pigmentation of lens:

- Nuclear cataract (most common): sclerosis of fibers in the lens w increased refractive index secondary to color changes.
- Anterior subcapsular: usually iritis leads to adherence to the lens, forming posterior synechiae and eventually, w epithelial cell proliferation, a subcapsular connective tissue plaque; lens is opacified and liquified until the entire lens cortex is involved, forming a "mature" cataract.

- Posterior subcapsular: formed by epithelial cells that migrate beneath the posterior capsule and enlarge.

Sx: Reduced visual acuity, although may report improved near vision (nuclear), distant or increased glare (posterior subcapsular).

Si: Opacities often visible on ophthalmoscopic exam; difficult to visualize fundus.

Crs: Develop after age 40, although almost anyone who lives long enough will develop them; painless progressive variable loss of vision.

Cmplc: R/o normal changes of aging: dark adaptation, decreased peripheral vision, diminished perception of low-contrast objects; advanced cataract may swell and the capsule may become leaky, causing secondary glaucoma.

Rx:

- 90% of extractions are extracapsular, leaving the posterior capsule in place, providing an anchor for the intraocular lens.
- Phacoemulsification (ultrasonic wave) used to pulverize the lens so it can be aspirated prior to placement of implant; less valuable for pts w hard sclerotic nuclear cataracts.
- Complications of rx: opacification of posterior capsule (50% over 3-yr period)—can use laser to correct this w improvement in 90% of pts.
- Pts w macular degeneration, also related to sun exposure, may also have cataracts; therefore, do not repair cataracts when there is coexistent severe macular degeneration (sometimes difficult clinical decision).
- Complication rates of surgery low: faulty wound closure w aqueous humor leakage and intractable secondary glaucoma; explosive choroidal hemorrhage that can cause blindness; endophthalmitis requiring hospitalization for iv antibiotics and corticosteroids (The Merck Manual of Geriatrics, 3rd ed., Beers MH, et al., eds. Whitehouse Station, NJ: Merck Research Laboratories, 2000).

- Second eye cataract surgery improves functional outcome, eg, reading normal print, engaging in activities previously precluded by vision impairment (Lancet 1998;352:925).

Glaucoma

Treat GuideL Med Lett 2007;5:1

Cause: Primary open-angle glaucoma (POAG): 70% of cases due to impaired aqueous drainage through the trabecular meshwork; POAG accounts for 90% of glaucoma in the elderly in the U.S.; narrow-angle (NAG): steroid-induced, traumatic, inflammatory, neovascular, low tension.

Epidem: Risk factors: increased age, females; weaker association with HT, cardiovascular disease, diabetes, smoking, UV light exposure and diet; POAG: 6 × more common in blacks, whereas NAG more prevalent among Asians, especially Chinese.

Pathophys:

POAG: Anatomically normal outflow channels but increased resistance to aqueous humor outflow from gradual meshwork occlusion.

NAG: As lens thickens, anterior chamber is made more shallow, especially in far-sighted pts w smaller eyes; elevated intraocular pressure occurs when the base of the iris is pushed forward, sealing off trabecular meshwork outflow; aqueous humor continuously produced by the eye circulating through the anterior chamber cannot leave through outflow channels, producing intraocular pressure of 50-60 mm Hg in hours (nl intraocular pressure = 20 mmHg), irreversible changes in 48-72 hr.

Crs:

POAG: 2% visual field loss/yr (Nejm 1993;328:1097).

Sx:

POAG: Asx till very late, gradual loss of visual fields over years; NAG: acute pain, blurred vision, halos from corneal edema, nausea.

Si:

POAG: Dx depends on the presence of optic nerve excavation (cupping), visual field defects, w or w/o intraocular pressure elevation (common, but not a diagnostic feature); if intraocular pressure < 21 mm Hg but no visual field deficit, then only ocular HT.

Rx:

POAG:

Preventive: Yearly intraocular pressure measurement w Schiøtz tonometer and ophthalmoscopic exam for optic head excavation increases detection rate to 80%, usually done by optometrist or ophthalmologist; stereoscopic equipment and formal visual field testing increase the accuracy of dx.

Therapeutic: Management falls largely to ophthalmologist and is directed toward lowering intraocular pressure (does not always stop progression of visual loss).

Topical: β-Blockers reduce the secretion of aqueous humor, watch for systemic side effects of β-blockers (bradycardia, CHF).

Adrenergics, eg, epinephrine, decrease aqueous humor production and increase outflow through the trabecular meshwork.

Miotics, eg, pilocarpine, carbachol, constrict pupil-stimulating longitudinal muscle fibers of the ciliary body, thereby opening the trabecular meshwork pores.

Oral: Carbonic anhydrase inhibitors, eg, acetazolamide, decrease production of aqueous humor, numerous adverse effects in the elderly—confusion, paresthesias, drowsiness, anorexia, calcium phosphate renal stones; prostaglandin analogue does not exacerbate asthma or cardiovascular sx (Sci Am 1998 IX;8:13).

Surgical: Filtration procedures designed to create drainage between the anterior chamber and the subconjunctival space; f/u q 6 mo.

NAG: Emergency pilocarpine 2%-4% q 5 min × 6, or acetazolamide 250 mg.

Surgical: laser iridotomy within 24 h, expect cure.

Macular Degeneration

UCLA Intensive Geriatric Review Course, 1/96; Am Fam Phys 2000;61:3035; Jags 2006;54:1130

Cause:

Epidem: The leading cause of irreversible blindness in U.S. elderly; among people > 55 yr in the U.S., 2.2% are blind in one eye from macular degeneration; increased w age, whites, females; weaker association with HT, cardiovascular disease, diabetes, smoking (Jama 1996;276:1141,1147), UV light exposure.

Pathophys: Degenerative changes in the macula lead to loss of fine central vision, but not peripheral vision; since macular changes such as pigment mottling and the appearance of drusen also occur in all older retinae, the label of acute macular degeneration is used only when there is accompanying loss of visual acuity; for both of these conditions the anatomic changes lie on a continuum; therefore the criteria for defining a diseased vs healthy eye in an older person is difficult.

Sx: Sudden or recent central vision loss, blurred vision, distortion, new scotomata indicate neovascularization; Amsler grid facilitates monitoring.

Si: Hard yellow-white pinhead-size drusen is localized disorder of retinal pigmented epithelium vs soft drusen w more widespread damage; 3 forms: dry or atrophic (80-90% w central loss of vision), subretinal neovascular membrane, retinal pigment epithelial detachment with drusen.

Rx:

Low Vision Aids: Magnifying devices, eg, magnified TV, special lighting (J Am Optom Assoc 1988;59:307; Geriatrics 1995; 50:51).

Photocoagulation (Arch Ophthalm 1994;112:489): indicated for symptomatic choroidal neovascularization outside foveal avascular zone (minority of pts), postpones visual loss. Complc: scar, if "runoff" beyond intended area of treatment.

Photodynamic rx w Verteporfin (Vis Dyne): For pts w age-related classic subflaval choroidal neovascularization (wet) (Med Lett 2000;42:81; 2007;5:5). Ranizumab (Nejm 2006;355:1419).

Iloprost: For nonexudative macular degeneration (Jags 2000;48:1350; 2002;50:780).

Team Management: Low vision aids, support group; improve function in bathroom for low vision persons using contrasting colors of cup, soap, and soap dish; install wall-mounted soap dispenser, mirror w extension arm; alphabetize medicine cabinet; keep cabinets closed; mark positions of cold and hot on faucet so same temperature settings can be selected each time; shampoo and other items in distinguishable shaped bottles; mark desired water level in bathtub (Am Fam Phys 2000;61:3035).

1.10 Diabetic Retinopathy

Cause: Diabetes neovascularization and hemorrhage.

Epidem: Third leading cause of adult blindness (7% of all blindness); increased prevalence (3%) with greater longevity, positively correlated with the duration of diabetes.

Pathophys: Selective loss of mural cells in the basement membrane of retinal capillaries; when glucose is converted by aldose reductase to sorbitol, water moves into the mural cells and they rupture; mural cells have contractile properties and their loss results in capillary dilatation, leading to increased volume of blood flow and resultant microaneurysms, which hemorrhage and lead to exudate formation.

Sx: Loss of vision, glaucoma in end stages.

Si:

Non-Proliferative: Hemorrhages in both the nerve fiber and mid retinal layers, cotton wool spots (nerve fiber layer infarcts), vascular dilatation and tortuousness, microaneurysms, macular edema.

Proliferative: Neovascularization at the disc and, elsewhere, preretinal/vitreous hemorrhage, traction retinal detachment, posterior retinal breaks, glaucoma, macular edema.

Crs: Early (3-5 yr) first see minimal visual loss from macular edema or clouding of vision from small vitreous hemorrhage, microaneurysms (> 5 in each eye); then non-proliferative changes; then proliferative changes.

Rx:

Preventive: Annual ophthalmologic exam; correlation between ACE inhibitor and postponement of diabetic retinopathy (Am J Med Sci 1993;305:280); tight diabetic control reduces progression.

Therapeutic: Aldose reductase inhibitor (Epalrestat) to decrease sorbitol; proliferative: laser photocoagulation early slows down visual loss; w non-proliferative, vitrectomy w impending retinal detachment.

1.11 Hearing Problems

UCLA Intensive Geriatric Review Course, 1/96

Cause:

- Sensorineural (most common): cochlear or auditory nerve damage due to loud noise (usually bilateral); ototoxic drug effects may be delayed in onset; aminoglycoside dose-related, hearing loss less common than vestibular disturbance and tin-

nitus; vestibular disturbance and tinnitus are often first signs, taking as much as 2 wk to abate after drug discontinued; aging (presbycusis: high-frequency loss); unilateral causes include trauma, infection, acoustic neuroma, Ménière's—also associated w peripheral vertigo.
- Conductive (less common): cerumen impaction, middle ear disease, otosclerosis.
- Central hearing loss: impaired speech discrimination beyond what would be expected based on threshold change (10% of cognitively impaired).

Epidem: Prevalence increases with age; in the Framingham cohort 41% > 65 yr had some level of impairment, only 10% had tried hearing aids; 80% of men between 85 and 90 yr reported having trouble hearing; in NHs prevalence ranges from 50%-100%.

Si: Whisper test from behind pt; observation of lip-reading ("intentness index"); types of hearing loss:
- Conductive: bone thresholds > air thresholds
- Sensorineural: both air and bone thresholds are elevated

Crs: Declines 2× faster in men than women; women have more sensitive hearing above 1000-Hz frequency, while men have more sensitive hearing at lower frequencies (J Acoust Soc Am 1995;97:1196); r/o acoustic neuroma-50% exibit dizziness or tinnitus.

Cmplc: Social isolation/withdrawal from conversations, frustration/resentment; mislabeled with dementia, depression; greater risk of falling, impaired mobility, cognitive impairment.

Lab: Audiometry tests and interpretation: measured in decibels at which the stimulus can be heard 50% of the time; test ability to understand words (speech discrimination); Audioscope set at 40 dB. Test tone at 60 dB delivered then four tones (500,100,2000,4000 Hz) at 40 dB. Fail if cannot hear 1000 or 2000 Hz both ears or both 1000 and 2000 Hz in either ear (Clin Ger Med 1999;15:153).

Rx:

Conductive: Amplification (for 45-60 dB loss): improvement in social function, emotional well-being, communication function, less depression; hearing aids are most helpful for understanding speech and listening to TV or movies, not as helpful in crowded or noisy situations. Barriers: cost (largest obstacle, not covered by Medicare); self-perceived handicap; difficulties with the small controls due to arthritis; excessive feedback from ear-mold fittings; if loss > 80 dB, only limited improvement w hearing aid.

Involvement of a hearing aid specialist for identification of appropriate equipment and training and counseling; adjustment may take weeks to months and is strongly influenced by motivation; cochlear implants w profound sensorineural deafness, if conventional hearing aid not feasible (Nejm 1993;329:1092).

Team Management: Physician-pt relationship: minimize background noise as much as possible; use good lighting; face the person at eye level; encourage pts to wear their hearing aids to an office visit; speak clearly from closer range and lower pitch if possible, rather than shouting; use gestures and write down important instructions; clinicians may purchase inexpensive, pocket-sized personal amplifiers with headphones that pts can wear during interview.

1.12 Incontinence

Urge Incontinence

Jama 2004;291:986,996; Nejm 2003;350:786; 1989;320:1; 1985;313:800; AHCPR Public No. 92-0039, U.S. Pub Health Service, 1992; Lancet 1995;346:94; Ann IM 1995;122:438; Michelle Eslami, UCLA Geriatric Review Course 9/02 *Urinary Incontinence*

Cause: Decreased CNS inhibition common in many normal elders; accentuated in dementia (voiding dysfunction in NPH results from paraventricular compression of frontal inhibitory centers leading to urge incontinence), Parkinson's, CVA, or cervical stenosis; or with parasympathomimetic drugs like bethanechol (Urecholine), cisapride; or irritation from cystitis, prostatitis, BPH, bladder tumor.

Epidem: One-third have urge incontinence (common in community-dwelling elderly). Of all women with some incontinence, black and Hispanic women are more likely to have urge incontinence (Am J Obgyn 2004;191:2).

Pathophys: Detrusor overactive instability may be due to CNS lesion, detrusor hyperreflexia or aging (Urol Clin N Am 1996;23:55) (90% is idiopathic).

Detrusor instability w (most common form in the elderly) or w/o impaired contractility (J Urol 1993;150:1668).

Sx: Little warning; leakage delayed or persists after cough volume of urine lost may be large or small; stained clothing; asking about diapers or accidents is insulting (Geriatrics 1999;54:22); inquire about degree of control.

Lab: Cystometrics show spastic contractions; office cystometry (Am Fam Phys 1998;57:2675); Ca, glucose, UA culture.

Rx:

- Antibiotics for any infection.
- If minimal in community-dwelling elderly: planned voiding, avoid caffeine, alcohol, carbonated drinks.
- Biofeedback (Jama 2004;291:986,996; Ann IM 1985;103:507); pelvic exercises; extend voiding intervals by half-hour increments once dry (Jama 1991;265:609; 1998;280;1995; Jags 1999;47:309); prompted voiding q 2 hr helps cognitively-impaired pts (Jags 1990;38:356) and is 25-40% effective (Dis Mo 1992;38:65).

- Behavioral plus meds added benefit in treating urge incontinence (Jags 2000;48:370).
- Oxybutynin (Ditropan) 5 mg po tid (anticholinergics, ie, parasympathetic inhibition), extended release oxybutynin, transdermal oxybutynin 10 mg qd (J Urol 2002;168:580) adding oxybutynin to prompted voiding more effective (Jags 1995;43:610) or propantheline 7.5-30.0 mg po tid; antimuscarinics less dry mouth like tolterodine (Detrol) 1-2 mg po bid (Med Lett 1998;40:101; 2001;43:28; Mayo Clin Proc 2001; 76:258; Jama 2004;291:991).
- Imipramine 25-50 mg po hs (∝-stimulation, parasympathetic inhibition).
- Flavoxate not effective.
- Tropsium chloride (Sanctura) poor absorption (Med Lett 2000;46:63).
- Trial of bladder relaxants; if urinary retention > 150 mL, suspect detrusor hyperreflexia coexisting w mild urinary outflow obstruction in males, or detrusor overactivity w impaired contractility; in pts w detrusor hyperreflexia and impaired contractility in which involuntary contractions are only provoked at higher bladder volumes, catheterize hs, avoid bladder relaxants (Jama 1996;267:1832).
- Estrogen (intravaginal) may ameliorate dyspareunia and reduce the frequency of recurrent cystitis (Nejm 1993;329:753, S. Cummings AMDA Annual Conference Mar 2000, Osteoporosis) but has not been found to prevent urge incontinence (J Obgyn 2001;97:116), with or without progesterone (Jama 2005;293:935); caution regarding systemic absorption.
- Refer for further urologic w/u if recurrent UTIs (Ann IM 1995;122:749), microscopic hematuria, failure to respond to pharmacologic or behavioral treatment, diagnostic uncertainty.

Overflow Incontinence

Cause: Bladder outlet obstruction, eg, BPH, uterine prolapse, large cystocele, ureteral stenosis (associated w atrophic vaginitis), constipation (up to 10% in hospitalized pts), stimulant drugs, neuropathy (impaired sensory input to sacral micturition center); or diminished detrusor strength (flaccid due to lower motor neuron disease); or herpes zoster (from pain); or neurosyphilis which causes detrusor sphincter dyssynergy (Urol Clin N Am 1996; 23:11); or meds (anticholinergics, calcium channel blockers, smooth muscle relaxants, opiates).

Epidem: Overflow incontinence less common than other forms of incontinence.

Sx: Obstructive w diminished urinary stream; leakage of urine, usually small amounts; frequency; if neuropathic, will have no sensation of bladder fullness.

Si: Prostate's palpated size correlates poorly w actual size; suprapubic and abdominal exam for distended bladder.

Lab: PVR >200 mL (easy office procedure); in women w large cystoceles, urine may "puddle" below catheter's reach, giving falsely low value for PVR; obtain renal function tests (Ouslander 1996, UCLA Intensive Geriatric Review Course, 1/96) and refer for cystometrics or voiding cystourethrogram; cystometrics show no contractions w 400+ mL when due to diminished sensation.

Rx:

- Stool softeners for constipation.
- Rx prolapse or BPH; finasteride modest and delayed benefits (Nejm 1992;327:1185); rx for 4 yr reduced probability of surgery, led to less extensive resection of prostate w local anesthesia in frail elderly men (Nejm 1998;338:557).
- Block sphincter constriction (∝-blockade) w prazosin (Minipress) 1-2 mg po tid or terazosin (Hytrin); finasteride

(∝-reductase inhibitor decreases BPH) not as effective (Ann IM 1995;122:438), but 2 drugs better than 1—finasteride plus doxazosin (Nejm 2003;549:2387).

- Bladder neuropathy from cobalamin deficiency reversible w vit B_{12} replacement (J Intern Med 1992;231:313); 60% of diabetics w incontinence do not have neuropathic bladder, they have constipation from autonomic neuropathy (Jags 1993;41:1130).
- Self-catheterization (Jags 1990;38:364) may be impractical in frail elderly (Ouslander 1996, UCLA Intensive Geriatric Review Course, 1/96); long-term catheters indicated in 1-2% pts.
- Increase detrusor strength w bethanechol (Urecholine) 10+ mg po tid, mostly useful in the setting of anticholinergic agents that can't be discontinued; or phenoxybenzamine (Dibenzyline) 10 mg po qd (sympathomimetics); monitor PVR.
- Wood pulp-containing absorbent undergarments superior to polymer gel; garments for women and men differ because different target zone of urinary loss (Urol Clin N Am 1996;23:11); substantial out-of-pocket expense (Geriatrics 1999;54:22).
- Indwelling catheter care: do not irrigate or clamp; leakage may be due to bladder spasm; therefore use smaller catheter; treat only symptomatic UTIs and do not use prophylaxis; consider acidification, if no urea-splitting organisms, and silicon catheter, if obstruction occurs frequently.
- Refer for urologic w/u if large cystourethrocele, markedly enlarged prostate (check PSA first), symptoms or signs of obstruction, and pt is a surgical candidate.

Stress Incontinence

Jama 2005;293:935

Cause: Estrogen deficiency effect on urethral mucosa; or pelvic relaxation after childbirth or urologic surgery; neuropathies.

Epidem: One-third have mixed stress and urge incontinence. Stress incontinence is four times more common in white women than black or Hispanic women (Am J Obgyn 2002;186:5). Risk is associated w vaginal delivery, increases w parity. Obesity also significantly included risk. Fibroid tumors do not contribute to risk (Am J Obgyn 2004;191:2).

Pathophys: Sphincter insufficiency.

Sx: Loss of urine w cough, sneeze, laugh.

Si: Cystocele on physical exam, if due to pelvic relaxation.

Lab:

- Voiding record kept for 48-72 hr useful; milder form of intrinsic sphincter deficiency occurs in older women resulting from urethral atrophy; they may leak urine at bladder capacity of 200 mL; therefore, if incontinent in morning after full night's sleep, then probably have volume-dependent stress incontinence.
- Urinary stress test: pt should tolerate 300-500 mL before becoming very uncomfortable; if tolerates < 250 mL, need further evaluation for interstitial cystitis (pain related to voiding without objective evidence of disease, which may be due to deficiency in bladder lining, autoimmune phenomena, r/o carcinoma-in-situ w cystoscopy) (Waxman J, Texas A+M Univ Health Science Center, Conference on Women's Health, 2/28/96, Cancun, Mexico).

Rx:

- Kegel exercises 20-200 qd (J Gerontol 1993;48:M167); postural maneuvers (Obgyn 1994;84:770); pre-contractions can reduce cough-related urine (Jags 1998;46:870); vaginal weights better than Kegel's; pessaries (Jags 1992;40:635), more effective in pts w concurrent sx of pressure due to uterine prolapse (Am J Obgyn 2004;190:4); 3 reps, 8-12 set, 8 sec duration 3 ×/w (Nejm 2004;350:786).

- Periurethral injection of collagen is not effective (Br J Urology Int 1999;84:966).
- For neuropathic types, imipramine 25+ mg hs (∝-stimulation, parasympathetic inhibition); or phenylephrine (∝-stimulation); or biofeedback (Ann IM 1985;103:507).
- Surgery (bladder neck suspension safe and effective, AP repair, sphincter repairs).
- Pessaries: foldable-recreate the urethrovesicular angle (Smith-Hodge); no incontinence but prolapse-use space occupying-doughnut, inflatable (Obgyn 2006;108:93).

Functional Incontinence

Cause: Difficulty getting to the toilet.

Si: All normal.

Rx: Schedules plus reinforcement of prompted voiding w 25%-40% response rate can be identified during a 3-d trial period (Jama 1995;273:1366).

1.13 Female Sexual Dysfunction

(Jama 2007;297:620; Nejm 2007;357:762)

Cause: Uterus not necessary for orgasm; radical procedures to remove part of the vagina do not affect ability to have orgasm (Obgyn 1993;81:357); quality of first sexual experience after breast cancer rx strongly influences later sexual recovery (CA 1988;38:154); women receive less sexual counseling after acute MI than do men; in couples who do not resume sexual activity, there is deterioration of their emotional relationships (Heart Lung 1987; 16:154); any major illness in self or partner can become "watershed point."

Epidem: Young people, especially physicians, underrate the extent of sexual interest of older people.

Pathophys: Androgens derived largely from the adrenal gland and a small amount from the ovaries sustain libido; however, coital activity is not correlated w blood levels of estradiol, testosterone, androstenedione, FSH or LH (Maturitas 1991;13:43).

Sx: Key screening questions: Are you sexually active? Do you have a healthy partner? Is there a change in your level of desire? Is there any discomfort w sexual activity? Is vaginal dryness a problem? Is there difficulty achieving orgasm?; dyspareunia (in 33% of women > 65 yr) associated w postmenopausal urogenital atrophy, including a feeling of dryness, tightness, vaginal irritation, burning w coitus, and postcoital spotting and soreness; w very old, explore from perspective of sexual feelings, thoughts, always ask about self-stimulation, masturbation; can be useful to start with "Sexual feelings continue to be important for many people during aging—this can sometimes surprise people as they get older—how would you describe this part of you?"

Si: Look for si of vaginitis (erythema introitus), atrophy (thinned, pallorous mucosa), depression.

Crs: Most significant determinant of sexual activity is unavailability of partner; rate of sexual activity earlier in life persists into old age; orgasm usually survives most illness and rx; sexual touching almost always continues to be pleasurable; most couples have resumed sexual activity 7 mo after acute MI; risk of death during sexual intercourse very low.

Rx:

Prevention: Let older women know that sexual fantasies, desires are normal, but be nonjudgmental about those who are satisfied w abstinence; open discussion of body image w couples (after breast removal, w placement of ostomy bags, incontinence, stroke); assumption of heterosexuality leads to a reluctance of older lesbians to interact w health system (J Gerontol Nurs 1990;16:35); staff attitudes and beliefs central problem for NH elderly who are categorized as having sexual problems (Jags 1987;35:331; Arch Sex Behav 1994;23:231); β-blocking agents decrease vaginal lubrication; ACE inhibitors and Ca-channel blockers do not cause sexual dysfunction; all psychotropic drugs associated w inhibition of sexual function; antidepressants can cause anorgasmia (J Clin Psychiatry 1991;52:66); alcohol causes sexual dysfunction, though very small amounts may help some people.

Therapeutic: Formal sex education yields more permissive attitudes (Int J Aging Hum Dev 1982;15:121); estrogen therapy reverses atrophic changes but may take as long as 6-12 mo; water-based lubricants better, eg, Astroglide, Replens; vaginismus (involuntary vaginal muscle contractions because of painful intercourse) responds to estrogen and voluntary contraction and relaxation of introitus w finger in the introitus, then w partner penetration in stages; androgen controversial (give progestational agent to avoid endometrial hyperplasia); masturbation (manual or w mechanical device); recommended reading for pts: Gershenfeld M, How to Find Love and Sex and Intimacy After Age 50: A Woman's Guide (Ballantine, 1991) Silverstone B, Growing Older Together: A Couple's Guide to understanding and coping with the challenges of later life (Pantheon, 1992).

1.14 Male Sexual Dysfunction (Impotence)

Jags 1987;35:1015; 1988;36:57; 1997;45:1240; Arch IM 1989;149:1365; Ger Rv Syllabus 3rd ed, 1996, p310; Jama 1993;270:83

Cause:

- Decreased libido due to psychological, social, physical (decreased testicular perfusion), and endocrine.
- Decline in androgen production secondary to testicular failure, as well as hypothalamic hyporesponsiveness and excessive

binding of testosterone in the plasma; morning peak of testosterone much lower in the elderly.

- Decreased erectile rigidity (hypothalamic-pituitary-testicular-autonomic dysfunction or inadequate nerve signaling of penile vessels seen in spinal cord injury, MS, radical prostatectomy, penile arterial occlusive disease, Peyronie's disease s/p radiation causing venous leakage).
- Decreased orgasm (decreased testosterone, retrograde ejaculation secondary to damage of proximal sphincter s/p TURP or from DM).

Epidem: 29% of men > 80 yr have sex 1×/wk; probability of erectile dysfunction in men > 70 = 67% (Arch Sex Behav 1993;22:545); there may be multiple causes, vascular or neurologic (48%), diabetes (17%), psychological problems (9%), drugs (4%), low testosterone (3%).

Pathophys: Atherosclerosis, clot, or vascular surgery lead to decreased arterial supply to penis; venous leakage; trauma to nerves of the penis from lumbar disc disease, rectal surgery, prostatectomy; diabetic neuropathy; alcoholic peripheral neuropathy; drugs, eg, β-blockers, alcohol, cimetidine, antipsychotics, antidepressants, lithium, sedative hypnotics, hormones.

Sx: Erectile dysfunction or lack of interest or decreased mobility; failure to reach ejaculation is very common and can be missed if not asked about.

Si: Gynecomastia, diminished male-pattern hair suggests endocrine etiology; abdominal/femoral bruits suggest vascular disease; penile size may prevent effectiveness of suction device; fibrous bands or plaques on penis suggest Peyronie's disease; penile-brachial index after 3-5 min bicycling w legs in air to dx pelvic steal; nocturnal tumescence not reliable; testicular atrophy suggests hypogonadism; absence of vibratory sense or neural reflex arcs suggests neuropathy; review meds; couple discussion helpful.

Crs: Intermittent course suggests psychogenic origin while progressive suggests organic; however, chronic illness course may cause intermittency also.

Lab: Hct, FBS, Lipid profile, HbA1c, Free Testosterone level, LH, if hypogonadal, prolactin level, TSH (Jama 2004:291:2994).

Dx: Intracavernosal injection of vasodilator papaverine or prostaglandin E_1(PGE_1). If neurogenic etiology suspected, 15 mg papaverine or 5mg PGE_1. If vascular etiology suspected, 30 mg papaverine or PGE_1-28 G needle inserted into side of penis 30-60 sec, response in 15 min w 20-40 min erection.

Rx:

Therapeutic: See Figure 1.2. Avoid drugs w adverse effects of sexual dysfunction: Ca-channel blockers and ACE inhibitors have the least effect of the antihypertensive meds; phenothiazine causes retrograde ejaculation; minor tranquilizers affect the limbic system, decreasing libido; MAO inhibitors, tertiary amine tricyclics, cimetidine, digoxin, progestational agents, heparin, estrogen, spironolactone, alpha adrenergics, GHRH antagonists.

Treat hypothyroidism, diabetes.

Mechanical: Have spouses of COPD pts assume the superior position in sexual intercourse.

Hypogonadism: Depressed mood, reduced energy, muscle mass, strength, reduced bone density, anemia, fatigue, impaired cognition, difficulty achieving orgasm, diminished intensity of orgasm, reduced sexual sensation in penis, reduced ejaculate volume. Common because testosterone levels decrease by 1%/yr. Testosterone gels much more expensive than injections. If PSA rise $\geq$ 1.0 ng/mL in 6 mo, bx. High-grade prostate Cancer, Gleason score 8-10 asociated w low testosterone (J Urol 2000;163:824). Monitor on testosterone w PSA, DRE, hgb 2-3×/yr and 1-2×/yr thereafter (Jama 2004;291:2994).

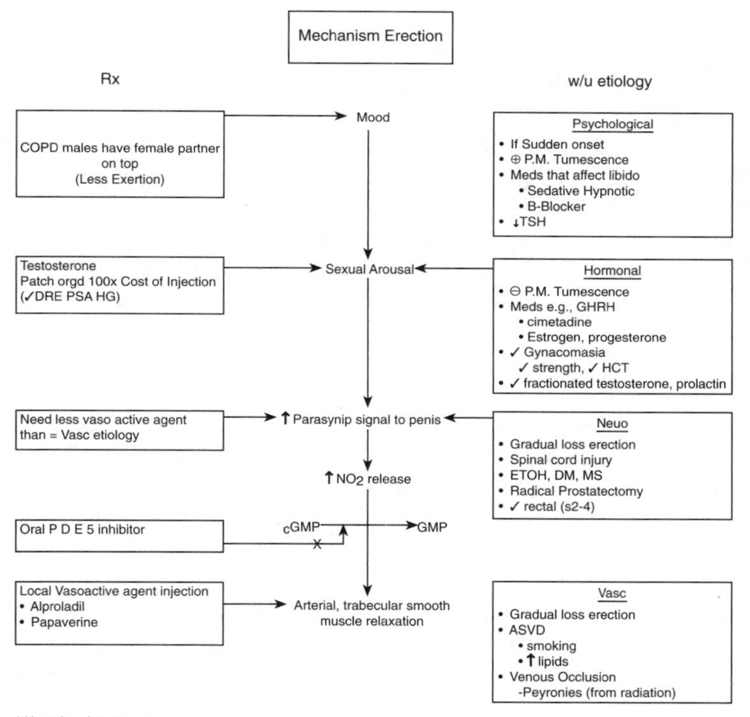

Figure 1.2 Algorithm for the Evaluation of Erectile Dysfunction (ED). ICI-intravernosal injection; LD = low dose; SAE = sleep associated erections; T = testosterone.

Replace zinc in pts w hyperzincuria: 70-mg elemental zinc/d (Jags 1988;36:57).

Vascular or neurologic etiology: alprostadil (Nejm 1996;334:873; 1997;336:1); topical prostaglandin E_1 (J Urol 1995;153: 1828; Clin Diabetes 1996;14:111). If unsuccessful, try penile prostheses (80% success rate): self-contained hydraulic

(Flexi-Flate and Hydroflex models) or cable spring (OmniPhase); low satisfaction w intracavernosal prostaglandin injection, avoid pain w slow injection PGE_1, pellets (rx prolonged erection > 4-6 hr, w aspiration 10-20 mL blood from corpora cavernosum 18 G, then inject w 0.5-1.0 mL of 0.5 mg/mL phenylephrine); angioplasty disappointing results. Vacuum erection devices: 70%-90% satisfaction rate.

Oral phosphodiesterase inhibitor for mixed etiology-sildenafil (Viagra) increases penile response to sexual stimulation and is well-tolerated (Nejm 1998;338:1397), inhibits cGMP metabolism—more smooth muscle relaxation and engorgement (Jama 2004;291:2994).

Don't use w nitrates-hypotension. Do not use w α-blockers. Can take with atenolol and HCTZ. Avoid in high-risk groups: unstable or refractory angina, uncontrolled HTn, high-grade CHF, MI within 2 wks, high-risk arrythmias, obstructive cardiomyopathy, moderate to severe valvular disease. Intermediate risk: moderate angina, recent MI < 6 wks.

Discussion of adaptation over time is warranted, since many men come to understand that sexuality and sexual intimacy are not dependent on capacity to perform intercourse alone.

1.15 Hypothermia

Geriatrics 1999;54:51; Conn Med 1995;59:515

Cause: Accidental: spontaneous decrease of core temperature to lower than 35°C (95°F) usually in a cold environment or dysfunction of hypothalamic thermoregulation from underlying illness (hypothyroidism, myxedema, hypoglycemia, hypoadrenalism, pancreatitis) or drugs; variety of age-related physiologic factors and disease states predispose older patients to hypothermia:

- Malnutrition
- Infections (most frequently missed)
- Social factors (isolation, poverty)
- Alcohol toxicity (Geriatrics 1999;54:51)
- Autonomic dysfunction: inability to vasoconstrict peripheral vessels or increase heart rate in response to cold; reduced ability to perceive cutaneous temperature changes; decrease in metabolic rate heat production and shivering response is reduced (Conn Med 1995;59:515).

Epidem: > 75 yr are 5 × as likely to die from hypothermia (Geriatrics 1999;54:51); 33% of elderly pts developed hypothermia in warm months; with sepsis, hypoproteinemia, cachexia, neuroleptic medication (most commonly thioridazine) (Arch IM 1989; 149:1521); 74% mortality rate (Conn Med 1995;59:515).

Pathophys: Decrease in O_2 delivery to tissue occurs due to increase in blood viscosity, decreased cardiac output, and leftward shift of oxyhemoglobin dissociation curve, respiratory alkalosis.

Depressed renal blood flow with a decrease in GFR by 50%, renal inability to resorb water, cold induced diuresis leading to intravascular volume depletion (Geriatrics 1999;54:51).

Sx:

- Decreased cold perception.
- Mild hypothermia may mimic cognitive decline, cerebral vascular accident, and hypothyroidism or myxedema coma; cerebral metabolism decreases 7% for each 1°C decline in temperature (Geriatrics 1999;54:51).
- Temperature < 32°C (89.6°F): skin is cold, violent shivering, chills, fatigue, confusion, hallucinations.
- Less than 28°C (82.4°F): unconscious; pronounce death if K > 10 or no spontaneous cardiac activity after rewarmed to 34°C (93°F).

Si: Hypothermia defined as core body temperatures lower than 35°C (95°F) by esophageal or rectal measurement of temperature. Hypothermia may be classified as:

- Mild 32.2°-35°C (90°-95°F): cerebral dysfunction begins to manifest with confusion, disorientation, introversion, and amnesia; tachycardia progressing to bradycardia; increase BP; bronchospasm; cold diuresis; shivering; ataxia.
- Moderate 28°-32.2°C (82.4°-90°F): depression level of consciousness; pupil dilatation; paradoxical undressing; pulse decrease of 50%; Afib, Aflut, ventricular ectopic beats, T-wave inversion, prolongation of PR/ST segments, Osborne J waves (Figure 1.3); hypoventilation; no insulin activity; hyporeflexia; diminished shivering; rigidity.

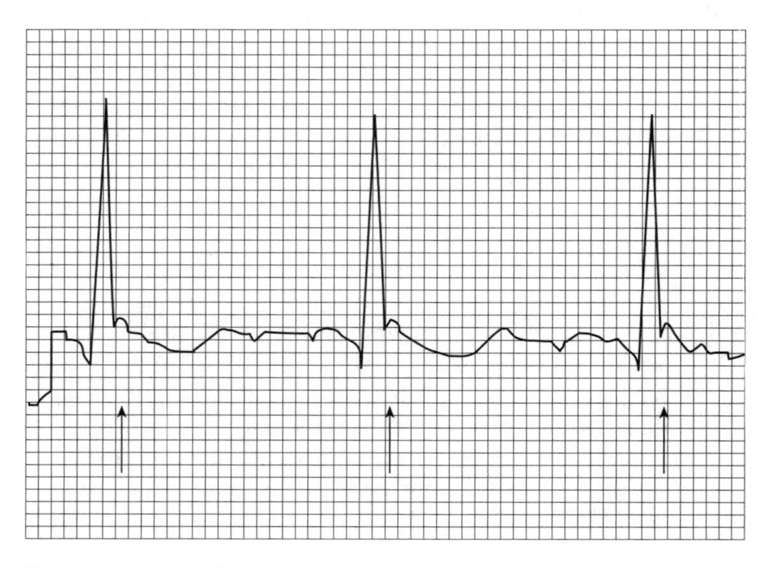

Figure 1.3 Osborne Wave

- Severe/profound < 28°C (82°F): coma; loss of ocular reflexes; decreased BP; ventricular dysrhythmias, asystole; apnea; extreme oliguria; peripheral areflexia
- At 19°C (66.2°F): EEG flat

Cmplc: Ventricular fibrillation, hypoglycemia, hyperkalemia, impaired drug clearance, acute renal failure, disseminated intravascular coagulopathy (DIC), upper gi bleed, respiratory failure; late cardiomyopathy due to multiple micro infarcts. Adverse reactions occur with rewarming:

1. Rewarming shock—sudden deterioration in cardiovascular status.
2. Continued fall of core temperature by up to 3°C after initiation of rewarming and resuscitation, probably due to reperfusion of cold extremities.

Labs:

- Continuous EKG monitoring; check for Osborne J waves (wide upright slur in terminal QRS) at < 27°C (80°F), may warn of impending Vfib.
- K^+ every 30 min
- Blood glucose
- CBC, coagulation profile due to incidence of cytopenia and DIC in this age group
- Toxicology screen
- Amylase/lipase
- ABG
- Digoxin levels

Rx:

- Gentle handling and moving essential, especially in profound hypothermia, to prevent Vfib or asystole (Geriatrics 1999; 54:51).
- Mild hypothermia: passive rewarming prevents further conduction, convection, radiation and evaporation losses; warm

sources such as radiant lights, forced warm air, electric blankets, warming mattress should be used at temperatures > 31°C (87.8°F); warming will occur gradually 0.5-2°C/hr (Geriatrics 1999;54:51).

- Consider broad-spectrum abx coverage for possibility of sepsis; thiamine (Conn Med 1995;59:515).
- Moderate to profound: do not do CPR as long as feel pulse, even if very slow, danger is that CPR may cause Vfib (Geriatrics 1999;54:51); CPR at half normal rate; active core rewarming:
  1. Heated, humidified O_2 mask (40°-46°C/104°-114.6°F) or endotracheal intubation; CO_2 retained in hypothermic state, therefore adjust vent for CO_2 level, not O_2.
  2. Thoracic, pleural lavage with 40°C (104°F) saline rewarms at 2°C/hr.
  3. Bypass rewarms at 4°C/hr.
  4. Glucose if indicated (Conn Med 1995;59:515); avoid insulin for hyperglycemia; insulin action delayed until normothermic, causing hypoglycemia.
  5. Try low dose catecholamines for low BP, if not responding to crystalloids and rewarming (Nejm 1994;331:1756).

Chapter 2

Health Care Maintenance

2.1 Arteriosclerotic Cardiovascular Disease

Blood Pressure

Jama 1995;274:570; U.S. Preventive Services Task Force, Guide to Clinical Preventive Services. Williams & Wilkins, 1996; Ann IM 1995;122:937; Arch IM 1997;157:2413; Canadian Task Force on The Periodic Health Examination, Ottawa, Canada Communication Group, 1994; Ann IM 2007;147:787

Issues: Systolic Hypertension in Elderly Persons (SHEP) study—treatment of systolic HTN significantly decreased the incidence of stroke in pts age 65–70 yo (Jama 1991;265:3255; Canadian Task Force 1994:943).

Benefits may not be demonstrable among the old-old (Jama 1994;272:1932; Lancet 1995;345:825; J Hypertens Suppl 1986;4:S642); mortality inversely related to elevated systolic and diastolic BP in those patients > 85 yr (BMJ 1988;296:887); however, higher rates of fatal MI in men w pharmacologically induced diastolic BP decrease from 90 to 86 mm Hg (J Hypertens 1994;12:1183); 20% of elderly whose antihypertensive meds withdrawn while normotensive remained normotensive for 3 mo to 1 yr (J Intern Med 1994;235:581).

Intervention: Screen NH pts for HT, but use caution in treating those > 80 yr; periodic trial off meds, particularly if become more sedentary (eg, pts w progressive disabilities, NH pts).

Table 2.1 Recommendations for Elder Screening

Maneuver Screening	Suggested Age
Blood pressure	Every exam, at least q 1-2 yr
Physical breast exam	Annually if life expectancy 5-10 yr
Mammogram	Q 1-2 yr if life expectancy 5-10 yr
Pelvic exam/Pap smear	Every 2-3 yr after 2 neg annual exams; can then decrease or discontinue after age 65
Cholesterol	Adults q 5 yr, > 75 with known CHD
Rectal exam, fecal occult blood test	Annually ≥ 50
Sigmoidoscopy	Every 5 yr ≥ 50 or colonoscopy q 10 yr
Test/inquire for hearing impairment	Periodically in older adults with questionnaire
Mouth, nodes, testes, skin, heart, lung exams	Annually
Glucose	Periodic in high-risk groups; q 3 yr starting at 45 TSH q 5 yr for women ≥ 50
Thyroid function (TSH)	Periodically > 40-50
Electrocardiogram	Periodically by eye specialist > 65
Vision/glaucoma screening	As needed; be alert for decline
Mental/functional status	If needed for treatment decision
Osteoporosis (BMD)	Annually ≥ 5 if >10 yr life expectancy NR esp > 70
Prostate exam/PSA	NR/as needed
Chest x-ray	
Prophylaxis/Counseling	
Exercise	Encourage aerobic and resistance exercise as tolerated
Influenza vaccine	Annual > 65 of chronically ill
Pneumococcal vaccine	23-valent at least once > 65, q 6 yr
Tetanus-diphtheria vaccine	Primary series then booster q 10 yr
Calcium; vitD	800-15-mg/d, 800 iU
Aspirin	With CHD risk factor men benefit more than women 80-325 mg qod
Vitamin E?, red wine?, NSAIDs?, Ginkgo?	May prevent/rx/slow progression of cardiovascular disease and dementia

Pulse

Ann IM 1988;108:70; Canadian Task Force on The Periodic Health Examination, Ottawa, Canada Communication Group, 1994

Issues: Risk of stroke for pts w Afib w at least one other risk factor (HT, DM, TIA, h/o stroke) is 8% annually.

Intervention: Check pulse in pts in whom aspirin or warfarin would be considered (Arch IM 1994;154:1443,1449).

Palpation Abdominal Aorta Width

Ann IM 1993;119:411; Canadian Task Force on The Periodic Health Examination, Ottawa, Canada Communication Group, 1994

Issues: Palpation for abdominal aortic aneurysm 80%-90% sens; elective non-emergent surgery risk for aneurysm > 5 cm = 5% as opposed to emergent 50%-70% mortality rate.

Intervention: Palpate abdominal aorta in pt in whom surgery would be considered (Prim Care 1995;22:731); men > 75 yr derive greatest benefit from screening (BMJ 2004;329:1259); US screening male smokers (age range 65-75) (BMJ 2005;330:750).

Carotid Auscultation

Issues: 55-> 60% reduction in relative risk results from endarterectomy in asx pts with > 70% stenosis (Circ 1995;91:566; Jama 1995;273:1421); both Canadian Task Force (1994) and European study (Lancet 1995;345:209; Ann IM 2007;147:860) do not advocate endarterectomy for asx pts; carotid bruit auscultation has low specificity for carotid stenosis.

Intervention: Where high-quality surgical services are available, auscultate carotids in high-risk pts < 80 yr who are good surgical candidates (American Academy of Family Practice recommendations, Prim Care 1995;22:731) vs consensus against both endarterectomy and routine screening for asx carotid artery stenosis (Arch Neurol 1997;54:25).

Cholesterol

Issues: High prevalence of hypercholesterolemia in asx elderly would require further lipid profiles in f/u, putting an enormous burden on the health care system (J Fam Pract 1992;34:320).

- Low HDL cholesterol predicts CHD mortality in older persons (Jama 1995;274:539); total cholesterol levels relate directly to CAD in elderly (Ann IM 1997;126:753).
- Prospective study of statins in elderly at risk for vascular disease: decrease in MI, - major benefit in elderly w LDL > 132 mg/dL and HDL < 43mg/dL (Lancet 2002;360:1623; Jama 2001;285:2486; Circ 2004;110:227), not in women (Jama 2004;291:2243).
- Inverse relationship between high cholesterol level and death from CAD by age 70-80 (Arch IM 1993;153:1065; Jama 1994;272:1335).

Intervention: Pts w >2 cardiac risk factors (Ann IM 1996;124:515); American Heart Association screen everyone into very old age. Those pts with a life expectancy < 3 yr should not be screened for hypercholesterolemia; statins extremely well tolerated in older cohort (Jags 1997;45:8) and effective in preventing CAD, MI (Jama 1998;279:1615; Ann IM 1998;129:681; Nejm 1998;339:1349; Geriatrics 2003;58:18; Jags 2003;51:717).

Risk stratification: 1 risk factor (HT, smoking, low HDL, advanced age, premature CHD in family member) – goal LDL < 160 mg/dL; 2+ risk factors – goal LDL < 130 mg/dL, CHD goal LDL < 100 mg/dL (Jama 2001;285:2486; Circ 2004; 110:227).

In NH setting, for LDL > 160mg/dL or LDL > 130 mg/dL w established CAD (Nurs Home Med 1997; supplement D: 1D); pts with decreased cholesterol may be at more risk than those with elevated cholesterol; low cholesterol indicates poor nutritional status and is associated with a high 6-mo mortality rate (Jags 1991;39:455).

Obesity

Issues: 42% female community dwellers overweight leading to medical comorbidities—DM type II, osteoarthritis knees, hyperlipidemia, sarcopenia, sleep apnea, CAD, stroke (Ann IM 2002; 162:2557).

Intervention: If obese lose 0.5 lb per week (Jama 2003;289:1747); pt ed (Am Fam Phys 2001;63:2185).

Electrocardiogram

Issues: Screening EKGs have low specif and poorly predict future cardiac events; U.S. Public Service Task Force recommends EKGs in pts with 2 or more cardiac risk factors, but does not specifically address the elderly; discovery of silent ischemia on screening EKG could lead to rx w significant side-effects (Ann IM 1989;111:489).

Intervention: Baseline EKG (comparison) for all NH pts and pts in continuity practices.

Counseling (Smoking, Exercise, Aspirin, Estrogen)

Issues: Cardiovascular benefits of smoking cessation do not diminish with age (Nejm 1988;319:1365); American College of Physicians, Canadian Task Force, and U.S. Preventive Task Force recommend smoking cessation; difficult to achieve in the NH setting where pt's rights to freedom of choice are invoked.

Increasing physical activity reduces the incidence of HT, NIDDM, colon cancer, depression, anxiety, and CHD in female pts as old as 69 (Jama 1997;277:1287; Clin Ger 2004;12:18; Jama 2003;289:2083); decreases cholesterol; may improve cognition and self-image (Ann Rv Pub Hlth 1987;8:253; Nejm 1986;314:605; 1991;325:147; Jags 1990; 38:123; Jama 1984;252:544); moderate-intensity aerobic training improves glucose tolerance independent of adiposity (Jags 1998;46:875); decreased episodes of CHF in elderly who walked 4 hr/wk at 75% of their maximum heart rate (Jama 1994;272:1442, Ann IM 1996;129:1051); older people who are already generally active start w increased volume of aerobic exercise or resistive training, eg, cycling, brisk walking, swimming (slow walking × 5 min and 5-10 min stretching before moderate exercise and after resistive training; free weights 70% of comfortable lift through a free range of motion one time increasing q mo; increase to 3 sets of 8-12 repetitions w 1-2 min rest between sets; exhale 2-4 sec w lift and inhale 4-6 sec w lowering weight (Jags 2000;48:318).

Intervention: Strongly encourage even the very old pt to quit smoking unless life expectancy is < 2 yr (J Fam Pract 1992;34:320); do not assume pts who have quit have done so forever, continue to counsel (Prim Care 1995;22:697); lung cancer screening with helical computed tomography in smokers expensive (Jama 2003; 289:313).

Walking programs for appropriately selected ambulatory pts; weight-bearing exercises that avoid flexion of the spine for osteoporotic pts; Tai Chi (Jags 1996;44:489,498); encourage wgt training.

U.S. Preventive Task Force recommends ASA for pts > 40 yr with at least 2 risk factors for CAD (1st degree relative, smoking, HT, DM, h/o stroke or peripheral vascular disease, obesity, low levels of HDL) (Jags 1990;38:817,933; Arch IM 2003;163:2006; Ann IM 2002;136:157), also decreased rate of adenomatous polyps (Nejm 2003;348:883,891); however, in the elderly the benefits may not outweigh the risks of ASA, ie, gi bleeding (J Am Board Fam Pract 1992;5:127), does not prevent stroke (Arch Neurol 2000;57:326).

2.2 Cancer

Consider life-expectancy estimates that account for comorbidity, functional status, age; physical and psychological risks of false-negative tests (Jama 2001;285:2750).

Breast Cancer

Issues: Breast cancer less aggressive than in premenopausal women; more poorly differentiated tumors with less organized cells (ie, no hormone receptors) are selected out by aging, resulting in the more differentiated tumors lasting into old age. According to actuarial statistics healthy 80 yr-old women will live 9 more yr, but most NH pts have medical problems that will shorten their life expectancy; greater risk if > 7 yr of hormone replacement therapy (Jags 2000;48:842). 40% of women > 80 yr don't need screening (Jags 2004;52:1688).

Morbidity: Fungating tumors, metastasis to bone, liver, lung, and 15% to brain; 50% of asx elderly women w breast cancer may have bony metastases (Ger Med Today 1989;8:27). Local complications develop in nearly half of untreated 85 yr-old women with a breast lump; a demented 85-yr-old woman has a 75% chance of dying before these complications develop (Jags 1995;43:282).

Tamoxifen has been used in lieu of surgery in frail elderly pts who develop breast cancer (Br J Surg 1991;78:591; Jags 2000;48:346); easily tolerated, and may also protect against osteoporosis.

Exercise ≥ 4 hr/wk decreases risk of breast cancer (Nejm 1997;336:1269).

Intervention: In selected pts in whom the likelihood of developing morbidity from breast cancer will precede death from other causes, screen for breast cancer into late life w mammogram, as well as breast exam (Lancet 1993;341:1973), annually or biennially until age 75 (Am Fam Phys 2002;65:2537). Biennially or at least q 3 yrs after that w no upper limit of age, as long as 4-yr life expectancy (NYFC III,IV CHF, DM w end organ damage, steroid or O_2-dependent COPD, severe dementia, malignancy) (Jags 2000;48:842; per AGS Clin Ger 2003;11:52). Medicare covers q 2 yr screening mammography.

In the frail NH pt w average life expectancy, limit screening to a breast exam (Ann IM 1995;122:539); low-risk rx (eg, tamoxifen) easily available for management.

Colon Cancer

U.S. Preventive Services Task Force, Guide to Clinical Preventive Services, 2nd ed., Williams & Wilkins, 1996; Lancet 1996; 348:1467; Am Fam Phys 2002;66:2287; Jama 2003;289: 1297

Issues: Two-thirds of new cases of colon cancer diagnosed each yr are found in people older than 65; time for polyp to become malignant ranges from 5-12 yr (Ann IM 1991;115:807); dx and rx of colorectal cancer is curative or palliative and may improve quality of life, though perioperative mortality does increase with age.

Digital rectal exam, fecal occult blood testing and sigmoidoscopy: 25% decrease in mortality associated with their use (Nejm 1993;328:1365; Ann IM 1993;118:1); well-designed case-control studies suggest protection remains unchanged for at least 10 yr after rigid sigmoidoscopy (U.S. Preventive Task Force, 1996); simple occult blood testing can lead to serial colonoscopies, expense and discomfort without necessarily increasing longevity in debilitated elderly; controversial one-time screening with colonoscopy has been suggested for those > 60 yr old (National Polyp Study—Am J Gastroenterol 1994;86:197; Nejm 1993;329:1977; Jama 1994;271:1011).

Interventions:

- General population of well elderly: screening with fecal occult blood tests yearly and sigmoidoscopies every 5 yr appropriate, q 10 yr colonoscopy (Jags 1999;47:122).
- Studies of colorectal screening targeting the growing NH population are needed to support more specific recommendations.
- Take advantage of low cost of fecal occult blood screening and use repeat screening as valuable diagnostic tool when clinical suspicion is high; abstain from ASA > 325 mg/d, substantial doses of NSAIDs, red meat, poultry, raw vegetables, fish, vit C for accurate study (Jags 2000;48:333).
- Medicare covers screening colonoscopy q 10 yr or every 2 yr if high risk.

Cervical Cancer

Issues: 40% of cervical cancer deaths occur in women > 65 yr; 15% of women > 65 yr have never had a Pap smear (Jags 2001;49: 1499), and an additional 25% have not had regular screening; women > 65 who have never had Pap smear have 2-3 × the risk of younger women for having abnormal Pap (Am J Obgyn 1991; 164:644); women > 65 would benefit more than any age group from cancer screening, with a 63% improvement in 5-yr mortality (Lancet 1990;335:97).

Canadian recommendations suggest that 2 neg pap smears are sufficient, even in women never previously screened who are > 65 (Jags 2001;49:655). Cervical cancer screening, according to these guidelines, is about one-sixth the cost of mammography screening per yr of life saved.

Women who have had any previous abnormal Paps should be screened q 2-3 yr late into life (U.S. Preventive Task Force, 1996); w regularly documented neg Pap smears, it is safe and cost-effective to stop screening at age 65 (Ann IM 1992; 117:529).

Pathophysiology of Cervix with Aging: As a woman ages, the transformation zone migrates further into the cervix and is more difficult for the clinician to visualize; estrogen reverses this change; in order to obtain optimally reliable cytology in high-risk elderly women, use intravaginal estrogen for 3 wk prior to Pap smear to avoid false-pos smears, because atrophic changes can be read as atypia on Pap smear (Ger Rv Syllabus 2002, 5th ed, p351).

Mechanical Barriers to Screening: Pelvic examination not only may be uncomfortable but also may lead to pain in severely arthritic, osteoporotic women; consider using "heels together, knees apart" position w assistant providing lateral knee support (rather than standard stirrups) for increased comfort. Demented pts may be unable to cooperate with the procedure; therefore may want to examine in left lateral decubitus position; decreased estrogen also makes vaginal introitus stenotic, shortened, narrowed.

Natural History of Disease: The natural hx of untreated cervical cancer usually involves local spread and subsequent ureteral and bowel obstruction causing death; rx options depend on the stage of the disease, progressing from cryosurgery, loop electrocautery excision procedure and laser, to surgery and radiation.

Intervention: Cost-effective schedule of cervical cancer screening can be limited to previously unscreened women and women w previous abnormal Pap smears who can tolerate the Pap smear, colposcopy and the various rx's for dysplasia and cervical cancer. High risk > 65 yr. Still screen nonmarried (Obgyn 2006;108:410).

Other Gynecologic Cancers: Routine screening for ovarian cancer not yet proven to reduce morbidity or mortality (Jama 1995; 273:491). A careful hx to elicit abnormal bleeding patterns requiring endometrial bx is the initial screening tool for endometrial cancer (J Fam Pract 1992;34:320).

Prostate Cancer

Issues: Most common cancer in men; 2nd leading cause of cancer death in men > 75 yr, after lung cancer (J Fam Pract 1992;

34:320); > 99% of men diagnosed with this disease die of other causes (Prog Clin Biol Res 1988;269:87). The American Cancer Society began recommending the PSA test along with digital rectal exam starting at age 50 for men with a life expectancy of at least 10 yr (CA 1993;43:42); PSA may be more sens for aggressive cancers than non-aggressive cancers, and may advance detection of early prostate cancer by 5.5 yr (Jama 1995;273:269).

Despite earlier detection of cancer and subsequent prostatectomy in the U.S., there has been no change in the incidence of advanced disease or overall mortality: 1% incidence of death with prostatectomy is about the same as the chance of dying of the prostate cancer itself for an older male (Lancet 1994; 343:251). Other risks of surgery include impotence and incontinence (often hidden by the pt). Benefit of screening offset by morbidity of treatment (Jama 1994;272:773). Long-term survival after conservative rx of localized prostate cancer not changed with low-grade tumors (Jama 1995;274:626) ; PSA velocity > 2.0 ng/mL increased mortality rate (Nejm 2004;351:125).

Interventions: Prostate cancer screening and rx are controversial even in otherwise well men and contraindicated in most NH pts whose average life expectancy is much less than 10 yr; rapidly developing literature demands attention by physicians and discussion w pts before screening; screening transrectal US not recommended (Ann IM 1997;126:480); PSA velocity identifies high-risk pts that might benefit from androgen suppression rx (Jama 2005;294:440). Not advised as screening for women > 75 yr (J Urol 2006;176:511; J Natl Cancer Inst 2006;98:1134).

Skin Cancer

Issues: Mortality from melanoma has increased by 50% in women > 65 yr and by 100% in men > 65 yr. High incidence of actinic keratoses combined w low incidence of conversion to squamous cell carcinoma; even basal cell carcinomas may rapidly disfigure, making early detection important to the pt.

Intervention: U.S. Preventive Task Force recommends yearly screening exam for people with increased sun exposure or with a family h/o of dysplastic nevi. Important for primary care provider to follow all abnormal lesions w serial exams for cost-effective management.

Oral Cancer

Issues: Tongue cancer most common (26%), then oropharynx (22%), then lip (19%), then gingiva (19%), then floor of the mouth (16%), then buccal mucosa (3%), then hard palate (2%). Speckled leukoplakia and erythroplakia carry more risk than leukoplakia. < 50% elderly survive oral cancer; 50% of elderly have undetected gum disease, which can have a systemic impact on health. Xerostomia common in NH elderly, especially those on anticholinergic drugs (Am J Nurs 1995;81:1135).

Intervention: Screen pts with a h/o tobacco or alcohol use for oral cancer, and other problems of the oral cavity as well; although there are no well-designed controlled, cohort studies that prove dental screening effective in the elderly, it is easy to screen yearly with an oral cavity exam (Gerodontics 1988;4:207).

2.3 Infection Control

Infection Surveillance

Clin Ger Med 1992;8:1821; Antimicrobial therapy in the elderly patient, Yoshikawa TT, Norman DC, eds; 1994; Clin Ger Med 1995;11:467; Nurs Home Med 1995;3:207

Issues:

Nursing Home: Endemic (UTI, URI, skin), and epidemic (influenza, tbc, gastroenteritis); approximately 1 infection/resident/yr; fever criterion should be lowered to 99° (rectal) or 100° (oral), and temperature rise of 2°F from baseline should be viewed as febrile response (Jags 1996;44:74). Atypical clinical manifestations:

anorexia, falling, incontinence, mental status change; MRSA infection: 10%-25% of NH pts colonized, but only 3%-5% infected. Just gloves needed for multi-bacterial resistance in NH (Jags 2004;52:2003).

Intervention:

Nursing Home: Develop daily reporting system that includes criteria for infection, for nursing staff to use, from which infection rates in the NH can be determined.

MRSA-colonized pts do not require isolation, but should not share room w pts w gastric feeding tubes, wounds, iv catheters, or immunosuppression (Am J Med 1993;94:313).

Vancomycin-resistant enterococci (VRE) (Nurs Home Med 1997;4:371; Nejm 1999;340:517,556; Inf Contr Hosp Epidem 1998;19:532). Contact precautions for colonized or infected pts include grouping pts in same room; wearing gloves and gowns if pt or environmental surface contact anticipated; dedicating frequently used equipment, and barriers for shared equipment, eg, exercise machines. VRE infection control includes surveillance stool cultures or rectal swabs of roommates of newly discovered VRE-colonized pts; may remove contact precautions when 3 neg VRE cultures separated by weekly intervals. Antimicrobial rx associated w prolongation VRE carriage (Jags 1998;46:157). New medication for VRE and MRSA-Linezolid (Zyvox) 600 mg iv q 12 hr (Med Lett 2000;42:45).

Tuberculosis

Issues: Declining immune system leads to reactivation of quiescent infection; chronic cough, weight loss incorrectly attributed to COPD, or malnutrition could result in unrecognized tbc epidemic.

Intervention:

Nursing Home: Screen new admissions with two-step procedure; screen staff yearly; screen pts yearly. For initial screening of NH admissions, if PPD < 10 mm after 48 hr, PPD booster in 2 wk.

- Use dermal controls for immunocompromised.
- F/u pos PPD w chest x-ray and screen for symptoms of active tbc; if positive PPD, CXR negative, no evidence of active tbc, and pt not a recent converter (< 2 yr), check risk factors (Am Fam Phys 2000;61:263); recent converter or regardless of duration of pos PPD if risk factors, then rx latent tbc (chemoprophylaxis).

Chemoprophylaxis: rx conversion from < 10 mm to ≥ 15 mm within 2 yr with INH 300 mg qd and pyridoxine 50 mg qd for 6 or 9 mo. Check AST q 3 mo, discontinue rx if AST rises to 3× nl, re-challenge once AST nl, with INH 50 mg, increasing by 50 mg weekly to 300 mg/d; do not re-challenge if AST rises again.

Pressure Ulcers

Issues: Prevalence in NH > 20-30%; incurs 4× risk of death.

Intervention: Norton or Braden scales (Decubitus 1989;2:44) (see pressure ulcers, 12.19).

Screen for risk of pressure ulcers, taking physical and mental condition, activity level, mobility, and incontinence into account. For pts at high risk: ensure adequate repositioning schedules, check albumin, and order high-protein diets (J Am Diet Assoc 1994;94:1301). (Table 2.2).

Table 2.2 Jen Scale for Predicting Pressure Sore Risk

Patient's Name		Evaluator's Name		Date of Assessment
SENSORY PERCEPTION Ability to respond meaningfully to pressure-related discomfort	1. Completely Limited: Unresponsive (does not moan, flinch, or grasp) to painful stimuli, due to diminished level of consciousness or sedation. OR limited ability to feel pain over most of body surface.	2. Very Limited: Responds only to painful stimuli. Cannot communicate discomfort except by moaning or restlessness. OR has a sensory impairment which limits the ability to feel pain or discomfort over 1/2 of body.	3. Slightly Limited: Responds to verbal commands, but cannot always communicate discomfort or need to be turned. OR has some sensory impairment which limits ability to feel pain or discomfort in 1 or 2 extremities.	4. No Impairment: Responds to verbal commands. Has no sensory deficit which would limit ability to feel or voice pain or discomfort.
MOISTURE Degree to which skin is exposed to moisture.	1. Constantly Moist: Skin is kept moist almost constantly by perspiration, urine, etc. Dampness is detected every time patient is moved or turned.	2. Very Moist: Skin is often, but not always moist. Linen must be changed at least once a shift.	3. Occasionally Moist: Skin is occasionally moist, requiring an extra linen change approximately once a day.	4. Rarely Moist: Skin is usually dry, linen only requires changing at routine intervals.

continues

Table 2.2 continued

Patient's Name		Evaluator's Name		Date of Assessment
ACTIVITY Degree of physical activity	1. Bedfast: Confined to bed	2. Chairfast: Ability to walk severely limited or non-existent. Cannot bear own weight and/or must be assisted into chair or wheelchair.	3. Walks Occasionally: Walks occasionally during day, but for very short distances, with or without assistance. Spends majority of each shift in bed or chair.	4. Walks Frequently: Walks outside the room at least twice a day and inside room at least once every 2 hours during waking hours.
MOBILITY Ability to change and control body position.	1. Completely immobile: Does not make even slight changes in body or extremity position without assistance.	2. Very Limited: Makes occasional slight changes in body or extremity position but unable to make frequent or significant changes independently.	3. Slightly Limited: Makes frequent though slight changes in body or extremity position independently.	4. No Limitations: Makes major and frequent changes in position without assistance.
NUTRITION *Usual* food intake pattern	1. Very Poor: Never eats a complete meal. Rarely eats more than 1/3 of any food offered. Eats 2 servings or less of protein (meat or dairy products) per day. Takes fluids poorly.	2. Probably Inadequate: Rarely eats a complete meal and generally eats only about 1/2 of any food offered. Protein intake includes only 3 servings of meat or dairy	3. Adequate: Eats over half of most meals. Eats a total of 4 servings of protein (meat, dairy products) each day. Occasionally will refuse a meal, but will usually	4. Excellent: Eats most of every meal. Never refuses a meal. Usually eats a total of 4 or more servings of meat and dairy products. Occasionally eats

	Does not take a liquid dietary supplement. OR is NPO and/or maintained on clear liquids or IV's for more than 5 days.	products per day. Occasionally will take a dietary supplement. OR receives less than optimum amount of liquid diet or tube feeding.	take a supplement if offered. OR is on a tube feeding or TPN regimen which probably meets most of nutritional needs.	between meals. Does not require supplementation.
FRICTION AND SHEAR	1. Problem: Requires moderate to maximum assistance in moving. Complete lifting without sliding against sheets is impossible. Frequently slides down in bed or chair, requiring frequent repositioning with maximum assistance. Spasticity, contractures or agitation leads to almost constant friction.	2. Potential Problem: Moves feebly or requires minimum assistance. During a move skin probably slides to some extent against sheets, chair, restraints, or other devices. Maintains relatively good position in chair or bed most of the time but occasionally slides down.	3. No Apparent Problem: Moves in bed and in chair independently and has sufficient muscle strength to lift up completely during move. Maintains good position in bed or chair at all times.	

©Copyright Barbara Braden and Nancy Bergstrom, 1988

For additional information on administration and scoring Braden BJ, Bergstrom N. Clinical utility of the Braden Scale for Predicting Pressure Sore Risk. Decubitus 1989;2:44-6, 50-1.

2.4 Immunizations

Influenza

Issues: Fourth leading cause of death pts > 75 yr: 70% NH residents contract influenza during outbreak, 10-20% in non-epidemic years; fatality rate 30% (Jama 2000;1:S25) effective in NH and community (Jama 2004;292:2089). Immunization rate is 20-40% because physicians do not communicate and pts do not understand seriousness of illness (Clin Ger Med 1992;8:183). Immunization is cost-effective.

Intervention: Vaccinate all elderly (Jama 1997;278:1333); efficacy debated (Lancet 1998;357:399);

Aim to immunize 80% NH pts (Jama 1994;272:1133); during outbreaks begin prophylaxis regardless of vaccination status to both ill and non-ill pts; rimantadine has fewer CNS side effects, more expensive than amantadine (Geriatrics 1994;49:30). Reduce side effects of amantadine by dosing according to calculated creatinine clearance and decreasing other anticholinergic meds. Vaccinations and swallowing evaluation prevent hospitalization of NH pts (Jags 2004;52:2010).

Pneumococcal Pneumonia

Issues: Increased incidence by 2-4 in pts > 65 yr. 20% vaccination rate, partially due to low Medicaid/Medicare reimbursement through 1989.

Intervention: Aim to vaccinate 60% NH pts; revaccinate q 6 yr in elderly w asplenia, nephrotic syndrome, or renal failure; revaccination w 23-valent vaccine should be considered for pts who were vaccinated w 14-valent vaccine (Am Fam Phys 1995;51:859). U.S. Task Force revaccinate q 6 yr (Jama 2000;1:S25) drug resistant pneumococci more common, therefore liberalize use of vaccine (Nejm 1998;338:1861,1915).

Tetanus

Issues: (Mmwr 1998;47:1)

Increased incidence with age because protective antitoxin levels decline; 28% have protective levels over the age of 70 (Nejm 1995;332:761); 10% pts are fecal carriers of *Clostridium tetani*, leaving pressure ulcers at high risk for contamination; case fatality rate 50%.

Intervention: Give tetanus immune globulin to pts with contaminated ulcers who have completed primary series, but have not had re-immunization within 10 yr. Give primary series to pts with unknown immunization status (Jags 2000;48:949). Pts in the military after 1941 have received at least one tetanus toxoid dose (Inf Contr Hosp Epidem 1993;14:591); primary immunization series consists of second dose 4-6 wks after the first, and third dose 6-12 mo later (Sci Am 2000;CE V).

Hepatitis B

Vaccinate for hep B in pts w chronic renal failure prior to dialysis, multiple sex partners, prolonged international travel to countries w high risk (Mmwr 2003;52:965).

2.5 Function

Functional Assessment

Issues: Emphasize quality of life issues over extension of life; screening emphasizes preservation of function. The Canadian Task Force and the U.S. Preventive Task Force recommend screening for functional assessment in the elderly.

Intervention

In Office and NH: Nurses perform a yearly functional assessment (Ger Rv Syllabus, 2002, 5th ed, 49, 404).

Katz functional assessment is one of the most common; assesses actual capacity and not performance and records loss of independence in 6 ADL skills in the order in which they are lost: bathing, dressing, toileting, transferring, continence, and feeding. Skills are usually regained in the reverse order.

2.6 Sensory—Hearing and Vision

Hearing

Issues: The Canadian Task Force and U.S. Preventive Task Force recommend screening for hearing loss in the elderly; particularly effective screen in the old-old pt (J Fam Pract 1992;34:320); 41% of pts > 65 yr are hearing impaired (Ear Hear 1990;11:247).

Intervention: (Am Fam Phys 1997;56:2057)

Whispered voice and otoscopy most sens and specif screens (86-96%) (Ann IM 1990;113:138; Canadian Task Force, 1994). Observation of listening behavior helpful. Obtain a continued h/o hearing loss, perform otoscopy for cerumen impaction, and f/u w portable audiometry for presbycusis where indicated. Pts sometimes refuse to wear hearing aids: ascertain the cause of their noncompliance, eg, poor fit, difficult to manipulate, change in hearing deficit, depression, dementia, rather than assuming indifference or stubbornness.

Vision

Issues:

Community:

- 9% > 65 yr, 50% > 75 yr have visual impairment, optical changes in aging (Mangione CM, Intensive Course in Geriatric Medicine and Board Review, 1/96).
- Increased light absorption by crystalline lens reducing intensity reaching photoreceptors.

- Senile miosis: Older pupils smaller, leading to less light getting to retina in low-light conditions.
- Increased intraocular light scatter, leading to heightened sens to glare.
- Decreased amplitude of accommodation of the lens (presbyopia) so by 60 or 70 yr most need glasses for near vision.
- Axis of astigmatism changes, requiring refraction.
- Neural change w loss of blue-yellow discrimination; no prospective studies to show that screening the elderly for visual acuity is worthwhile, however.

Nursing Home:

- 17% of pts in NHs blind and another 19% have <20/40 vision; 20% of blindness, and 37% of impairment remediable with adequate refraction (Nejm 1995;332:1205); Baltimore eye study: un-operated cataracts accounted for 27% of all blindness in blacks, suggesting that elderly with less access to eye care would benefit from screening for cataracts (Nejm 1991; 325:1412; Mangione CM, 1996).
- Macular degeneration leading cause of blindness among whites (3% of all whites > 80 yr); early treatment w laser effective in slowing progression in minority of patients who have neovascularization (see Macular Degeneration under Common Geriatric Problems); referral to low vision services may help pt to maximize peripheral vision.
- Diabetic retinopathy most treatable in presymptomatic phase when neovascular changes have just begun.
- Impaired visual acuity linked to falls and hip fractures; thus screening the eldery may be beneficial (Nejm 1991;324:1326).
- Screen using combination of visual field exam, tonometry, and direct ophthalmoscopy by ophthalmologist, w pt's eyes completely dilated (2.5% phenylephrine w tear duct occlusion to decrease systemic absorption). Long asx and potentially treatable phase before irreversible vision loss (UCLA Intensive

Board Review, 1/96). However, reliable screening tests for glaucoma are not available and early treatment does not improve pt outcome (Surv Ophthalmol 1983;28:194).

Intervention: Screen for visual acuity yearly; visual acuity screening criteria for referral to specialist: best eye < 20/40 (wearing correction), > 2 Snellen lines difference between two eyes. H/o night driving problems helpful for accident prevention vs vision screening no apparent benefit, many causes untreatable (BMJ 1998;28:316).

2.7 Mental Health Issues

Dementia

Nejm 1990;322:1212, Jama 2007;298:2409, Lancet 2007;7:734.

Issues: Screening recommended by the American College of Physicians, Canadian Task Force, and U.S. Preventive Task Force. Mini-Mental State Exam (MMSE) has a broad range; moderate, but not mild deficits can be picked up; Wechsler identifies subtle deficit, but lengthy to administer; 4-7-yr delay in presentation to health care provider. Exit interview screens for subcortical dementias by testing executive function

Intervention: Use MMSE (Folstein, Bar Harbor, ME, 6/96) to pick up attention span deficit associated with the reversible dementias (and delirium), ie, thyroid disorders, other metabolic abnormalities and acute infections; MMSE helps identify the type and stage of dementia; prevent unnecessary agitation in demented pts by providing stage-appropriate challenges without overstimulating them with activities that are too difficult for them; careful spouse and family hx probably undervalued as dx tool.

Depression

Issues: 10-15% of general geriatric population depressed; 60% of NH elderly may be depressed. Masked depression more common among the elderly presenting w agitation, jealousy, or somatization.

Intervention: Asking single question, "Have you been feeling depressed?" may be just as effective as Geriatric Depression Scale (GDS) (Jags 1994;42:1006). Anhedonia (failure to enjoy usual pleasures) can be sensitive sx; GDS only requires yes/no answers, has a shortened form, but may lack specif among medically ill pts. Beck, Zung, and Hamilton depression inventories rely heavily on somatic complaints and, therefore, are less useful in the elderly; nonverbal depression scale developed by Hayes and Losche is useful in more debilitated NH pts (Clin Gerontol 1991;10:3).

Alcohol Problems

Jags 1995;43:415

Issues: Prevalence of alcohol problems = 10% in community; in the NH ranges from 2.8-15%; 33% of pts who enter a NH will return to their community, thereby making alcohol rehabilitation more relevant (Ger Rv Syllabus, 2002 5th ed, p 101). Knowledge of ETOH hx may add to understanding of family-pt interactions; behaviors exhibited with the staff such as "dry drunk" spells will take on new meaning as well; move to retirement communities associated w increased ETOH use.

Intervention: Screening with either a CAGE or MAST-G (see alcohol misuse) yields 82/90 and 93/65 sens/specif percents, respectively (Ger Rv Syllabus 1996). CAGE not reliable as only screening tool in outpatients > 60 yr. Clinicians should directly ask about number of drinks per week (Jama 1996;276:1964). Watch for reluctance to appropriately modify ETOH use w illness, new meds;

HEALTH CARE MAINTENANCE

pointing out percentage of daily calories provided by 1, 2, 3, etc drinks may help to improve nutrition.

2.8 Falls

Issues:

Community: Lower extremity dysfunction predicts subsequent disability (Nejm 1995;332:556); one-leg balance important indicator of injurious falls (Jags 1997;45:735); slowed timed chair stands, decreased arm strength, decreased vision and hearing, high anxiety or depression score also predictors for falls (Jama 1995;273:1348).

Nursing Home: Increased fall rates in NH residents after relocation in a new facility (Jags 1995;43:1237); pts who fall infrequently are at most risk for injury; they tend to be going at faster speeds at point of impact; these pts, as well as those who fall frequently, can be helped by an intervention that determines the etiology of their falls; fear of falling leads to functional decline (Gerontol 1994;40:38), and should be considered important part of all fall management.

Intervention: Screen all outpatients and ambulatory NH pts with an assessment of balance and gait (see osteoporosis, hip fracture). Tinetti assessment tool (Jags 1986;34:119) evaluates normal and adaptive ability to maintain balance when arising from a chair, standing with eyes closed, turning and receiving a sternal nudge; also evaluates several components of gait (step height, postural sway, path deviation). Abnormalities in particular parts of the exam point to specific intrinsic etiologies of falling, eg, "uses arms to assist in standing—may have proximal muscle weakness and might be helped by strength training for hip and quad muscles"; foot scuff during swing phase—anterior tibial muscle weakness, which might be aided by an ankle/foot orthosis or reconditioning; observational gait analysis.

Prevent falls by using both intrinsic and extrinsic approaches: increased muscle strength is associated with decreased falling (Jags 1994;42:953); exercise training decreases falls (Jama 1995;273:1341); work w physical therapist to develop a care plan; use antigravity exercises that do not flex the spine to avoid vertebral compression fractures in severely osteoporotic pts.

Osteoporosis likely in pts whose height has decreased on yearly screening; high risk: white, Asian, thin, nulliparous, sedentary, kyphotic women, with past or family h/o fracture, both men and women who smoke, have COPD or take steroids chronically; pts who take bisphosphonates (see Osteoporosis, Chapter 10.1). Vit D 800 IU qd (Jama 2004;291:1999) calcitonin via intranasal route is a costly option for pts with fracture pain (Ann IM 1992; 117:1038).

Hip fractures reduced by 23% when adequate Ca supplementation prescribed (1.2 gm/d) with 800 IU of vit D (Osteoporosis Int 1994;4:7); unless elderly women have a h/o renal stones, should have total Ca intake = 1.2 gm/d and add vit D, if they are not exposed to direct sunlight for at least ½ hr qd; a serving of broccoli or dairy product equivalent to 1 regular strength Tums tab (calcium carbonate), which is 0.2 gm of elemental Ca; use this as a guide to decide Ca tab supplementation.

Extrinsic approaches: hip pads and chariot ambulators maintain independent walking, prevent serious injury (Lancet 1993;341:11); fall-proofing house, proper footwear (handouts www.americangeriatrics.org). Restraint reduction does not increase serious falls (Jags 1994;42:321,960; Arch IM 1992; 116:368). Evaluate meds: sedatives, narcotics, neuroleptics, and antihypertensives.

Table 2.3 Useful Questions on Sexual History

What actually happens when you try to have sex?
Is the penis ever firm enough to go inside your partner?
Does your penis ever become firm?
Upon awakening?
With masturbation?
How long has this been a problem?
Did anything happen, medically or socially, around the time that this problem began?
Any new medications around the time that the problem began?
What do *you* think is causing the problem?
How has this affected you? Your partner? Your relationship?
Are you interested in treating the problem?
Are you able to have an orgasm?
Is there any new curve when you have an erection?
What treatments, if any, have you tried so far?

Box 2 Jama 2004;291:2997.

2.9 Incontinence

Urinary Incontinence in Adults: Clinical Practice Guideline, AHCPR Public No. 92-0038, Rockville, MD, Urinary Incontinence Guideline Panel, Agency for Health Care Policy and Research, Public Health Service, U.S. Dept of Health and Human Services, 3/92.

Issues: 50% of NH pts incontinent of urine resulting in social embarrassment and medical complications such as skin infections; high hidden prevalence in both men and women in community.

Intervention: (See Incontinence, Chapter 1.12) Screen for reversible causes of incontinence:

- Local causes: bladder infection, atrophic vaginitis, stool impaction
- Functional causes: delirium, depression, immobility
- Systemic illnesses: CHF, hyperglycemia
- Meds: Anticholinergic and adrenergic agents
- Diet: excess caffeine, soda, alcohol (all "bladder irritants").

Collaborate with nurses to determine the etiology of incontinence, obtaining significant pos hx for urge, stress, overflow, or functional incontinence; fluid intake, voiding pattern, PVR volume, and UA complete the w/u necessary for empiric rx. Screening in this way will allow for identification of a select number of pts who are likely to respond to bladder retraining, an intervention requiring significant staff time and commitment; careful management of early dx and management (change of habits, exercise, meds) of community elderly can be rewarding.

2.10 Sexual Function

Nurs Home Med 1995;3:56

Issues: 70% of male NH residents and 50% of female NH residents have thought about being close or intimate (Arch Sex Behav 1988;17:109); sexual contacts often casual and involve manual or oral genital stimulation, rather then coitus; privacy rooms often lacking or ill-equipped for a couple engaging in a mutual sexual act, even for an able-bodied couple; private space infrequently made for heterosexually wedded couples, almost never made available for gay, lesbian, or bisexual couples; public masturbation may occur when pts seek out stairwells or alcoves, attempting to avoid the scrutiny of the staff.

29% of men > 80 yr have sex 1/wk; primary reason older women do not have sex is unavailability of partner (Arch Sex Behav 1993;22:543; 1994;23:231) (see Common Geriatric Problems).

Intervention: See Table 2.3. Remove barriers to sexual expression by encouraging privacy (do-not-disturb signs, closed doors), allowing conjugal or home visits, evaluating complaints of sexual function and changing meds that may affect sexual function. Counsel interested pts about sexuality, assess decision making capacity of impaired elderly, and provide staff education (Am Fam Phys

1995;51:121); situation capacity: voluntariness, avoidance of harm, avoidance of exploitation, avoidance of abuse, ability to stop and start an interactive behavior when desired, appropriateness of time and place (Elder Abuse: Assessment and Intervention. Hamilton, Ricker, LMSW Presentation May 26, 2005 Maine Med Ctr Portland, Maine).

Outpatient: Educational counseling to increase pt's comfort in addressing sexual issues and enlarge views of sexuality to link w larger intimacy issues and wide variation a "healthy" sexual adaptation.

2.11 Other Anticipatory Measures

Driving

Screening tools correlated with behind-the-wheel performance: Trail making test part B, MMSE, grip strength, reaction time (Jags 2004;52:1326).

Advance Directives

Ouslander JG, Osterweil D, Morley J, Ethical and legal issues, in: Medical Care in The Nursing Home. New York: McGraw-Hill 1991:358. Ann IM;2008;148:141.

Issues: Definition of medical futility nebulous; pts > 69 have a 5% chance of surviving CPR, but physicians underestimate what pts consider futile; some pts would consider these odds encouraging and preferable to death (Jama 1995;273:156; Ann IM 1989; 111:199); demented pts may be capable of making some decisions about their health care (Jama 1995;273:124; 1988;260:797), eg, options regarding a gangrenous leg may be more difficult to comprehend than whether or not to do CPR (J Am Board Fam Pract 1992;5:127).

Pts and families may fear that advance directives are not readily carried out in many hospitals; failure of pts to review advance directives w adult children may lead to conflicts within the family at the time of health crisis; strength of documents can depend on regular reiterations of values and wishes to personal physician recorded in medical record.

Intervention: End-of-life decisions should be discussed with the pt or guardian and family members; include discussion of the following: CPR, ventilator support, hospital or ICU admission, blood transfusion, iv therapy, tube feeding, antibiotics; values questionnaires may be useful to help facilitate discussions (Arch Fam Med 1994;3:1057); early discussions (time of dx of terminal illnesses, including dementia) helpful.

2.12 Medications

Nurs Home Med 1995;3:6

Issues: Risk of adverse drug reaction directly proportional to number of meds pt is on (Ger Rv Syllabus, 2002, 5th ed, p 40); The Omnibus Budget Reconciliation Act of 1987 (OBRA) mandates strict review of psychotropic meds. Psychotropic usage has decreased by 50% since OBRA implementation; use same principles for nonpsychiatric drugs.

Intervention:

Community: If pt has multiple physicians, use "brown bag" strategy to determine complete med list (Prim Care 1995;22:697).

Nursing Home: Avoid excessive dosing frequency, prolonged duration of med, duplicate therapy, and side effects that outweigh the benefits of the drug. Do not add a med to relieve the side effects of another medicine, except perhaps when using anticholinergics to treat extrapyramidal side effects, bowel regimen to prevent constipation on narcotics, or misoprostol to prevent NSAID gastritis. Consider cost. Interdisciplinary teams, including consultant pharmacists, can review drug-drug and disease-drug interactions regularly; consider all drugs candidates for regular re-evaluation.

- NSAIDs: Check BUN, Cr Hct q 2 mo
- Diuretics: BUN, Cr q 4 mo (Ann IM 1994;121:584)

2.13 Elder Abuse

Prim Care 1993;20:375; Nejm 1995;332:437; Jags 1994;42:169; 1996;44:65; Clinics in Ger Med 2005;21:279

Issues: Prevalence not well-documented; family, caregivers, and other neighbors (Jags 1998;46:885) of community-dwelling elderly, other NH residents, NH staff, or visitors may be implicated in acts of abuse; stressed caregiver, especially of pts w significant functional disabilities, represent the overwhelming majority (Patterson C. Secondary prevention of elder abuse. Canadian Task Force on the Periodic Health Examination. Canadian Guide to Clinical Preventive Health Care. Ottawa: Health Canada, 1994;922); also associated w child abuse and low income (Jags 2000;48:513).

Nursing Home: Inadequate and inconsistent training of caregivers may contribute to abuse. In one study 10% of nursing assistants admitted to at least one act of physical abuse and 40% admitted to at least one act of psychological abuse in the preceding year.

Poor hygiene, signs of dehydration, multiple skin lesions with various degrees of healing, wrist or ankle restraint bruises, and pain with occult fractures; may be subtle: unjustified chemical restraint, verbal and emotional attack or failure to follow an appropriate care plan. Pts with cognitive and physical impairment and violent, disruptive or annoying behavior are at particular risk for abuse.

Assess Environment Early: Baseline physical exam and long-term perspective may allow the physician to perceive changes in demeanor, such as withdrawal, depression, or injuries that suggest abuse.

- Question capable residents directly to clarify any concerns of abuse or neglect:
  Has anyone ever tried to hurt you?
  Has anyone ever made you do things you didn't want to do?
  Has anyone ever taken anything away from you without your consent?
- Evaluate mental status to validate the hx, check driving status
- Address spiritual concerns
- Interview family members, close friends, and staff to determine general social, psychological status and support; differences in details of unlikely explanations of events from various parties may heighten suspicions of abuse.

  Document physical abuse with photographs when possible (Public Health Service, U.S. Dept. of Health and Human Services, AHCPR Publc No. 92-0038, 3/92).

  In most states it is mandatory to report suspected abuse (U.S. Preventive Services Task Force, Guide to Clinical Preventive Services: An Assessment of the Effectiveness of 169 Interventions. New York: Williams & Wilkins 1996).

Intervention:

Community: Home care agencies, volunteer organizations, adult day-care, other forms of respite.

Nursing Home: Weekly decompression groups for staff to discuss their feelings of frustration in caring for challenging pts provide a forum for creative and constructive changes in care plans. Staff training in behavioral modification techniques.

Chapter 3

Endocrinology

3.1 Diabetes Mellitus

Am Fam Phys 1995;1:1; Sci Am Med 1995;9:VI; Clin Ger Med 1999;15; Ger Rv Syll 2002, 5th ed; Am J Ger Soc 2000; 51:s265)

Cause: Resistance to effects of insulin peripherally, as well as impaired insulin release w aging (Diabetes 1991;40:44); secondary causes: glucocorticoids, hydrochlorothiazide, β-blockers, estrogen, hemochromatosis, Cushing's, acromegaly, pheochromocytoma.

Epidem: At least 20% of pts over 65 have diabetes; in 1998, 12.7% of age 70 or older had a dx of DM, and 11% of U.S. population ages 60-74 had untreated DM (Diab Care 1998;21:518; 2000;23: 1278); 18% prevalence, Mexican Americans 3 × risk of whites and 3 × risk of severe retinopathy (Diabetes 1988;37:878); Native Americans 5 × risk of whites (Diabetes 1987;36:523); end-stage renal disease 4.3 × higher in blacks and 6 × higher in Mexican Americans (Nejm 1989;321:1074); associated w 5-10-yr loss of life. DM associated w smoking (BMJ 2006;332:1064).

Pathophys: Glucotoxicity leads to both insulin resistance and decreased insulin production (Diabetes 1985;34:222); genetic peripheral insulin resistance in the obese pt, and increased levels cause eventual β-cell exhaustion (Ann IM 1990;113:9050); impaired/delayed insulin release response to glucose load also allows hepatic neogenesis to persist 1-2 hr, then insulin overshoot occurs (Nejm 1992;326:22); DM-like aging 10 years, causing increased collagen crosslinking-wrinkles, increased capillary basement membrane thickening, increased cataracts, atherosclerosis, decreased cognitive funtion, decreased bone density; amylin increased in aging leading to increased glucose; lystin decreased w aging leading to increased adiposity (Morley, David, Diabetes at AMDA Annual Conference 3/5/99 Orlando, Fla); elderly w type II DM at risk for hyperglycemic hyperosmolar nonketotic coma (HHNC), secondary to stress, steroids, tube feeding; failure to replace water because of impaired thirst and mental status increases osmolarity.

Metabolic Syndrome: Hyperinsulinemia, hyperglycemia, hypertriglyceridemia, decreased HDL, and HT caused by nitric oxide synthetase, which is inhibited by metformin and troglitazone (Ger Clin 1999;15:211).

Sx: Usually atypical presentation in elderly, eg, slowly resolving infection, weight loss, fatigue, weakness, acute confusional states, depression.

Si: Necrobiosis lipoidica = pigmented skin plaques with white lipid center, irregular, atrophic; fatty hepatomegaly; retinopathy w hard exudates, microaneurysms and hemorrhages (see photos in Nejm 1993;329:320); neuropathy w decreased sensation, vibratory sense, position sense; acanthosis nigricans.

Crs: Years before onset of type II diabetes, pts have hypertriglyceridemia, low HDL, and HT. Factors affecting diabetes control in the elderly: decreased vision, altered taste, poor dentition, arthritis, tremor. Living alone impairs food preparation and consumption, as well as med administration.

Cmplc:

- Glucotoxicity leads to increased infections, and increased pain perception.

- HHNC: Hyperglycemia > 600 mg/dL without ketosis or ketoacidosis, w severe volume depletion 25% body weight; serum osmolality > 350 mOsm/kg usually compounding an illness; steroid therapy or tube feeding w concentrated carbohydrate solutions.
- Cardiovascular disease 2-3 times greater in type II DM than general population; MI and peripheral vascular disease cause 60% of deaths from type II DM, glucose control decreases risk of MI, half of nontraumatic amputations due to type II DM (Therapy for Diabetes Mellitus and Related Disorders. 2nd ed, Lebovitz HE, ed. American Diabetes Association 1994).
- Retinopathy: After 15-yr duration, HgbA1c < 7 decreases risk of retinopathy (Jags 1994;42:142), proliferative in 25% of type II DM on insulin and 5% of those on diet and oral agents (Diabetes Metab Rev 1989;5:559); nonproliferative most common. Loss of supporting cells of the retinal vasculature leads to microaneurysms, especially at the macula, affecting central vision and visual acuity; when microaneurysms leak, they form punctate "dot-and-blot" hemorrhages that then form hard exudates, which can cause macular edema if they accumulate near the macula. With progression of retinopathy, terminal capillaries become obstructed and the retina becomes ischemic; infarctions of the nerve layer cause soft "cotton-wool" exudates. New vessels proliferate in response to ischemia; these new vessels can bleed into the vitreous, which can lead to scars that can retract the retina, leading to retinal detachment and permanent loss of vision. Type II diabetics also prone to glaucoma, cataracts, corneal abrasions, recurrent corneal erosions, presbyopia.
- Nephropathy: Highest mortality of all the complications; 20% of pts w type II DM develop nephropathy (Arch IM 1989; 111:788); begins w microalbuminuria 30-300 mg/24 hr; risk factors for nephropathy include duration of DM and HT (Nejm 1988;318:140); inherited tendencies toward ASHD (Nejm 1992;326:673) and w higher infection rates.

- Neuropathy: Symmetric sensorimotor peripheral neuropathy most common—"stocking-glove"; dysesthesias progress to more severe anesthesia, and neuropathic foot ulcers.
- Asymmetric mononeuropathies affecting both peripheral and cranial nerves secondary to nerve infarcts.
- Entrapment syndromes such as carpal tunnel syndrome.
- Autonomic neuropathy leading to gastroparesis (delayed gastric emptying, early satiety, fullness, nausea, and vomiting), postural hypotension, atonic bladder; polyneuropathy more common in pts w Type II DM and hypoinsulinemia (Nejm 1995;333:89).
- Associated w cognitive decline (Diabet Med 1999;6:93; Arch IM 2000;160:174; Neurol 1999;52:97; Lancet 1998;352:837; Jama 2004;292:2237).
- Decreased visceral pain perception, therefore risk of silent angina and MIs (Ann IM 1988;108:170); hyperglycemia lowers pain threshold producing more pain with peripheral neuropathy (Morley, Diabetes in the Nursing Home at AMDA annual meeting 3/5/99 Orlando, Fla).
- Increased risk of hip fx in elderly men and women with DM, especially those using oral medication or insulin (Am J Ger Soc 2004;52:1778).
- Diabetic cystopathy: Decreased bladder sensation, increased bladder capacity, impaired detrusor contractility; generally presents as overflow incontinence, though can also have elements of urge incontinence (detrusor overactivity); no effective pharmacological tx (Ger Nurs 2003;24:138).
- DM associated with reactive tbc.
- Depression is lethal w sulfonylurea OD. Increased prevalence of depression with DM.

Lab:

- ADA criteria: Provisional diagnosis with FBG ≥ 126 mg/dL, 2 hr OGTT (75 gm load) ≥ 200, or symptoms of polyuria,

polydipsia, unexplained weight loss with random glucose ≥ 200; all must be confirmed with repeat testing on a different day; use OGTT if FBG < 125 with high suspicion of DM; use of HgbA1c for diagnosis not recommended; FBS 100-125 or OGTT 140-199 indicative of "pre-diabetes" (ADA 2004 Guidelines).
- Monitor HbA1c q 6 mo if stable, quarterly if poor control; goal < 7% in relatively healthy persons with good functional status; goal < 8% for frail elderly, life expectancy < 5 yr, or when treatment risks outweigh benefits. HbA1c increased by Fe deficiency, decreased by sickle cell disease.

Rx:

Preventive: Annual exams to detect early retinopathy; foot care, careful foot examination every visit; wgt and BP every visit; detect neuropathy early, monofilament sensory exam; screen for microalbuminuria with diagnosis, then annually if no previously demonstrated macro- or microalbuminuria; w tight control of blood sugars, there is less progression (J Am Ger Soc 1994; 42:142). BP goal less than 140/80; with microalbuminuria, goal is 130/80; some evidence for increased benefit from BP less than 130/80 in all elderly with DM, but HT needs to be treated gradually to avoid complications (Am J Ger Soc 2003;51:5269).

Therapeutic: (see Table 3.1)
- Any lowering of blood glucose reduces rate of complications (BMJ 2000;321:405).
- Minimally impaired (≥ 8 yr life expectancy): euglycemia the goal; dementia, or significant life-limiting comorbidities: control DM w pharmacologic management, minimize hypoglycemia; terminal (< 1 yr life expectancy): goal postprandial BS < 200 mg/dL, unrestricted diet (table of standing NH orders in Ann Long-Term Care 2002;6:100)

ENDOCRINOLOGY

- For the 85% of diabetics who are obese: low-fat, low-cholesterol diet has best risk-benefit ratio; aim for fasting total cholesterol < 200 mg/dL, fasting LDL < 100 mg/dL, fasting triglycerides < 150 mg/dL, and HDL > 40 mg/dL (ADA, 2004); check lipids at least annually, and more frequently if targets not met (exception for NH residents and/or pts with significantly reduced life expectancy
- Wgt loss of 5-10 lbs. is adequate (BMJ 1975;3:276); diabetic pts have more difficulty losing weight than those without; 20% of pts initially control their diabetes by diet alone (Diabetes 1995;44:1249); avoid diabetic diets in NHs where pts at risk for malnutrition because not eating unappetizing foods on restricted diets
- 20 min exercise 3×/wk decreases risk type II diabetes (Nejm 1991;325:147); exercise 1×/wk decreases risk developing DM by 40%, 60% for overweight men; progressive resistance training decreases insulin resistance, and may be more feasible than aerobic exercise regimens in the elderly (Diab Care 2003;26:1580)
- Stop hyperglycemic-producing meds, eg, estrogen, thiazides (or try low dose thiazides =12.5 mg qd), glucocorticoids, sympathomimetics (see list in Ann IM 1993;118:536)
- Conditions requiring drug therapy: sx secondary to hyperglycemia not controlled by diet alone, hyperglycemia leading to risk of dehydration, ketones are present; weight loss is rapid and uncontrolled; hyperlipidemia-hypertriglyceridemia; in elderly, main goal to prevent sx of hyperglycemia, these sx usually begin to occur at glucose concentrations 200-250 mg/dL (Nejm 1996;334:574).

Medications:

- Autonomic warning of hypoglycemia (sweating, palpitations) decreased in elderly, especially those on β-blockers.
- Most oral diabetic agents provide 75% or more of maximum effect at 50% of the maximal dose—submaximal doses of two medications more effective than a maximal dose of one; if

HgbA1c > 8-8.5% on two oral medications, addition of insulin is preferable to addition of another oral medication (Med Clin N Am 2004;88:851).

2nd Generation Sulfonylureas: Glipizide, glimiperide, glyburide; stimulate endogenous insulin; 2nd-generation sulfonylureas have fewer interactions with other meds than the 1st generations but more frequently cause hypoglycemia, especially the longer-acting ones; glyburide more hypoglycemia than glipizide (J Am Ger Soc 1996;44:751); therefore start w low doses and increase every 4-7 d; sustained-release glipizide qd; 20% primary failures.

Insulin has more beneficial effect on lipids (Ann IM 1988;108:134); hypoglycemia from insulin less prolonged than with oral agents.

Insulin + Oral Hypoglycemic: Need only 5%-20% of insulin dose required if insulin used alone (Ann IM 1991;115:45). Combination therapy using insulin more succesful and cost-effective, with newer oral agents—metformin and glitazones (Med Clin N Am 2004;88:869).

Biguanides: Metformin (Glucophage) inhibits gluconeogenesis and increases insulin-mediated glucose uptake, does not cause weight gain (Nejm 1995;333:550); good 1st choice (Ann IM 2007; 147:386). Metformin decreases mortality (Lancet 1998;352:854); start with 500-850 mg po hs or bid; increase by 500 mg q 1-2 wk, not exceeding 2500 mg; give w meals; decreased likelihood of hypoglycemia; give after failure of diet therapy or add if monotherapy with sulfonylurea fails; moderate decrease in triglycerides and LDL, moderate increase HDL; only oral agent shown to reduce macrovascular complications of Type 2 diabetes (Lancet 1998; 352:854); gi side effects (diarrhea, nausea, anorexia, abdominal discomfort, metallic taste, decreased absorption of vit B_{12}, folate); lactic acidosis, especially w liver and renal impairment (abnormal LFTs, Cr >1.5). Avoid metformin in patients > 80 yr old, vs ? metformin ok w CHF (Diab Care 2005;28:2345), and avoid in the following: baseline Cr above nl for gender, cardiac or respiratory problems that could lead to hypoxia, severe infection, alcohol abuse; hold for radiographic contrast agents (Nejm 1996; 334:577); generally held in the inpatient setting.

Thiazolidinediones: Pioglitazone (Actos) 15-45 mg max qd monotherapy and max 30 mg qd in combination therapy; rosiglitazone (Avandia) 4 mg qd bid, 8 mg qd max in monotherapy or w Metformin, 4 mg qd w insulin or sulfonylurea; improve insulin resistance w/o stimulating insulin secretion; may also help w HT, dyslipidemia (increases HDL, decreases TG), atherosclerosis (Clin Diabetes 1997;15:60); Am Fam Phys 1997;56:1835); increases risk of CHF, contraindicated in NYHA class III or IV heart failure, stop if any decline in cardiac status; CV effects uncertain (Ann IM 2007;epub), ALT increased 3× (Nejm 1998; 338:861); check liver function q 2 mo × 1 yr; stop if abnormal liver function > 2.5 nl; rosiglitazone plus metformin improve glycemic control in type 2 DM within 2 mo (Jama 2000;283: 1695); h/o liver injury w rosiglitazone (Ann IM 2000;132:118), accelerated bone loss (J Clin Endocrinol Metab 2007;92:1305).

Meglitinides: Repaglinide (Prandin) and nateglinimide (Starlix) (nonsulfonylurea insulin secretagogues), act directly on Ca channels stimulating insulin secretion, rapid acting, give 30 min ac, potential for drug interactions, caution if renal or hepatic insufficiency, decreased frequency of hypoglycemia (Sci Am 1998); short half life so do not use in NH where meals can be delayed.

α-Glucosidase Inhibitors: Acarbose (Precose) and miglitol (Glyset) decrease digestion and absorption of disaccharides 25-100 mg po ac tid (Ann IM 1994;121:928); take with first bite of meals; gi side effects may be troublesome (diarrhea, abdominal pain, flatulence); may not want to use w metformin because of additive gi effects; treat hypoglycemia w glucose not sucrose because sucrose may not be adequately hydrolyzed or absorbed (Med Lett Drugs Ther 1996;38:9) (Table 3.2); avoid if Cr >2 mg/dL; monitor LFTs on acarbose, but not needed with miglitol.

Types of Insulin: See Table 3.3. Lispro (Humalog, Novolog) onset 5-15 min, peak 0.5-2 hr, duration 6-8 hr; Regular onset 15 min-1 hr, peak at 2-4, duration 8-12 hr; NPH—onset in 1-1.5 hr, peak at 4-12 hr, duration 12-24 hr; Insulin glargine (Lantus)—onset in 1-2 hr, continuous level without peak for 24 hr in most (decreased duration in those with significant insulin resistance), 45% decrease in nocturnal hypoglycemia compared to NPH (Diab Care 2003;26: 3080); insulin pumps becoming more popular; even in elderly, basal insulin levels (infusion or scheduled long-acting insulin) highly preferable to "sliding scale" insulin in hospitalized pts.

Newer Drugs:

Sitagliptin (Januvia): DPP-04 enzyme inhibitor. For type 2 DM. Enhances endogenous incretin hormones. 100 mg once daily as monotherapy or in combination with metformin or thiazolidinedione. 50 mg/d if crcl 31-50 ml/min, 25 mg/d if crcl < 30 ml/min. (Diab Care 2006;29:2638, 2632; Drugs 2007; 67:587).

Exenatide (Byetta): For type 2 DM. Incretin mimetic, glucoregulatory activities similar to GLP-1. SC inj 5-10 mcg bid. Avoid if crcl < 30 ml/min. (Diab Care 2005;25:1092). Severe GI SE, limit to morbidly obese elderly (Jama 2007; 8:421).

Pranlintide (Symlin): Amylin analog for type 1 and type 2 on insulin. 60 mcg sq immed before meals. Nausea & hypoglycemia common. Reduce premeal dose of short acting insulin by 50%. (Diabetes Med 2004;21:1204; Diab Care 2003;26:784).

Apidra (insulin glulisine): Rapid acting. Onset 20 min, peak 0.5-1 hr, duration 3-4 hr. (Diab Care 2004;27:2363).

Exubera (inhaled insulin): Rapid acting. Bioavailability ~ 10%. Pulmonary spirometry before beginning, at 6 mo and annually thereafter. If decline in FEV1 is = or > 20%, repeat PFT. If confirmed, DC. Not rec for pt w underlying lung dz (eg asthma, COPD).

Table 3.1 Special Considerations for Diabetes Management in the Elderly

Diagnosis

Recognition of worsening glucose tolerance with aging that contributes to the increasing incidence of type 2 diabetes in the elderly population

Use of screening guidelines to help uncover diabetes at its earliest, asymptomatic stages

Treatment

Use of diet and exercise to help improve insulin resistance and maintain lean body mass

Avoidance of hypoglycemia when choosing drug therapy

Prevent mental status change and adrenergic discharge during low blood glucose

Thiazolidinediones are safe and well-tolerated in the elderly (best studied with rosiglitazone).

α-glucosidase inhibitors are safe but limited by potential gastrointestinal side effects.

Use of metformin will also avoid hypoglycemia; however, loss of glomerular filtration with aging and decline in renal function needs to be considered.

If employed, short-acting insulin secretagogues and newer agents (repaglinide, glimepiride) are safest; avoid chlorpropamide and other insulin secretagogues with long half-lives.

Adapted from Clinical Geriatrics 2000;8(7):54.

Table 3.2 Insulin Types and Blood Glucose Monitoring

Insulin Types and Actions

Insulin Type	Action	Onset (hours)	~Peak	~Clinical Duration
Lispro	Ultrafast	¼	1 hour	3-4 hours
Regular	Fast	½-1	3 hours	6-8 hours
NPH & Lente	Intermediate	2-3	6-8 hours	14-16 hours
Ultralente (human)	Long	4-8	6-16 hours	18-24 hours
Glarginc	Basal/Very Long	?	None	>24 hours

Time of Blood Glucose Monitoring

	Before Breakfast	Before Lunch	Before Dinner	Bedtime
Insulin dose affecting blood sugar level	Bedtime NPH OR Evening NPH	Breakfast Reg OR Breakfast Lispro	Morning NPH OR Lunch Regular/ Lispro	Dinner Regular OR Dinner Lispro
Meal affecting blood sugar level	N/A	Breakfast	Lunch	Dinner

Tom Bartol, RN-C, MN, CDE, 2000.

ENDOCRINOLOGY

Table 3.3 Titrating Lispro Insulin

Start with 10 IU/day bedtime basal insulin and adjust weekly	
Mean of Self-Monitored FPG Values From Preceding 2 Days	**Increase of Insulin Dosage (IU/day)**
≥180 mg/dl (10 mmol/l)	8
140-180 mg/dl (7.8-10.0 mmol/l)	6
120-140 mg/dl (6.7-7.8 mmol/l)	4
100-120 mg/dl (5.6-6.7 mmol/l)	2

The treat-to-target FPG was ≤100 mg/dl. Exceptions to this algorithm were 1) no increase in dosage if plasma-referenced glucose <72 mg/dl was documented at any time in the preceding week, and 2) in addition to no increase, small insulin dose decreases (2-4 IU/day per adjustment) were allowed if severe hypoglycemia (requiring assistance) or plasma-referenced glucose <56 mg/dl were documented in the preceding week.
Diabetics Care, 2003;26:3080-3086

Special Considerations:

- ACE Inhibitor or ARB if HT, cardiovascular risk factor, albuminuria; check Cr when 1 week after start, with any dose increase, or at least yearly.
- ASA 81-162 mg qd, if not contraindicated.
- Supplementation with vit D may correct mild DM.
- Metabolic control of diabetes decreased risk of CHD (Diabetes 1994;43:960), but associated with more driving accidents (J Am Ger Soc 1994;42:695).
- Hyperglycemic hyperosmolar nonketotic coma (HHNC): look for precipitating infections; replete volume deficit w normal saline until corrected sodium normalizes, then one-half NS (add dextrose when glucose < 250); low-dose insulin infusion; 50% mortality; usually insulin rx not required in long-term if pt recovers; bicarbonate therapy usually not recommended, reserved for pH < 7.

- Retinopathy: proliferative retinopathy and macular edema respond to laser rx (Ophthalm 1991;98:766); vitrectomy for vitreous scarring may restore sight (Arch Ophthalm 1985; 103:1644).
- Nephropathy: control HT, PO_4 restriction (Nejm 1991;324:78), low-protein diets (BMJ 1987;294:295), intensive diabetes rx (Nejm 1993;3329:977); ACE inhibitors prevent proteinuria (Nejm 1993;329:1456; Jama 1994;271:275; Med Lett Drugs Ther 1994;36:46; Arch IM 1994;154:625). Carvedilol significant improvement in HbA1c compared with metoprolol (Jama 2004;292:2227). Recent studies show ARBs equally effective in preventing proteinuria (Nejm 2004; 351:1934); end-stage renal disease: peritoneal rather than hemodialysis because increased risk of cardiovascular event, and retinal bleed w BP fluctuations and anticoagulation; if renal failure occurs in the absence of proteinuria or retinopathy, search for other etiologies, eg, NSAIDs or UTI.
- Neuropathy: gabapentin 100 mg qHS up to 600 mg tid.

Team Management:

- Antioxidants, vit C and E, enhance glucose-induced insulin release (Clin Ger Med 1999;15:239).
- Mediterranean diet superior to low fat diet (Ann IM 2006;145:1).
- Exercise (Jama 1999;282:1433).
- Occupational therapy: magnifiers to wrap around syringes, spring filling devices that click, "talking glucose meters"; family or nurse may need to do weekly supply setup.
- Foot ulcers/infections (Nejm 1994;331:854) w anaerobes and Pseudomonas; rx w parenteral imipenem or ticarcillin-clavulanate (Timentin), or oral fluoroquinolone plus clindamycin po 10-14 d, or if mild, not limb-threatrening and previously untreated, clindamycin, cephalexin or amoxicillin/clavulanate; r/o osteomyelitis (Jama 1995;273:712). Avoid barefoot walking, get good shoes, rx calluses, check water temperature when

bathing feet, toenails clipped straight across; zinc 220 mg tid (70 mg elemental zinc) (Morley 1999 AMDA Annual Meeting, Orlando, Fla.) risk of dyspepsia.

- Medicare B covers one pair of depth-inlay shoes, and one pair of custom-molded shoes, and 2-3 shoe inserts annually for diabetics w: h/o partial or complete foot amputation; h/o previous foot ulceration; h/o of pre-ulcerative callus; peripheral neuropathy with evidence of callus formation; poor circulation; foot deformity.

3.2 Thyroid

Hypothyroidism

Clin Ger Med 1995;11:231,239; Jama 1995;273:808; Jags 1993; 41:1361; 1994;42:984; 1995;43:592

Cause: Autoimmune thyroiditis; iodine-containing drugs decrease thyroid hormone secretion (Nejm 1995;333:1688), eg, radiographic contrast agents; amiodarone (Br J Clin Pract 1993;47:123); cough medicines, eg, codeine phosphate-dextromethorphan hydrobromide (Tussi-Organidin); antiseptic solutions, eg, povidone-iodine (Betadine); long-term lithium (South Med J 1993;86:1182); cholestyramine; aluminum hydroxide; sucralfate (Carafate) decreases T_4 absorption; rarely tumors of pituitary, hypothalamus.

Epidem: 2-5% prevalence; F/M = 5:1; risk factors for thyroid failure: family h/o any thyroid disease, h/o hyperthyroidism, subacute thyroiditis, postpartum thyroid disease, radiation (head, neck, chest), other autoimmune disease, eg, Addison's, pernicious anemia; 50% pts with PMR developed hypothyroidism (BMJ 1989; 298:647).

Sx: Neither pt nor family aware of changes over number of years; debilitation and apathy (66%); falls (17%); frequently subclinical (14%).

Si:

- Skin: Myxedematous infiltration of dermis loosening interface dermal-epidermal layers causing shiny tissue paper appearance; hair loss in scalp.
- Head/neck: Goiter rare, hoarse voice (0.8%), hypothyroid facies (3.3%) (Jags 1995;43:59); ophthalmologic—primary open-angle glaucoma (Ophthalm 1993;100:1580; Can J Ophthalm 1992;27:341).
- Neurologic: Decreased hearing, carpal tunnel syndrome, paresthesias, positional vertigo, myopathy (1.7%).
- Mental status: Withdrawn, confused (3.3%), psychotic (Int J Psychiatr Med 1990;20:193), cognitive deficit (Jags 1992; 40:325), treatable dementia (Am J Phys Med Rehab 1992; 71:28).
- Cardiovascular: Pleural effusions (11%), angina (8%), CHF (5.2%), pleural CVA (3.3%), CPK-MB elevated, bradycardia, infrequent HT.
- Respiratory: Airway obstruction secondary to swollen tongue, pharynx
- Metabolic: SIADH, hypothermia (1.7%).
- Anemia may be only manifestation; screen for hypothyroidism in pernicious anemia (Arch IM 1982;142:1465).

Cmplc: Myxedema coma (lethargy, confusion, psychosis, sometimes frontal/occipital headache) associated with severe infection, cold exposure, psychoactive meds (Ger Clin N Am 1993;222:279).

Lab:

- TSH > 10 mU/L; TSH may be increased by dopamine blocker; there may be an acute elevation of TSH in non-thyroidal illness, recheck 4-6 wk after illness resolves; associated w elevated cholesterol.
- R/o hypothalamic-pituitary axis damage: look for DI, acromegaly, hypogonadism, adrenal insufficiency.

- If no sx, check antimicrosomal antibody; if increased, likely that subclinical hypothyroidism will convert within 5-yr period to clinical hypothyroidism, monitor free T4 q 6 mo for TSH 5-10 mU/L (Clin Ger 2005;13:43)

EKG: Sinus bradycardia, low-voltage, prolonged QT, AV block, intraventricular conduction delay.

X-ray: Pleural effusion.

Rx:

Preventive: Screen all older women recommended by some groups, but U.S. Preventive Services Task Force does not find evidence for or against screening (USPSTF, 2004); some advocate "aggressive case finding," low threshold for ordering in pts w nonspecific complaints (Jags 1996;44:50), and in all pts w cognitive, medical, or functional deterioration, vs do not use as widespread screen (Jama 2004;292:2591).

Therapeutic:

- L-thyroxine (Synthroid) 0.025 mg/d, increase by 0.025 mg/d q 4-6 wk until TSH normal; in elderly pts w heart disease may start as low as 0.0125 mg/d, due to risk of precipitating ichemia.
- Switching from desiccated thyroid preparation, which has variable bioavailability, to L-thyroxine may lead to iatrogenic hyperthyroidism.
- Hypothyroid pts with angina can undergo surgery without replacement; do not delay emergent CABG in hypothyroid pts w unstable angina; be careful of CNS-active meds that are cleared more slowly in hypothyroidism (Ann IM 1981;95:456; Am J Med 1984;77:261).
- Thyroid replacement does not affect bone density, unless over replace.
- Of Myxedema coma: Initial T_4 100-500 μg iv; subsequent dose 100 μg iv qd × 10 d, then po.

- Pts w profound hypothyroidism requiring emergency general surgery should receive preoperative L-thyroxine 300-500 μg slow iv infusion + hydrocortisone 300 mg iv; Swan-Ganz monitoring; watch for prolonged ileus and infection (altered febrile response) (Clin Ger Med 95;11:251).
- Some argue that if TSH mildly elevated and T_4 nl, treat to slow atherosclerosis and lower cholesterol (Solomon D, Thyroid Disease Intensive Geriatric Review course, UCLA 1996; Jama 2004;291:228). Rx sx and antithyroid antibodies, increased LDL-C, goiter or repeated TSH > 10 (Jama 2004;4:335).

Hyperthyroidism

Clin Ger Med 1995;11:181; Jama 1995;273:808

Cause: Most common cause is toxic nodular goiter; Graves or diffuse nodular goiter less common in late life; iatrogenic: takes T_4 5-6 half-lives to reach steady state in the elderly, or 6-7 wk in pts 80-90 yr old; therefore may induce hyperthyroidism if do not wait appropriate amount of time before increasing dose; T_4 may be suppressed in T_3 toxicosis (almost exclusively seen in the elderly). Due to paucity of complaints, important to screen q 2 yr w TSH (Jags 1996;44:50).

Epidem: 15-25% of cases occur in the elderly; 0.47% prevalence in community-based elderly.

Pathophys: Apathetic thyrotoxicosis diminished postreceptor responsiveness to thyroid hormone w age.

Sx: Rarely report loose stools, but may note a correction of constipation, reduction in appetite, consumption of fewer calories, wgt loss; inability to rise from chair due to proximal muscle weakness; apathetic hyperthyroidism.

Si: Coarse tremor; less common in elderly; most frequent cardiac manifestation is sinus tachycardia; Afib.

Cmplc: Accelerates bone turnover, leading to osteoporosis; causes insulin resistance (2-3% of thyrotoxic pts develop clinically significant diabetes); CHF (60% of elderly persons w hyperthyroidism develop CHF). High-output failure leads to widened pulse pressure. 50% have Afib; 20% have angina (Nejm 1992;327:94). Thyroid often largely substernal.

Lab: TSH < 0.1 mU/L, lowered by dopamine agonists and coricosteroids (GRS 5th ed, 2002, p 336); monitor free T_4 q 6 mo for TSH 0.1-0.4 mU/L (Clin Ger 2005;13:43).

X-ray: Diagnosis confirmed by increased uptake of radioactive iodine.

Rx:

Preventive: If asx but TSH low w nl T_3, T_4, monitor more frequently for sx and increase in T_3, T_4 and treat.

Therapeutic: I^{131} for toxic multinodular goiter requires 2-3 × the radioisotope dose for diffuse toxic goiter. For Graves: irradiation (Table 3-4), propylthiouracil (PTU) for 3 wk before radioactive iodine therapy to eliminate the possibility of radiation-induced thyroiditis; major complication of radiation is hypothyroidism: 50% develop hypothyroidism within 20 yr.

Table 3.4 Thyroid Carcinoma

	Papillary	Follicular	Medullary	Anaplastic
Cause	Graves: LATS	—	—	—
Epidem	75% of thyroid cancers	15%	5%	3%
Pathophys	—	—	Associated w MEN IIA, hyperparathyroidism, pheochromocytoma	—
Sx	30% present as occult tumors; lymph node enlargement, hoarseness, dysphagia, neck pain	Slow-growing goiter; lymph node not as common as papillary; 50% metastatic at presentation; occasionally thyrotoxicosis	—	Sudden increase in size of goiter; difficulty breathing
Si	Bilateral	—	Mostly bilateral	Firm, tender w soft areas of hemorrhage, necrosis

Table 3.4 Continued

	Papillary	Follicular	Medullary	Anaplastic
Crs	Good prognosis if < 1.5 cm despite lymph node involvement; 55% 10-yr survival; enters more malignant phase after 10 yr w metastases to lung, bone (lytic), brain, and soft tissue	High mortality w vascular invasion	To lymph node, liver, bone, adrenal	Mortality 6 mo to 1 yr
Lab	Psammoma bodies pathognomonic on histology	—	Calcitonin $>$ 250 pg/mL indicates cancer	—
Rx	Surgery: total thyroidectomy w excision of suspicious lymph nodes, ablate postoperatively w ^{131}I; watch calcium levels postoperatively; f/u T_4 q 6 mo, if elevated, check radioiodine scan and rx recurrent disease w ^{131}I	Radioactive iodine; replace w T_3 because shorter-acting and can discontinue for only 2 wk when checking radioactive scan yearly	Not responsive to radioiodine; rx w surgery	Radiation shrinks tumor (4-5000 rads); may cause tracheal obstruction; undifferentiated cancer fatal in 1 yr; rx doxorubicin (De Vita VT, Cancer principles and practice of oncology, 4th ed, Lippincott, 1993; 1333)

LATS = long-acting thyroid stimulator; MEN = multiple endocrine neoplasia.
Source: Gupta KL. Neoplasm of the thyroid gland. Clin Geriatr Med 1995;11:271-290.

- Methimazole (Tapazole): When TSH low, T_3,T_4 normal but pt is sx (Jags 1996;44:573; Nejm 2005;352:405).
- Graves: β-blockers: For heat intolerance, anxiety, myopathy; adverse effects: cardiac, pulmonary, memory, mood, sleep disorders, fatigue.

  PTU 100 mg or methimazole (Tapazole) 10 mg q 6-8 h blocks hormone synthesis. Large goiters may require twice as much, rarely up to 1000 mg/d of PTU; euthyroid in 6 wk, then can begin maintenance 50-300/d 1 yr; > one-third respond permanently. Adverse effects include hypothyroidism, agranulocytosis (0.5%) (early in rx, w large doses, reversible w withdrawal, baseline WBC and repeat w signs of infection—fever), skin rash, arthralgia, myalgia, neuritis, SLE, psychosis.

  Prior to surgery on those with untreated hyperthyroidism: iv loading dose of PTU 1000 mg or ipodate sodium 500 mg po qd × 5 d prior to surgery; or propranolol 1 mg/min iv during surgery.

Thyroid Nodules

Epidem: More common in elderly and more frequently malignant, and when malignant more aggressive than in younger pts; more common among women. Differentiated tumors more aggressive at age > 45 yr; anaplastic exclusively at age > 65 yr.

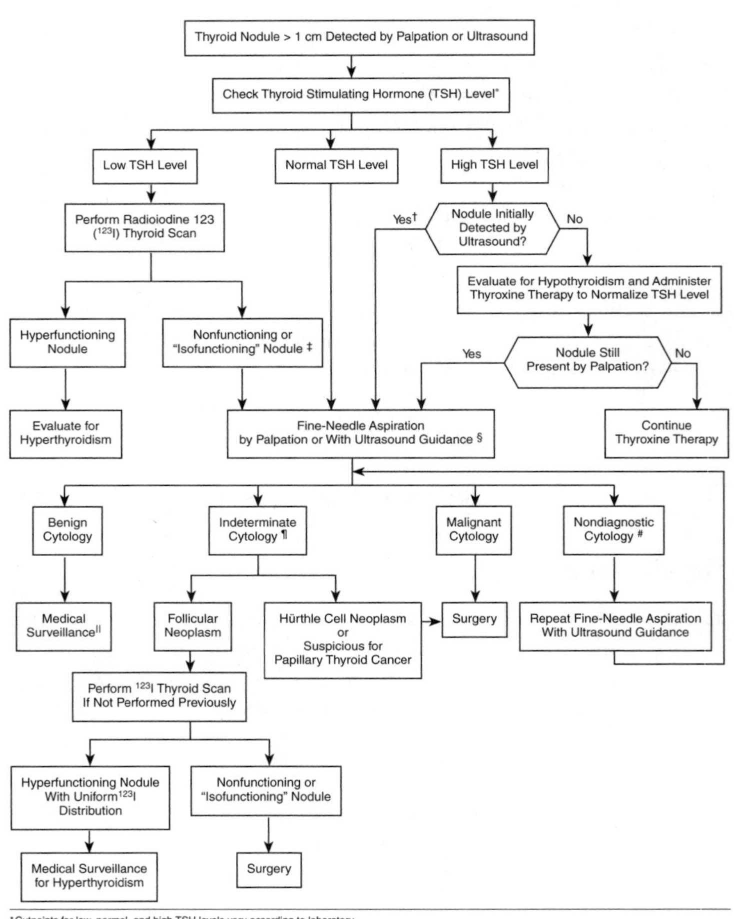

*Cutpoints for low, normal, and high TSH levels vary according to laboratory.
†Evaluate for hypothyroidism.
‡Evaluate for hyperthyroidism.
§Indications for fine-needle aspiration guided by ultrasound include palpable nodule greater than 50% cystic, difficult to palpate or nonpalpable nodules, and nondiagnostic cytology on previous fine-needle aspiration.
||Perform diagnostic thyroid ultrasound if not previously performed.
¶Follicular neoplasm, Hürthle cell neoplasm, suspicious for papillary thyroid cancer.
#Insufficient quantity of follicular thyroid cells.

Figure 3.1 Evaluation of Thyroid Nodules (Jama 2004;292:2636).

Sx: Dysphagia, pain suggests cancer.

Si: Hard nodules, enlarged lymph nodes, rapid growth should raise suspicion of cancer.

Crs: Variable and dependent on pathologic grade.

Cmplc:

Of Multinodular Goiter: Thyrotoxicosis, subclinical thyrotoxicosis (Clin Endocrinol 1992;36:25), vocal cord paralysis, tracheal compression (Am J Med 1988;84:19).

R/o Benign: Colloid (60%), adenomas (30%); carcinoma (see Table 3-4), lymphoma frequently in persons w underlying Hashimoto's thyroiditis.

Lab:

- Pathologic: Fine-needle aspiration (FNA) bx—malignant reports in 5% of specimens, and an indication for surgery (except w lymphoma or anaplastic carcinoma); false pos rate of 5-7%; bx several areas of multinodular goiter (larger, harder ones, those that are cold on scan).
- X-ray: Both US and radionuclide scan more sens than palpation; nodules frequently cold and solid.

Rx:

Therapeutic:

Thyroid replacement: If TSH elevated, reassess nodule after 2 mo of thyroid replacement; multinodular goiters do not respond, as well to suppressive therapy as Hashimoto's thyroiditis or simple diffuse goiters.

Treatment of hot nodules: Older pts w hot nodules, nl T_4, but suppressed TSH (subclinical thyrotoxicosis) have increased risk for osteoporosis and possible underlying heart disease; should have lower threshold for radioactive rx, solitary autonomously functioning nodule 200-400uCi/gm and 80-100uCi/gm for toxic multinodular goiter, surgery if rapid decompression vital structures (Nejm 1998;338:1438).

ENDOCRINOLOGY

If benign FNA and nodule < 2 cm: Use suppression rx; if benign FNA and > 2 cm, surgery indicated (larger nodules not as responsive).

Preoperative cardiac screening indicated for pts undergoing thyroid surgery w following risk factors: Q-wave MI on EKG, angina, DM, ventricular ectopy requiring rx, advanced age (Ann IM 1989;110:859).

Chapter 4

Neurology

4.1 Stroke

Am Fam Phys 1994;49:1777; Clin Ger Med 1993;9:705; Ger Rv Syllabus, 5th ed, 2002, p88; Am J Med 1996;100:465; Circ 1996;94:1167; Arch Neurol 1995;52:347; Clin Ger 2004;12:27; Jags 2006;54:674

Cause: Carotid or aortic arch (Nejm 1992;326:221), basilar system plaque and/or platelet emboli, cardiac emboli, vascular spasm, hypercoagulable states, idiopathic.

Risk Factors: HT, DM, CAD, MI, Afib (14% risk embolic stroke at onset and 5%/yr), peripheral vascular disease (PVD), smoking, lipids, homocystinemia (Jama 1995;274:1526; 1997;227:1775; Ann IM 1995;123:747; Nejm 1995;372:286,328); cholesterol associated positively with ischemic stroke risk and negatively with hemorrhagic stroke (Jama 1997;278:316).

Hemorrhagic Stroke: 50% are due to HT, 17% from amyloid angiopathy, 10% from anticoagulation rx, 5%-10% from brain tumors, 5% from smoking (Nejm 1992;326:1672; Curr Concepts Cerebro Dis 1990;25:31; 1991;26:1).

Epidem: 75% of pts w CVA are > 75 yr; 2% incidence/yr for elderly; 35,000 pts/yr in NH; 100,000 pts/yr at home.

Pathophys: Occasionally is vasospastic and can rx w Ca-channel blocker (Nejm 1993;329:396).

Sx:

- TIA: most resolve < 24 hr, 70% < 1 hr.

- Infarct: h/o TIA (80%); 60% onset in early morning hours awakens w stroke.
- Anterior circulation sx: amaurosis fugax (Stroke 1990;21:201); weakness of arm > face > leg paresis (middle cerebral artery affected pattern); leg > arm > face paresis (anterior cerebral artery pattern); depression; abulia; delusions; aphasia if dominant hemisphere.
- Posterior circulation sx: diplopia, numbness in face and mouth; slurred speech; loss of consciousness; crossed signs CN vs body; headache; vomit; dizzy; ataxia.
- Lacunar: pure motor w internal capsule; pure sensory w thalamus; dysarthria and clumsy hand w pons; ataxia and hemiparesis w base pons, genu and internal capsule.
- Embolism: 75% mid cerebral, 90% maximum loss at onset, loss of consciousness (LOC) common, seizure.
- Hemorrhagic infarct (see Table 4.1): during physical activity, most commonly from berry aneurysm or microaneurysm from HT; decreased alertness, vomiting; hemiparesis w putamen or thalamus bleed; bilateral signs and coma w brainstem; headache, vertigo, ataxia, gaze, and facial palsy w cerebellar.

Table 4.1 Stroke Types and Mortality

Cerebral Infarct (75%)	Intracerebral Hemorrhage (15%)	Subarachnoid Hemorrhage (10%)
40%	80%	50%

Si:

- Nl changes w aging: decreased arm swing 30%, decreased toe vibratory sense 20%, decreased nasolabial fold, absent pupillary response, pos Babinskis or decreased toe position 10%, reduction arm strength 5%.

- TIAs: in elderly, asx bruit present in 10% and does not correlate with CVA rate in or out of affected carotid distribution.
- Infarct: specific occlusion patterns.
- Middle cerebral: face and arm motor; expressive aphasia (Broca's).
- Carotid watershed: parietal aphasias, weakness arm > face > leg.
- Posterior cerebral: homonymous hemianopsia, hemisensory loss, memory loss (Curr Concepts Cerebro Dis 1986;21:25).
- Lateral medullary plate syndrome (PICA: posterior inferior cerebellar artery); (Curr Concepts Cerebro Dis 1981;16:17): ipsilateral pain and temperature loss on face, contralateral for rest of body, hoarseness, swallowing dysfunction, Horner's, hiccups, ipsilateral cerebellar si's.
- Subarachnoid hemorrhage: HT, stiff neck.
- Cerebellar hemorrhage: awake, alert even with ophthalmoplegias; acute hypotonia; conjugate gaze paresis.
- Cerebral hemorrhage: seizure (13%) w onset or within 48 hr.
- Brainstem hemorrhage: early loss of consciousness, brainstem si's, quadriplegia.

Crs:

- 20% of pts w TIAs will have CVA within 1 mo; 50% in 1 yr; 50% of pts w TIAs die of CAD while 36% die of CVA; association of TIA w MI as strong as MI and 3-vessel CAD.
- Infarct: if there is even slightest voluntary twitch within 7 d of stroke onset, full upper extremity recovery may be expected; voluntary hip flexion predictor of ambulation, spasticity resolves, hyperreflexia persists.
- Embolic stroke: 15% 30-d mortality; 12% w cardiac embolic stroke have 2nd embolus within 2 wk of first event.
- Hemorrhagic stroke: over 1 mo 33% die, 33% are impaired and 33% are OK (Nejm 1993;311:1547).

Cmplc:

- TIA: r/o migraine, subdural, hematoma, seizures, hypoglycemia, tumor, MS.
- Stroke: r/o MI w EKG.
- CVA: seizures, 33% of which occur within 2 wk after infarction; depression occurs in 40% of L-hemisphere infarction; probably physiologic not psychological phenomenon (Stroke 1994;25:1099). Arthritis of shoulder after hemiplegia, despite passive ROM exercises; pulmonary emboli; pneumonias; UTIs.
- Reflex sympathetic dystrophy: burning pain, vasomotor instability, trophic changes to skin, bony demineralization of hand or foot secondary to abnormal stimulation of sympathetic nervous system; dx w 3 phase bonescan; rx: short course high dose steroids, physical therapy, sympathetic nerve block (Lancet 1993;342:1012).

Lab:

Noninvasive: Carotid duplex US, carotid Doppler US, MRA all about 85% sens and 90% specif (Ann IM 1995;122:360; 1988;109:805,835); CBC w platelets, PT/PTT; VDRL; EKG (r/o MI, arrhythmia), which often shows abnormal "anterior MI" patterns (Nejm 1974;291:1122; J Neurosurg 1969;30:521); MRI white matter lesions predict stroke (Jama 2002;288:67).

- Hemorrhagic Stroke: LP preferably only after CT to r/o mass lesion; CSF: some intracerebral bleeds and all subarachnoid bleeds show grossly bloody tap w > 1000 rbc/dL (100% sens, 80% specif), protein > 1 gm/dL; xanthochromia present in 90% (centrifuge immediately to avoid false-pos); rbc decrease 10-fold from 1st to 3rd tube (Ann IM 1986;104:880).

X-ray: W/u TIA w US Doppler; CT best for acute bleed vs MRI just as good (Jama 2004;292:1823); MRI for lacunar—not good for acute bleed; old strokes often found during acute CT in elderly; MRA as good as angiography; videofluoroscopy to determine aspiration and subsequent pneumonia risk (Arch Phys Med Rehab 1996;77:707).

- Hemorrhagic Stroke: 25% of subarachnoid bleeds won't show blood on CT.

Rx: Insert table modifiable risk factors (Jama 2002;283:1385).

Preventive:

- Decrease systolic BP to 140 even in pts > 80 yr; decreases long-term incidence of CVA by 3% and MI by 5.5%; prefer thiazides and β-blockers, ACE inhibitors (for acute BP management). If initial BP < 155/70 mortality increases in ischemic stroke (Neurol 2005;65:1178).
- Control blood sugar in diabetic pts.
- If smoke > 20 cigarettes/d, have 6 × increased risk for CVA; incidence falls significantly after 2 yr of not smoking and falls to risk of nonsmokers after 5 yr of not smoking.
- ASA after TIA reduces recurrence of nonfatal stroke, MI and vascular death by 20%-25% (BMJ 1994;308:81,1540; Curr Opin Neurol 1994;7:48), not at increased risk of intracranial bleed w head injury (J Neurosurg 2003;99:661). Adding dipyridamole to ASA decreases recurrence (Lancet 2006;367:1665).
- Warfarin for all Afib unless contraindications (Ann IM 1994;121:41,54; Nejm 1995;332:238; 1995;333:5; Jama 1995;274:1839), worse outcome stroke w afib (Stroke 2001;23:392); INR > 3.5 assoc w incr bleeding in pts > 85 yrs (Ann IM 2004;141:745).
- Patients w nonvalvular Afib can be rx w ASA if low risk, eg, don't have CHF or EF < 25, previous thromboembolism, systolic blood pressure > 160mm Hg (Jama 1998;279:1273), DM, thyrotoxicosis (Jama 2002;283:1385); LA peak velocity < 20 cm/sec independent risk fx future thrombosis ✓ TEE.
- Warfarin for patients w 60% carotid stenosis (Jama 1995; 243:1421; Nejm 1995;332:238).
- Statins to reduce risk of nonhemorrhagic stroke (Ann IM 1998;128:89; Nejm 2000;343:317).

- Folic acid 1 mg po qd to reduce risk of ASCVD (Jama 1998;279:359; Nejm 1998;338:1009).
- Adding ASA to clopidogrel increases bleeding without decreasing ischemic vascular events in high-risk pts (Am Coll Phys J Club 2004;141:68).

Therapeutic: TIA: evaluate rapidly (BMJ 2004;328:326), endarterectomy if > 70-80% stenosis (Nejm 1991;325:445; Jama 1995; 273:1421; Lancet 1998;351:1373,1379), older men w > 70% stenosis not as likely to benefit (Lancet 2004;363:915), consider if combined cmplc rate of angiography and surgery at your hospital is < 3%, since often morbidity is 14% in community hospitals, but only 1% in big centers, perform 1 mo after stroke (J Vasc Surg 2006;44:480); more risk of MI s/p endarterectomy in pts > 70 yr old (Cardiovasc Surg 1993;1:30); ETT if any cardiac risk factors; warfarin 3 mo course. If risk of bleeding, ASA 300 mg; if risk of bleeding ticlopidine (Ticlid) better (Med Lett Drugs Ther 1992;34:65); adverse effects of ticlopidine: diarrhea, abdominal cramps, rarely neutropenia (monitor blood counts q 1 mo for 3-4 mo) (Ann IM 1994;121:45).

Stroke in Evolution: Iv TPA within 3 hr of onset of stroke results in 30% improvement in clinical outcome, but increased incidence of intracranial hemorrhage within 36 hr (6.45% vs 0.6%) (Nejm 1995;333:1581; Jama 1996;276:961) in pts up to 85 yr (Circ 1996;94:1826); alteplase (Activase) (Med Lett Drugs Ther 1996; 38:99). Poor px at 3 mo, if BS was high, cortical involvement or if increased time to rx (Jama 2004;292:1839).

Nonhemorrhagic Infarct: Use anticoagulant only w CVA in evolution, TIA in pt on ASA or ticlopidine; otherwise risk of bleeding too great (Stroke 1994;25:1901). Wait 48 hr before anticoagulation in large embolic stroke middle-cerebral or middle cerebral and anterior cerebral (Ger Rv Syll 2002; p296).

Acute Care (Curr Concepts Cerebro Dis 1989;24:1): rx diastolic BP > 140 or systolic > 230 acutely with iv nitroprusside. If diastolic persists > 105 or systolic > 180 for 1-2 hr, then rx with labetalol iv or po, mannitol 25-50 gm as 20% soln over 30 min q 3-12 hr and/or furosemide iv, and/or nifedipine sl or po (sl nifedipine may lower BP too abruptly) (Stroke 1994;25:1901); keep PCO_2 at 25-30 mm Hg if on respirator; monitor; give 100-125 mL/hr of Ringer's or D5S.

Supportive Care: Heparin sc to prevent DVT, which occurs in 70% (Ann IM 1992;117:353); pneumatic compression further prevents DVT in stroke pts (Neurol 1998;50:1683); post-stroke depression: SSRIs (Stroke 1994;25:1099) or nortriptyline (Lancet 1984;1:297) may try trazadone, or citalopram, better than other SSRIs (Jama 1997;278:1186; 2000;283:1607).

Follow-up Care: Embolic stroke: decreased by 86% if anticoagulate 2 yr; annual bleeding rate 2.5% (Ann IM 1992;320: 352,392). Maintain INR 2-3; warfarin, if abnormal echocardiogram; anticoagulate > 60% occluded asx carotid stenosis w intermittent or chronic Afib to decrease embolic stroke, NNT = 16 (Jama 1995;273:1421); surgically fix > 70% carotid stenosis (Nejm 1995;332:238; Lancet 2003;36:107).

Hemorrhagic Infarct: Prevent aspiration; use caution w hydration; do not lower BP aggressively; supratentorial > 5 cm size, bad px; pontine > 3 cm, bad px.

Rehab (Clin Ger Med 1999;15:819,833): Px for pts w CVAs > 65 yr: 10% no dysfunction, 40% moderate dysfunction, 40% severe dysfunction, 10% institutionalized. Begin physical therapy right away after stroke w progression to full program as able. Good prognostic signs: motivated to participate in rehab, follows one-step commands, memory to learn, little neglect, less sensory deficits, bowel and bladder control, feeding and grooming skills, strong social support. Successful rehab not associated w size or site of infarction (Arch Phys Med Rehab 1989;7:100) or age alone.

- 6 mo to regain motor function w continuous gains for 2-3 yr; 2-3 yr to regain language function.
- Upper extremity motor skills can improve despite residual spasticity (Stroke 1998;29:75); whole-task and meaningful-task better than part-task practice (Am J Occup Ther 1997; 51:508); 2- or 4-wheeled walker most popular with pts, must have good control, hemi-walker when more support needed, 3- or 4-pronged cane may be useful outside, straight cane only if good balance. Cane should come to wrist and there should be a 20°-30° elbow bend, use on uninvolved side. Lower wheelchair after stroke, so pt can use good leg.

Reimbursement from Medicare for rehab requires multidisciplinary approach: documentation of goals, documentation of improvement; goal cannot be maintenance.

Criteria for Admission to Acute Rehab Facility: expected rapid rate of improvement, eg, 3-4 wk; tolerate 3 hr/d of combined therapy 6-7 d/wk; minimal dementia; may want to use methylphenidate HCl (Ritalin) for severely depressed pts to ensure their candidacy for rehab but would try SSRIs first; Ritalin good prior to SSRI because of rapid onset of action.

- To obtain rehab in the home, must need two therapies daily, as well as daily nursing and 24-hr physician availability. Location of rehab program may vary w managed-care programs.

Team Management (Dreshem GE, Duncan PW, Stason WB, et al. Post Stroke Rehabilitation Assessment, Referral and Patient Management Clinical Practice Guideline. Quick Reference Guide for Clinicians, No. 16 Rockville; MD: US Department of Health and Human Services, Agency for Health Care Policy and Research. May 1995. AHCPR Publc No. 95-0663, 1995. Clinical Practice Guidelines, Jama 1997;45:881)

Physical Therapy: Return of function 3-12 mo: start brace when have "en masse" flexor or extensor synergism of all joints and 4 out of 5 strength and can balance on good leg; then work on selective flexion and bed access; metal brace for spasticity.

Shoulder pain common and has many possible causes: adhesive capsulitis, shoulder subluxation, rotator cuff injury, tenosynovitis, rarely reflex sympathetic dystrophy (cutaneous sens and swelling of hand and arm); rx w ROM exercises, hot and cold contrast baths; if unresponsive, can try high-dose corticosteroids, stellate block; rx spasticity w baclofen, dantrolene or tizanidine (D_2-adrenergic agonist, expensive), all of which cause sedation.

Occupational Therapy: Diagnose and rx perceptual, cognitive losses and ADL deficits, and help pt begin to engage in social activity again.

Swallowing Evaluation: Oral preparatory phase where tongue places food between tongue and palate assessed by being able to say "mi, mi, mi"; oral phase where food received into pharynx assessed by being able to say "la, la, la"; and pharyngeal phase where tongue and pharynx push food into esophagus assessed by being able to say "ga, ga, ga." (Am J Nurs 1995;95:34).

Six nerves and 25 facial and oral muscles involved; 40%-50% of stroke pts have some degree of dysphagia, which can carry up to a 40% risk of aspiration. Transit time is measured by placement of examiner's index and third fingers at the top and bottom of the thyroid cartilage while pt swallows; delay > 10 sec is associated w a significant risk of aspiration (Am Fam Phys 1994;49: 1777). Methylene blue dye test useful for pts w tracheostomy, dye in tracheal secretions after oral intake of dye in foods indicates aspiration (Am J Nurs 1995;95:34).

Feeding Recommendations:

1. 30-min rest before eating.
2. Observation of eating essential until degree of risk established.

3. Call button, if eating without assistance.
4. Allow 30-40 min for pt to eat meal.
5. Juice better than water because taste helps locate food in mouth; the pulp in citrus juices may pose a problem.
6. Avoid sticky, dry foods and mucus-producing foods, such as milk products; just because pt has gag reflex does not mean will not aspirate; small amounts of food may not stimulate a gag reflex; may need to thicken fluids; chopped better than puree.
7. Have pt clear throat before swallowing, say "ah," and if sound is gurgly, may have aspirated; pt can perform finger sweep between swallows.
8. Straws deposit food too far back in the throat; if pt has a weak swallow reflex, keep drinking glass three-fourths full, so pt doesn't have to tilt head too far back.
9. Keep patient upright 45-60 min after eating.
10. Pt education re: risk factors (Jama 1998;278:1324).
11. Cabergoline (dopamine agonist), ACE inhibitors improve silent aspiration (Jags 2003;51:1815; Lancet 1998;352:115; 1999;353:1157).
12. If decreased salivation but they can still swallow, gum chewing recommended (Jags 2006;54:867).

4.2 Parkinson's Disease

Robbins L, UCLA, 1/96; Neurol 1994;44; Ger Rv Course UCLA 9/02 Jeff Bronstein, Parkinson's Disease

Table 4.2 Parkinson's Disease and Other Disorders

	Bradykinesia	Tremor	Automatic Dysfunction	Dementia	Depression	Downward Gaze Paralysis/PDD	Other Neurologic Signs	Response to Dopaminergic Rx
Parkinson's 130/100000	Facial Psychomotor slowing (cog wheeling) Slowed gait, decreased arm swing, forward flexion of neck and trunk Decrease turning (truncal rigidity) Decrease stride, step height (festonating gait) Drooling Hypophonic speech Micrographia	Alt. flexion ext fingers; resting, disappears with action; 4-8 c/sec; 70%	Hypotension Constipation (Shy-Drager) Increased salivation Increased sebum Dysphasia	40% increased SE with meds	60%	Absent/absent	Absent	Yes
Supranuclear palsy	Axial rigidity Neck extension posture	Absent	Absent	Decreased cognition Decreased memory	Present	Present/present	Speech swallow problems	Poor

continues

NEUROLOGY

Table 4.2 continued

	Bradykinesia	Tremor	Automatic Dysfunction	Dementia	Depression	Downward Gaze Paralysis/PDD	Other Neurologic Signs	Response to Dopaminergic Rx
				Decreased abstract thought				
Lacunar infarct	Present	Absent	Present	Early	Emotional lability	Absent/ present	Gait Difficulty	None
Hypothyroid	Delayed response Slowed movement	Absent	Absent	Present	Present	Absent/ absent	Wide-Based Shuffling	
Hypopara-thyroid	Present	Absent	Absent	Absent	Absent	Absent/ absent	Present, cerebral dysfunc-tion	
Drugs Methyl-dopa Diazepam Lithium Reserpine	Present symmetric persists for months after drug stopped	May be present symmetric	Absent	Delirium	May be present	Absent/ absent	Absent	Makes sx worse
Choliner-gics Pheno-thiazines Excess vit B_6	Present	+/–	—		+/–	–/–	—	

Other AIDS Neoplasia Trauma Creutzfeldt-Jakob Viral postencephalitis Hydrocephalus	Present	—	—	—	—	Absent/absent	—	
Lewy Body Dementia	+/–	rare	+	Improves without Exelloan	–	–/–	Psychosis REM sleep Disorder	Worsens psych. symptoms
Corticobasal Degeneration	+/–	asymmetric	–	Cortical	–	–/–	Limb Dystonia apraxia corticospinal signs	Poor
Multiple System Atrophy	+/–	+	+	–	–		Cerebellar signs corticospinal signs Respiratory stridor +/–	Poor

Alt = alternating; ext = extension; SE = side effects; PDD = pseudobulbar dysarthria, dysphagia

Cause: Environmental factors (blacks in America have 5 × risk of blacks in Nigeria); genetic cause, chromosome 4 (Science 1996;274:1197); drugs w antidopaminergic properties: haloperidol (Haldol), metoclopramide (Reglan), prochlorperazine (Compazine), amoxapine (Asendin), lithium, methyldopa (Aldomet); drug-induced Parkinson's possible in first 3 mo of therapy.

Epidem: 50,000 new cases annually; 1:100 elderly vs 1:1000 general population; prevalence second only to Alzheimer's among degenerative neurologic diseases: cigarette smoking associated w decreased risk of Parkinson's (Neurol 1995;43:1041). High intake of caffeine associated w decreased incidence of Parkinson's (Jama 2000;283:2674). NH pts w Parkinson's undertreated: lacking in physical therapy, rx of depression, adequate social interaction (Jags 1996;44:300; Nejm 1996;334:71).

Pathophys: Loss of pigmented neurons in substantia nigra and brainstem, Lewy bodies (concentric hyaline cytoplasmic inclusions); dopamine reduced in substantia nigra and corpus striatum; clinical sx when 80% depletion of striatal dopamine. Neurotoxins: manganese toxicity; copper in Wilson's disease destroys dopaminergic neurons (Onion DK, The Little Black Book of Primary Care. Malden, MA: Blackwell Science, 1996).

Table 4.3 Clinical Classification of Tremors

Feature	Parkinsonian	Exaggerated Physiologic	Essential	Cerebellar
Frequency (Hz)	4-7	6-12	6-12	3-5
Amplitude	Coarse	Fine	Variable	Variable
Tremor at rest	++++	+	+	+
Tremor with action				
Postural	++	++++	+++	+++
Intention	++	++	++	++++
Distribution	Limbs, jaw tongue	Limbs	Hands, head	Limbs, head

Si: Bradykinesia, rigidity (no loss of muscle strength), dystonia less common (Neurol 1988;38:1410), tremor (3-7 Hz), pill rolling tremor (not as common in drug-induced Parkinson's or atherosclerotic Parkinson's) (Lancet 1984;2:1092) and bilat 50% (Neurol 1988;38:1410), hypophonia, micrographia, depression 15%-40% (serotonin pathway may be affected, too), drooling, constipation, seborrheic dermatitis.

Crs: Average life expectancy = 12.3 yr, some live 20+ yr. More rapid course in elderly, declining 5 yr after diagnosis.

Cmplc: (See Table 4.2) Sleep disturbance, common problem (Jags 1997;45:194).

- Shy-Drager seen w bradykinesia, autonomic dysfunction, and cerebellar ataxia due to degeneration of sympathetic preganglionic nerves of thoracic and upper lumbar spinal cord, and not responsive to levodopa. Hypotension resulting from rx of Parkinson's can be treated w high-salt diet or fludrocortisone or midodrine (Geriatrics 1999;54:44).

- Hallucinations associated w Parkinson's dementia (see Subcortical Dementia) chief reason for admission to NH for Parkinson's patients (Jags 2000;48:938).
- R/o essential tremor, which is sporadic or hereditary w onset at early age; interferes w volitional movements, eg, writing, eating, highly skilled occupations; alcohol helps. β-blockers (propranolol 40-320 mg/d) significant improvement in one-half pts; primidone (Mysoline) (125-750 mg/d) also effective; clonazepam third choice.
- R/o vascular Parkinson's: Gait and balance problems out of proportion to rigidity, tremor does not respond to meds.
- R/o Lewy Body disease: sx of dementia preceded by depression/sleep disorder, drug-induced hallucinations. May respond to levodopa in early stages.
- R/o drugs/toxins causing tremor: methylxanthines, β-agonists, valproate, thyroid hormone, corticosteroids; also heavy metals (Hg, Pb, As), multiple environmental toxins, methylphenyltetrahydropyridine (MPTP).
- R/o: progressive supranuclear palsy (axial rigidity, vertical and later horizontal gaze paralysis, very little in the way of tremor); nortriptyline 100 mg/d to rx depression of SNP (Jags 1997; 45:1034).

Lab: CBC, routine chemistries, albumin (nutritional assessment), thyroid profile, VDRL, Pb level.

- *X-ray:* CXR—baseline for aspiration changes.
- Flow sheet for medications for Parkinson's disease (see Figure 4.1).

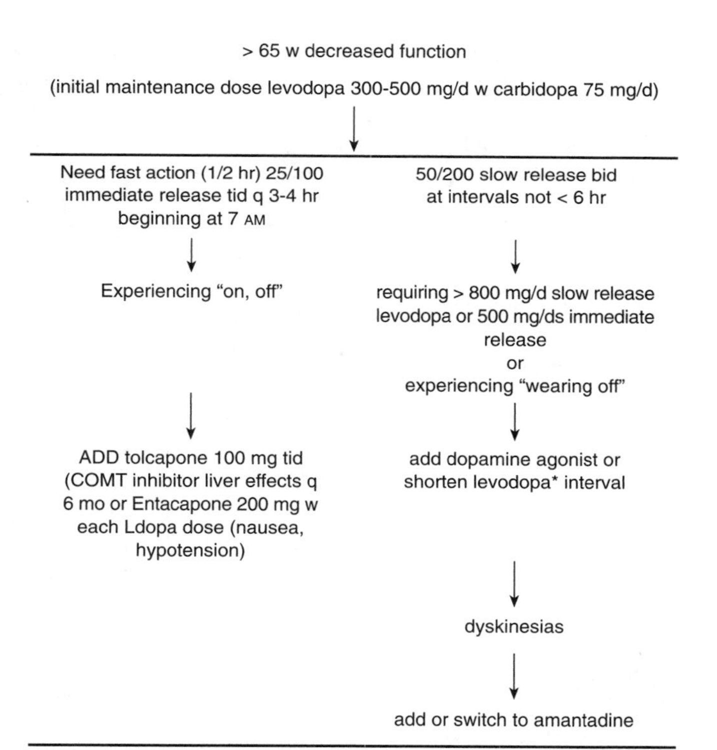

Figure 4.1 Flow Sheet for Medications for Parkinson's Disease. (Adapted from Stacy M. Parkinson's disease: Therapeutic choices and timing decisions in patient management. Interview by Wayne Kuznar. Geriatrics 1999;54:44-9)

Therapeutic: Begin treatment when function is impacted; Parkinson's sx fluctuate from hour to hour and day to day; therefore, evaluate med adjustments over days to weeks. Seek family, staff observations over 24-hr periods.

- Levodopa: Effective, but because of adverse effects sometimes saved for more advanced disease; carbidopa/levodopa precipitates oxidation that further damages the substantia nigra and eventually spreads disease progression (Jags 1997;45:233); give w carbidopa (Sinemet) to limit breakdown (need at least 75-100 mg/d of carbidopa and do not exceed 200 mg/d); start with 25/100 one-half tab bid, increasing daily dose every week by one-half to 1 tab (2-8 tabs/d); levodopa requirement for most pts is 500-1000 mg, therefore may need to add 10/100 mg tabs to increase levodopa, but keep down carbidopa. Painful dystonia upon awakening is a good indication that levodopa should be increased. Give 2nd dose in afternoon to avoid insomnia. Major side effects: Hypotension, hallucinations, psychosis. Dyskinesias usually mean there is too much dopamine; take controlled release (CR) with food and increase total dose of levodopa by 30% because not as bioavailable as short-acting (Nejm 1993;329:1021); CR 50/200 mg bid 8 AM and 3-4 PM (J Am Board Fam Pract 1997;10:412); breaking tablets in half speeds absorption and action, tid or qid; combine dosing CR night with multiple small doses during day (25/100 mg CR); use 50/100 mg CR for motor fluctuations (Am Fam Phys 1996; 53:1281). Avoid supplements that contain high doses of vit B_6 (50-100 mg) because reduces activity of carbidopa.
- Dopamine agonists: May want to start rx w dopamine agonist to delay or minimize use of carbidopa/levodopa and also to avoid anticholinergic drugs. Pramipexole not as effective as levodopa in initial rx of Parkinson's (Jama 2000;284:1931). Pt does not need to avoid protein in diet because does not affect absorption of dopamine. Titrate slowly; may be neuroprotective (Mayo Clinic Proc 1966;71:659; Med Lett 2001;43:57; Jama 2004;291:358); may increase risk of sudden somnolence (Arch Neurol 2005;62:1242); increase regurgitation in cardiac valvular dz (Nejm 2007;356:6,29,39).

- Bromocriptine (Parlodel): At 20-30 mg moderate effects on bradykinesia; can be added to levodopa to reduce the dose needed of levodopa: start at 1.25 mg/d and increase over several days to weeks (every week by 1.25-2.50-mg/d increments). Side effects: nausea, vomiting, dry mouth, orthostasis, confusion, hallucinations. Ropinirole and pramipexole not expected to have side effects of bromocriptine. Alter overall symptomatic course of Parkinson's by binding selectively to D_2-like receptors; (Med Lett 1997;39:102; Jama 1997;278:125).
- Pergolide (Permax): When bromocriptine not effective, both expensive (Mayo Clin Proc 1988;63:969). Pergolide better than bromocriptine (Neurol 1995;45:522). Transdermal dopamine agonist Rotigotine (Med Lett 2007;49:69).
- Selegiline (Deprenyl): MAO-B inhibitor may delay onset Parkinson's by 1-3 yr (Nejm 1989;321:1364); may not be so good for early Parkinson's (multicenter British study-BMJ 1995;311:1602). Cost: $1400-1500/yr. Not active in gut, so no tyramine effect. Selegiline in doses of 2.5-10.0 mg/d blocks metabolism of CNS dopamine, thus enhancing levodopa, may also be antioxidant. Sometimes used in advanced disease for reducing wearing-off effect; adverse effects include insomnia, confusion, dyskinesias, gi distress. Do not combine w tricyclic antidepressants. Selective serotonin reuptake inhibitors because of severe risk of hypertensive reaction. Serious drug interactions w meperidine (Demerol). Selegiline acts as MAO-A at > 10 mg/d.] 2nd gen MAOI Rasayiline (Agilect) adjuvant to Levodopa (Lancet 2005;365:847).
- Other newer agents may act in similar manner, eg, catechol O-methyltransferase (COMT) inhibitors, which in conjunction with levodopa/carbidopa lengthens levodopa's duration of action by inhibition of the conversion of levodopa to 3-OMD; best for wearing off phenomenon; better in setting of confusion (Jags 2000;48:692); may be better than dopamine agonists (Lancet 1997;350:712); can be adjusted downwards if dyskinesias appear (Tolcapone 100-200 mg/d). Metabolized by liver,

monitor liver function q 6 mo). Allows reduction of levodopa dose (Ann Long-Term Care 1998;6f:1).

- Propranolol: 160 mg/d (controlled release) first choice for tremor (Arch Neurol 1997;44:921).
- Parkinson's tremor may be coexistent with familial tremor—propranolol-responsive (20-320 mg) (Arch Neurol 1986; 43:42). High dosing may worsen depression and sleep disturbance.
- Anticholinergics: Generally toxic and minimally useful. Benztropine 0.5 mg/d, increasing slowly to 2 mg bid; trihexyphenidyl 2 mg/d increasing slowly to 5 mg tid; ethopropazine HCl (Parsidol) 50 mg/d, gradually increasing to 600 mg/d for tremor.
- Amantadine: Influences the release of dopamine. Adverse effects: confusion, hallucinations, edema, livedo reticularis (purplish mottling of skin); modest short-lived efficacy. Pts may respond again when reintroduced. More effective for rigidity and bradykinesia than tremor.
- Antioxidants (vit E): Selegiline might help.

High drug costs and variable drug effectiveness over time mandate regular reviews, including trials off drugs, with careful, comprehensive, detailed observations to ascertain drug effectiveness implied.

- Clozapine: 12.5 mg qd hs (Clozaril) for hallucinations, so can keep on using levodopa and selegiline. Drug-induced psychosis typified by visual hallucinations w insight. Psychotic depression or dementia associated w auditory hallucinations. Fewer extra-pyramidal side effects on low dose olanzapine or quietapine than other anti-psychotics; risperidone may worsen sx; can try cholinesterase inhibitor for hallucinations.
- Confusion and disorientation may be best remedied by decreasing Parkinson's meds.
- Depression responsive to nortriptyline—mild anticholinergic effects, also helps movement disorder, sialorrhea, tremor; sero-

tonin reuptake inhibitors helpful as well, but have also been known to cause akathisia (β-blockers rx of choice for this side effect); paroxetine (Paxil), citalopram (Celexa), mirtazapine (Remeron) for problems w sleep. Mirtazapine can cause wgt gain. Buproprion (Wellbutrin) less risk impotence, but lowers seizure threshold. Zolipidem (Ambien) or zaleplon (Sonata) short-term for sleep. Both tricyclics and serotonin reuptake inhibitors can cause myoclonus, which can be controlled w clonazepam. Identify and monitor specific "target" depression sx; may not require chronic antidepressants—review useful.

- Risk of polypharmacy with treating one medication side effect with another medication.

Sexual Dysfunction: Sildenafil (Viagra).

Seborrheic Dermatitis: May be relieved by levodopa, ketoconazole (Nizoral) plus careful attention to hygiene.

Stereotactic Pallidotomy: Long-term risks/benefits not established, complications include visual field deficits, contralateral paralysis, and speech problems (Med Lett Drugs Ther 1996;38:107).

Fetal cell transplantation: Post-op sleep disturbance and mental status change more common and profound in older pts (Ann Neurol 1988;24:150).

Team Management:

- Front-wheeled walker for Parkinson's avoids retropulsion and tripping.
- Restricted protein diet—limit to protein meal at dinnertime; investment in long-term work w family and staff education vital to quality management; pain, fatigue, depression, strained family relationships—referrals to home health, social service, counseling, Parkinson's Disease support groups (Jags 1997;45:844).
- Nausea: diphenidol 25mg q 6 hr does not block dopamine receptors as other antinausea medications do (Chlorpazine, metoclopramide), but may cause confusion and ataxia.

- Constipation: Senna 1-2 tabs hs.
- Daytime sleepiness: stimulants, eg, methylphenidate (Ritalin), dextroamphetamine (Dexedrine), pemoline (Cylert) (J Am Board Fam Pract 1997;10:412).

4.3 Seizures

Nurs Home Med 1995;3:4b; Nejm 1990;323:1468; Jags 1998;46:1291; Mayo Clin Proc 2001;76:175; Am Fam Phys 2003;67:325; Jama 2004;291:606

Cause: In 85%-90% of new-onset seizures in the elderly, there is identifiable brain lesion; vascular disease 50% of time (33% occur w onset embolic event that is predictive of future epilepsy (Neurol 1996;46:35), 33% occur during rehab phase, 33% are recurrent); focal seizure usually caused by brain tumor (cause of seizures in 12% of elderly population); brain abscess; previous head trauma; generalized seizure associated w h/o meningitis, encephalitis; 25% of pts w late-stage Alzheimer's have generalized seizures; metabolic; hypoxia; abrupt withdrawal from benzodiazepines; other drugs lower threshold, eg, phenothiazines, tricyclics, meperidine, new generation quinolones, theophylline.

Epidem: Occur 2-3× more frequently than in younger pts; complex partial seizures common; fewer than 20% of NH pts on anticonvulsants actually have a seizure diagnosis (Nurs Home Med 1995;3:4b).

Sx: "Don't feel myself, something's happening."

Si:

- Generalized tonic-clonic motor (grand mal) most common type of seizure in elderly.
- Complex partial seizure: "tune out": intermittent confusion, disorientation, staring; repetitive motor acts: patting, rubbing, smacking lips, rarely wandering or disrobing.

Cmplc:

- Fx, states of confusion (Arch Neurol 2006;63:529), aspiration pneumonia.
- R/o early dementia or late dementia behaviors can be confused w partial complex seizures (behaviors ranging from mutism to hallucinations); focal seizures can be confused w TIAs.

Lab:

- CBC, BUN, Cr, electrolytes, Ca, magnesium glucose, LFTs.
- No LP unless suspect meningitis.
- Noninvasive: EEG, if confusing differential; most diagnostic value during event, periodic epileptiform discharges (occur in elderly w any acute CNS injury), possibly EKG.
- *X-ray:* MRI best for small structural lesions; CT only in emergency r/o bleed or MRI contraindicated; contrast with both.

Rx:

Therapeutic:

(Treatment Guidelines 2008;6:37)

Table 4.4 Treatment of Seizures

Type	
• Simple partial, complex partial, secondarily generalized	Rx Carbamazepine, phenytoin, lamotrigine, levetiracetam, oxcarbazine (Mayo Clin Proc 2001;76:175)
• Absence	Rx Ethosuximide
• Myoclonic	Rx Valproic acid
• Primary generalized tonic-clonic	Rx Valproic acid, phenytoin
• Atonic	Rx Valproic acid, clonazepam

Table 4.5 Advantages and Disadvantages of Antiepileptic Drugs

Antiepileptic Drug	Advantages	Disadvantages
Felbamate	Broad spectrum of coverage Efficacy	Serious idiosyncratic side effects Expensive
Gabapentin 300-600 mg tid	Few side effects No drug interactions Easy to dose Renal excretion	Limited efficacy Multiple daily doses Expensive
Lamotrigine 100-300 mg bid	Broad spectrum of coverage Well tolerated Twice a day dosing	Slow to initiate Rash Expensive Increases PR interval (GRS 2002)
Topiramate 25-100 mg bid	Broad spectrum of coverage Twice a day dosing Limited drug interactions Mostly renal metabolism	Cognitive adverse effects Expensive
Tiagabine 2-12 mg bid-tid	Well tolerated Limited drug interactions	Multiple daily doses Cognitive adverse effects Expensive
Vigabratin	Well tolerated No drug interactions Renal excretion	Multiple daily doses May exacerbate underlying psychiatric disorder Expensive

Reproduced with permission from Sirven JL. Epilepsy in older adults: causes, consequences and treatment. J Am Geriatr Soc 1998;46:1291-301. Only felbamate, lamotrigine, oxcabazepine approved for Mono Rx (Jama 2004;291:606)

Because of high rate of recurrence of seizure in elderly, start antiepileptic drug after first seizure, unless obvious metabolic cause (Lancet 1988;1:721). More likely to be recurrent if partial seizure, post-ictal paralysis, FH, positive EEG, abnormal neurological exam. Adverse effects of neuroleptics: gait disturbance, sedation, tremor. Folate deficiency predisposes pts to neurotoxicity. Gabapentin, lamotrigine tolerated better than carbamazepine (Neurol 2005;64:1868).

- Valproic acid: For generalized seizures, 250 mg -750 mg bid-tid. Inhibits hepatic drug metabolizing enzymes, so raises levels of benzodiazepines: pts may develop increased bleeding time, gi side effects; monitor LFTs and platelets.
- Carbamazepine (Tegretol): for focal seizures, 100 mg bid-tid; anticholinergic side effect; pts with heart block can have conduction abnormalities; induces cytochrome P-450 system, so interacts with drugs metabolized with this system, eg, antidepressants. Can cause hyponatremia, neutropenia.
- In pts w long-standing epilepsy already on phenobarbital (> 60 mg not usually tolerated, resulting in severe mental, behavioral effects; may also get osteopenia secondary to altered vit D metabolism) or phenytoin (Dilantin, 200-300 mg qd usual dose), drug may not need to be changed, unless experiencing side effects (hirsutism, gum hyperplasia, folate deficiency, osteopenia secondary to impaired calcium absorption); but not first choice meds to start in elderly.

Effective phenytoin level = phenytoin level/[0.2 (albumin + 0.1)]

- The lower the albumin, the more free drug fraction, the higher the effective level of phenytoin; therefore, NH pts usually have a 25%-50% higher "effective" phenytoin level than serum level indicates.
- Many psychoactive meds (especially phenothiazines and antidepressants) lower seizure threshold, especially w h/o alcoholism.
- CNS stimulants such as methylphenidate (Ritalin), pemoline (Cylert), oral decongestants, pentoxifylline (Trental), theophylline can provoke seizures (Nurs Home Med 1995;3:4b)
- Rimantidine may lower seizure threshold.
- Enteral feedings, milk, supplements, and antacids reduce absorption of phenytoin, and should be dosed several hours away from antiepileptic drugs.

- Diarrhea can reduce the amount of anticonvulsant.
- Consider discontinuation of seizure med if long seizure-free period and normal EEG (Ger Rv Syllabus Suppl 1994;1:127S).
- Gabapentin (Nejm 1996;334:1583; Neurol 1994;44:787) (GABA agonist) for partial seizures; lipid-soluble; doesn't affect concentrations of other seizure meds.
- Lamotrigine (Lamictal, a phenyltriazine derivative): Decrease the dose if given w other seizure meds (Nurs Home Med 1996;4:6b).
- Some advantages to newer drugs: less drug interaction; lamotrigine less ataxia and cognitive impairment.
- Withdraw seizure med slowly over months (reduce phenobarbital by 30 mg/mo).

Team Management: Educate family and staff on recognition and responses.

4.4 Sleep Problems

Am Fam Phys 1994;51:191; 2000;62:110; Alessi C, Sleep Problems in Elderly Geriatric Intensive Review Course UCLA 1/96; Sleep Med Rv 2000;4:5

Cause: Transient: Stress, new bed, change time zone; chronic: depression, fear of death, substance abuse, pain, paresthesia, dyspnea, GE reflux, anxiety, delirium, myoclonus, restless legs, sleep apnea; drugs (15%): alcohol, antihypertensives, antineoplastics, β-blockers, caffeine, diuretics, levodopa, selegiline, SSRIs (Jags 2006;54:1508), nicotine, oral contraceptives, phenytoin (Dilantin), serotonin reuptake inhibitors, protriptyline (Vivactil), corticosteroids, stimulants, theophylline, thyroid hormone.

Types:

1. Difficulty initiating or maintaining sleep (insomnia or dyssomnias).
2. Excessive sleep.

3. Sleep-wake cycle problems.
4. Parasomnias occurring during sleep-wake transitions; characterized as behaviors that intrude into sleep but do not change sleep architecture, eg, nocturnal leg cramps.
5. Sleep disorders associated w Alzheimer's: increased duration, increased frequency of awakenings; decreased REM, stages 3 and 4 sleep; daytime napping; sleep apnea in later stages.
6. REM sleep behavior disorder—drug-induced (SSRI, venlafaxine, MAO inhibitors, TCAs, caffeine, drug or alcohol withdrawal), Parkinson's, psychiatric illness.
7. Sleep disorders associated w depression: more nighttime wakefulness and decreased slow-wave sleep; early morning awakening; more REM sleep earlier in night; community-dwelling elderly have decreased latency (number of min to fall asleep).
8. Sleep apnea: repeated cessations for ≥ 10 sec w oxygen saturation ≤ 80%
   - Central: simultaneous cessation of breathing effort and nasal and oral airflow, as well as cessation of effort by diaphragm muscles
   - Obstructive: airflow stops while thoracic respirations persist (Jags 2005;53:S272)
   - Mixed: (features of both) most common
9. Periodic leg movements: characterized by debilitating, repetitive, stereotypic leg movements occurring in non-REM sleep.
10. Restless leg syndrome: uncontrollable urge to move one's legs at night, "creepy-crawling" sensation.

Epidem: 50% of community have sleep problems, 90% of NH pts; 70% of caregivers cited sleep problems as reason for admitting relatives to NH; NH residents awake on average q 20-25 min during the night; psychoactive meds dampen normal diurnal variation in sleep, eg, sleep during day, not at night. Pts who have taken 30 prescription sleeping pills in the last mo have same mortality risk as smoking 1-2 ppd (Sleep Med Rv 2000;4:5).

Increased mortality when oxygen saturation < 85% and > 20 episodes apnea/night.

Pathophys:

- Normal changes in sleep pattern with age: sleep latency increased; sleep efficiency decreased (ratio of time asleep to time in bed); earlier bedtime; earlier morning awakening; more arousals during night; more daytime napping.

  Changes in sleep structure w age:
  - Stages 1 and 2 (light sleep) remain the same.
  - Stages 3 and 4 (deep sleep, slow high-amplitude delta-wave sleep) decreased.
- Total REM sleep decreases. Earlier-onset REM sleep and it does not increase in duration throughout the night as in young people.

Sx: Loss of concentration and memory, dysphoria, malaise, irritability, daytime napping, fatigue, interference w ADLs, headaches on awakening.

Si: Sleep apnea: consider if pt has unexplained right-sided heart failure, decreased cognitive function; most severe episodes occur in REM sleep.

Cmplc: Pulmonary HT, RV failure.

Lab: Noninvasive: Polysomnography in a sleep laboratory if sleep apnea, narcolepsy, periodic leg movements.

Rx:

Preventive:

- Screening questions: Is pt satisfied w his/her sleep? Does sleep or fatigue intrude w daytime activities? Does bed partner notice snoring, interrupted breathing, leg movements?
- Sleep hygiene: Bed at same time each night; bedroom environment conducive; avoid excessive napping or before bedtime

exercise. Early day exercise helps in community dwelling elderly, but not in NH elderly (Jama 1997;277:32; Jags 1995; 43:1098). Comfortable levels—temperature, light, noise. If a pt can't get to sleep in one-half hr, get out of bed, participate in non-stimulating activity, and return to bed when sleepy; light snack; relaxation techniques for those who ruminate; light therapy if a symptom of seasonal affective disorder (Jama 1997;277:990).

Therapeutic:

Table 4.6 Benzodiazepines—Onset and Elimination Characteristics

Examination	Fast Onset	Intermediate Onset	Slow Onset
Past (6 hr)	Zolidem (Ambien) Zolipdem Zaleplon	Triazolam (Halcion), oxazepam (Serax)	—
Intermediate (15 hr)		Lorazepam (ativan), alprazolam (Xanax)	Temazepam (Restoril)
Slow (30-72 hr)	Diazepam (Valium), clorazepate (Tranxene)	Chlordiazepoxide (Librium), flurazepam (Dalmane), clonazepam (Klonopin)	Prazepam (Centrax)

- Chronic insomnia: Intermittent dosing (2-4 × per week) (Nejm 1997;336:341).
- Most OTC hypnotics are antihistamines w sedating properties; they also have anticholinergic properties and should be discouraged in the elderly.
- Sedating antidepressants, such as trazodone and nortriptyline, may help w sleep, especially w underlying depression, bruxism,

and fibromyalgia; eg, trazodone 25 mg qd hs, mirtazapine (Remeron) single dose hs, not just for depressed pts (J Clin Psychiatry 1999;60:28).

- Nonbenzodiazepines (for short-term use only):
  - Zolpidem (Ambien): No anticonvulsant or myorelaxant properties; as yet very few side effects reported: no withdrawal effects, no rebound insomnia, no tolerance. Effectiveness lasts a year; rapid onset; half-life 1.5-4.5 hr, longer in liver disease. Can use w warfarin; fewer falls; start at 5 mg dose (cognitive impairment at higher doses). Side effects: nightmares, agitation, headache, dizziness, daytime drowsiness, confusion, impaired memory, and unsteady gait in the middle of the night (Med Lett 2000;42:71).
  - Zaleplon (Sonata): an imidazopyridine, does not decrease premature awakenings or increase total sleep time, but appears to have a low risk of next-day residual effects, even w middle-of-the-night use (Med Lett 2000;42:71) start at 5 mg qd hs, half-life 1 hr, do not take with alcohol.
  - If elderly pt on low-dose barbiturates, glutethimide, or chloral hydrate for years, may be reasonable to continue if pt very resistant to stopping it or may need to consult w psychiatrist (Ger Rv Syllabus 1996;175).
- Choral hydrate: 500 mg/hypnotics for 2-4 wk; tolerance develops unless dosed q 3 nights; increases warfarin metabolism; gradual tapering rather than abrupt discontinuation following prolonged use of agent (Drugs 1993;45:44). Fatalities have occurred w as little as 4 gm ingestion of chloral hydrate (Med Lett 2000;42:71); contraindications: significant renal, hepatic, or cardiac conditions.
- Benzodiazepines (not for long-term use): work on GABA pathway, highly protein-bound; highly lipid-soluble; active metabolites prolonged in obese pts, except oxazepam (Serax) and lorazepam (Ativan), which are altered to inactive metabolites. Many undergo oxidative hepatic metabolism, so avoid in el-

derly: alprazolam (Xanax), chlordiazepoxide (Librium), clorazepate (Tranxene), diazepam (Valium), prazepam (Centrax); levels are increased by meds that inhibit liver metabolism: cimetidine, contraceptives, disulfiram, fluoxetine (Prozac), INH, valproic acid.

- Clonazepam (Klonopin): For nocturnal myoclonus.
- Flurazepam (Dalmane): Has long half-life (85 hr); accumulates; do not use in elderly.
- Temazepam (Restoril): Effective for 6-8 hr but has 2-3 hr onset, and daytime drowsiness.
- Triazolam (Halcion): Psychosis and violent behavior in doses over 1 mg (maximum dose for elderly = 0.125 mg).
- When withdrawing from short-acting benzodiazepines, decrease drug by 50% first week and then by 12% for each of the next 4-8 wks.

- Alleviation of insomnia w timed exposure to bright light (Jags 1993;41:829).
- Melatonin mg 2 po improves sleep efficiency 75-85% (Lancet 1995;346:541), possible vasoconstrictive effects (Ger Rv Course UCLA 2002).
- For obstructive sleep apnea: tricyclic antidepressants reduce REM sleep and therefore ameliorate apnea; progesterone helps by increasing respiratory drive (Nejm 1990;323:520); dental prostheses; tracheotomy.
- For central and mixed sleep apnea: CPAP (5-20 cm H_2O 50-70% successful).
- For nocturnal myoclonus: avoid caffeine, tricyclics; clonazepam 0.25 mg hs, increasing by 0.25 mg q 2 wk to maximum of 2 mg; trazodone 50-150 mg hs; levodopa 100-200 mg, carbamazepine.
- For restless leg syndrome, avoid caffeine, alcohol, tricyclics, SSRIs, lithium, antipsychotics, and antihistamines. R/o iron deficiency: treat with sleep hygiene, self-massage, baths; meds to treat. Levodopa or dopamine agonist, carbamazepine, gabapentin, clonidine, clonazepam, temazepam, if nothing else

effective (Am Fam Phys 2000;62:110)—cautious use of narcotic analgesics.

Team Management: Nonpharmacologic sleep protocol in NH w massage, relaxation tapes, warm drinks (Jags 1998;46:700); delayed sleep phase: 2 hr 2500 Lux bright light in AM, advanced sleep phase: 2 hr 2500 Lux bright light PM.

4.5 Neuroleptic Malignant Syndrome (NMS)

Med Clin N Am 1993;77:185; Neurol Clin 2004;22:389

Cause: Idiosyncratic reaction involving dopamine blockade, neuroleptic-induced hyperthermia via dysregulation of hypothalamus and basal ganglia and muscle rigidity related to myonecrosis (Med Clin N Am 1993;77:185).

Epidem: Rare with incidence 0.02%-3.23%; risk factors: increased age, high-dose/high-potency neuroleptics, eg, haloperidol, thiothixene, fluphenazine, and trifluoperazine. May also see increased incidence with depot meds, lithium, antidepressants or multiple neuroleptics (low-dose/low-potency), carbidopa/levodopa and withdrawal of amantadine. Increased incidence in pts with h/o NMS, dehydration, electrolyte imbalance, thyrotoxicosis, elevated ambient temperature (Med Clin N Am 1993;77:185), underlying CNS impairment (Jags 1996;44:474).

Pathophys: Precipitated by any med that acts as D_2 dopamine receptor antagonist; severe dopamine blockade-induced parkinsonism with resulting muscle rigidity, then myonecrosis; autonomic thermogenic dysregulation via dopaminergic input also postulated (Dis Nerv Syst Clin Neurobiol 1992;62:831).

Si: Hyperthermia w diaphoresis in 98% of pts, but can be lacking in elderly; rigidity 97%; other movement disorder less often; mental status changes vary from clouded consciousness to coma; autonomic instability, tachycardia, hypotension 97%; tachypnea secondary to metabolic acidosis, pneumonia or pulmonary embolism

(Med Clin N Am 1993;77:185; Clin Pharmacol Ther 1991; 50:580).

Crs: High mortality if untreated; 10-20% mortality with rx; usually occurs soon after initiating neuroleptic rx or with dose increases; recovery usually within 10 d, but up to 30 d (Med Clin N Am 1993;77:185).

Cmplc: Cerebellar or other brain damage secondary to hyperthermia; fatal arrhythmias; metabolic acidosis; pulmonary emboli; pneumonia; respiratory arrest.

R/o encephalopathies, tumors, CVA, seizures, infections, endocrinopathies (thyrotoxicosis, pheochromocytoma), SLE, heat injury, toxins, drugs (Med Clin N Am 1993;77:185; Psych Ann 1991;21:130), polymyositis, mesenteric vascular occlusion, RA; cancer of prostate, colon, lung (small cell); chronic renal disease; myoglobinuria (67%).

Lab: EKG, CBC (leukocytosis common), CPK occasionally extremely elevated, TSH, LDH, transaminases, and aldolase may also be elevated from myonecrosis; metabolic acidosis and hypoxia may be present; cardiac monitoring.

Rx: Discontinue all neuroleptics and other centrally acting antidopaminergics. Bromocriptine 7.5-60.0 mg qd po or via NG tube; dantrolene, initially 1-2 mg/kg iv, then 10 mg/kg qd, may have synergistic effect. Other useful meds: amantadine; benzodiazepines, to lessen agitation. Electroconvulsive therapy for refractory cases, but can also lead to NMS when given to pts exhibiting extrapyramidal adverse effects.

Team Management: Observe carefully for early signs in elderly when using neuroleptics.

Chapter 5

Psychiatry

5.1 Depression/Mood Disorders

Am J Ger Psychiatry 2002;10:233; 2005;13:88; 2002;10:256; 1993;1:421; 1994;2:193; J Clin Psychiatry 2004;65:5; Am J Psych 2002;159:1119; Nejm 1989;320:164; 2002;287:1568; Jama 1997;278:1186; Clin Ger 2004;12:51; BMJ 2002;325:991

Cause:

Primary Depression:

1. Biologic vulnerability, especially in early adult onset depression that recurs into old age;
2. Reaction to severe stress;
3. In late onset depression, cortical vascular changes. (J Affect Disord 2001;65:19).

Secondary Depression: Due to medical conditions, especially thyroid dysfunction, diabetes, B_{12} deficiency, cardiovascular-cerebrovascular disease or cancers; or due to substances of abuse; or due to medication effects (Psychother Psychosom 2004;23:207), especially corticosteroids, benzodiazepines or other sedatives, interferon alpha, interleukin-2, GnRH agonists, and possibly propranolol. β-blockers are considered less of a depressant than previously (Jama 2002;288:351).

Epidem: Lifetime prevalence around 20% in older women and 10% in men (Arch Gen Psychiatry 2000;57:601) and 30-45% in the medically ill and in NHs (Jama 1997;228:1186). Prevalence of major depression in community samples actually decreases with age, but subsyndromal or minor depression is more common. Disability is proportional to depressive symptomology (Am J Ger Psychiatry 2002;10:233). However, on inpatient psychiatric ward, persons > age of 70 are 8 × more likely to be depressed than those < 30 (Int J Geriatr Psychiatry 2004;19:487). Depression is under-treated in elders across races, but particularly in black populations: 16.7% of older blacks with depression treated vs 32% of depressed white elders (Am J Ger Psychiatry 2004;12:531). Bipolar Disorder: 10% diagnosed < age 50, but 50% of first manic cases occur > age 50, and 25% > age 65. Geriatric mania is more likely to be secondary to a medication, neurologic, cerebrovascular, or infectious disease. (Am J Ger Psychiatry 1999; 7:188).

Risk Factors: Female gender, disability, bereavement, disturbed sleep, previous h/o depression (Am J Psych 2003;160:1147). Cerebrovascular risk factors (Am J Ger Psychiatry 2002;10:592). Poverty, burden of co-morbid medical illness, institutionalization; active alcohol or substance abuse. For suicide, older white male w comorbid medical problems; substance abuse; presence of firearms in the home. In homicide-suicide, controlling man tends to be perpetrator, often in caregiver role for debilitated wife, and feels overwhelmed (Am J Ger Psychiatry 2001;9:49).

Pathophys: Hypothalamic-pituitary-adrenal axis and circadian rhythm disruption; theorized that monoamine transmitters and neural pathways involving prefrontal cortex, amygdala, and hypothalamus axis are involved; MAO activity is increased in brains of elderly (Am J Psych 1984;141:1276); proinflammatory cytokines involved in increased cortisol production and immune system activation (Am J Psych 2003;160:1342). Vascular burden (Am J Ger Psychiatry 2004;12:93).

Sx: DSM-IV criteria for dx of major depression (may miss significant depression in geriatric age group) requires 2 wks of either depressed mood or anhedonia and 2 wks of at least 4 of the following additional sx: impaired sleep often w early morning awakening, depressed mood, decreased interest in usual sources of pleasure (anhedonia), feelings of guilt, decreased energy, altered concentration, decreased appetite, psychomotor retardation or agitation, suicidal ideation. Less typical presentations: hypochondriasis, pain syndromes, shoplifting, alcoholism, depressive dementia, malnutrition, passive suicide, nondysphoric depressions (Jags 1997;45:570), anxiety/agitation (Jags 1989;37:458). Executive function is impaired in geriatric depression leading to impairment in tasks involving initiation of novel responses, problem solving and set shifting (Am J Psych 2002;159:1119.) A recent increase in aggression may indicate increased risk of suicide (Am J Ger Psychiatry 2004;12:37).

Bipolar illness in the elderly: Compared to pts age 40, bipolar manic pts over age 60 have comparable symptomology, although they have a higher risk for cognitive dysfunction (Am J Ger Psychiatry 1999;7:188); greater duration of episodes; mortality rate higher for bipolar than unipolar.

Si: Tearfulness, stooped posture, frequent sighing, increased response latency, low volume of speech, poor eye contact, poverty of movement, hand-wringing, weight loss, restlessness. Always ask directly about depressed mood; current elderly cohorts may resist dx because of ageist expectations, sense of shame, or self-blaming.

Dx: Clinical diagnosis per DSM-IV. Depression scales (see tables) (J Psych 1983;17:37), 5-question geriatric depression scale validated in hospital, community, NH (Jags 2003;51:694). Cornell Depression Scale for use in dementia (see Figure 5.1) (Biol Psychiatry 1988;23:271).

Cornell Scale for Depression in Dementia

Name__________________________ Age ______ Sex ______ Date _________

Inpatient Nursing Home Resident Outpatient

Scoring System

A = unable to evaluate 0 = absent 1 = mild or intermittent 2 = severe

Ratings should be based on symptoms and signs occurring during the week prior to interview. No score should be given in symptoms resulting from physical disability or illness.

A. Mood-Related Signs

1. Anxiety: anxious expression, ruminations, worrying	A 0 1 2
2. Sadness: sad expression, sad voice, tearfulness	A 0 1 2
3. Lack of reactivity to pleasant events	A 0 1 2
4. Irritability: easily annoyed, short-tempered	A 0 1 2

B. Behavioral Disturbance

5. Agitation: restlessness, handwringing, hairpulling	A 0 1 2
6. Retardation: slow movement, slow speech, slow reactions	A 0 1 2
7. Multiple physical complaints (score 0 if gi symptoms only)	A 0 1 2
8. Loss of interest: less involved in usual activities (score only if change occurred acutely, ie, in less than 1 month)	A 0 1 2

C. Physical Signs

9. Appetite loss: eating less than usual	A 0 1 2
10. Weight loss (score 2 if greater than 5 lb in 1 month)	A 0 1 2
11. Lack of energy: fatigues easily, unable to sustain activities (score only if change occurred acutely, ie, in less than 1 month)	A 0 1 2

D. Cyclic Functions

12. Diurnal variation of mood: symptoms worse in the morning	A 0 1 2
13. Difficulty falling asleep: later than usual for this individual	A 0 1 2
14. Multiple awakenings during sleep	A 0 1 2
15. Early morning awakening: earlier than usual for this individual	A 0 1 2

E. Ideational Disturbance

16. Suicide: feels life is not worth living, has suicidal wishes, or makes suicide attempt	A 0 1 2
17. Poor self-esteem: self-blame, self-depreciation, feelings of failure	A 0 1 2
18. Pessimism: anticipation of the worst	A 0 1 2
19. Mood congruent delusions: delusions of poverty, illness, or loss	A 0 1 2

Figure 5.1 Cornell Scale for Depression in Dementia

Diff Dx: Alzheimer's or subcortical dementia; grief reaction (beginning within 3 mo of loss and lasting a year); dysthymia (not free of depression for > 2 mo over a 2-yr period); secondary dysthymia (from chemical dependency, anxiety, post-traumatic stress disorder, distress, or physical illness). Apathy due to dementia, stroke, or schizophrenia.

Crs: If untreated, lasts 6-14 mo; relapse rate is increased compared to younger (Jags 1987;35:516; Convuls Ther 1989;5:75). Poorest prognosis: recent bereavement, delusions (50% of the time in the elderly), panic disorders; will respond better to antidepressants if have early AM awakening or shorter period of depression. Late life depression w cognitive impairment reversed by antidepressants may predict development of irreversible dementia (Jama 1997;278:1186); depression w first appearance in late life often becomes chronic and often has vascular neuropathology; executive dysfunction predicts greater risk relapse (Arch Gen Psychiatry 2000;57:285). Watch especially for depression as earliest presentation of mild cognitive losses of Alzheimer's.

Cmplc: Increased 1-yr mortality rates (8-15% vs 5%); major depression increases risk for MI and risk of death from ischemic heart disease (Circ 1996;943:3123; Ann IM 1999;130:563). Suicide fastest growing rate in U.S.; completed suicides M > F; suicide—20% fatal. Rate of suicide in white men > 84 is 6 × higher than general population; depression increases functional disability and reduces rehab effectiveness; longer hospital stays; multiple depressive sx are associated with 2 × increased mortality. Women w depression are at increased risk of falling (Sci Am Med 2000;13:2).

Lab: TSH, B_{12} level, lytes, CBC; UA.

Rx:

General Considerations re Medications:

- Start LOW, Go SLOW, But Go ALL the way
- Begin 1/2 usual adult doses (demethylation is decreased in the elderly), increase monthly, and use smallest effective dose.
- Outpt rx f/u 1-2 wks, assess adverse effects; f/u 5-6 wks, assess response; f/u 8-12 wks, assess if in remission (Jama 2002; 289:1569).
- Post-stroke depression: tricyclics, SSRIs, trazadone—all equally effective (J Ger Psych Neurol 2001;14:37).
- Biologic sx may improve before mood (insomnia may improve in first few days).
- Familial response may be good predictor of individual success w an antidepressant.
- May discontinue antidepressant after 9 mo, if no previous episode of depression in 2.5 yrs; reduce the dose by 1/2, then taper weekly to avoid serotonergic hyperactivity w abrupt withdrawal (dizziness, nausea, fatigue, anxiety, irritability malaise, chills, muscle aches); maintenance doses of antidepressants should be as high as doses for acute rx; if seasonal affective disorder (SAD) pattern, take into consideration when planning discontinuation; if recurrent episode, rx for 12 mo; if 2 episodes, or dysthymia may need indefinite maintenance rx.
- Efficacy is similar within class; most decisions based on side effect profile and h/o prior response.

Mood Stabilizers: Very few randomized controlled studies in geriatric age group. Consensus opinion (J Clin Psychiatry 2004;65:5):

1. Agitated, non-psychotic Major Depressive Disorder (MDD)
    - First line: antidepressant alone
    - Second line (after failure of 2 antidepressants):
      antidepressant + antipsychotic
      antidepressant + mood stabilizer
      antidepressant + benzodiazepine
      ECT

2. Psychotic MDD
   - First line: antipsychotic (× 6 mo) + antidepressant
   - ECT
3. Bipolar Disorder
   - Depression—mood stabilizer
   - Mania
   - Mild—mood stabilizer
   - Severe
     Stop antidepressant
     Mood stabilizer
     +/− antipsychotic (× 3 mo)
     - Rx with Psychosis: Mood stabilizer + Antipsychotic

Mood Stabilizers: Lamotrigine (Lamictal) for bipolar depression; depakote, carbemazepine; lithium (with caution).

Antipsychotics: For mood disorders,

- Risperidone 1.25 mg-3 mg d total
- Olanzapine 5-15 mg/d total
- Quetiapine 50-250 mg d total

PSYCHIATRY

Table 5.1 SSRI Antidepressants

Name (Generic Name)	Starting Dose (mg)	Typical Daily Dose (mg)	Max Dose (mg)	Dosing Schedule	Typical Side Effects	Special Considerations/ Dangers	Elimination Half Life
Selective Serotonin Reuptake Inhibitors (SSRIs)					Sleep Disturbance GI Sexual Headache Restlessness Weight gain	–Switching to Mania in bipolar patients –Hyponatremia –Serotonin Syndrome (rare) –OK to use low dose TCA for pain –Don't take St. John's Wort, too	
Citalopram (Celexa)	20	40	(40 may be top)	qd	SSRI ?less sexual side effects?	Few drug interactions	35 hr
e-citalopram (Lexapro)	10	10	20	qd			27-32 hr
Fluoxetine (Prozac/ Sarafem)	10-20	20	80	qd (a.m.)	SSRI	–long half life, so S.E. may linger even after med is stopped –CYP 2D6, 3A4 –watch warfarin levels	24-96 hr
Prozac Weekly	90 mg q wk						

Fluvoxamine (Luvox)	25-50	150-200 (divided)	300	tid	SSRI	–labeled for OCD Drug interactions: CYP 3A4 eg, alprazolam, cyclosporin, HIV, antivirals, phenytoin, theophyllne, carbamezepine, warfarin	17-22 hr
Paroxetine (Paxil)	10-20	20-40	60	qd (HS)	SSRI Constipation	–CYP 2D6 drug interactions, eg, TCA's.	18-24 hr
Paroxetine controlled release (Paxil CR)	25	25-62.5	62.5	qd (a.m.)		–reduce dose if Cr Cl < 30 ml/min	15-20 hr
Sertraline (Zoloft)	25-50	50-150	200	qd	SSRI Diarrhea	Prescribe 100 mg and break in half for 50 mg dose—cuts cost –mild CYP 3A4	26 hr

PSYCHIATRY

Selective Serotonin Reuptake Inhibitors (SSRIs): (See Table 5.1) Considered first line treatment; safer than and efficacy similar to tricyclics: 60-80% respond, risk of falls in frail elderly may be similar to tricyclics despite decreased hypotension (Nejm 1998; 339:875; Lancet 1998;351:1303), but may not be as effective as tricyclics in melancholic elderly hospitalized pts (Am J Psych 1994;151:1735); not sedating. Do not produce anticholinergic side effects, are not cardiotoxic (Jama 2007;297:411), and do not cause hypotension. Useful in OCD, panic attacks as well. Some may cause overstimulation and worsen anxiety sx, but are being used in low doses for anxiety; not effective in neuropathic pain (Nejm 1992;326:1250).

Adverse effects are nausea, diarrhea, headache, anxiety, more sexual dysfunction than other antidepressants (Geriatrics 1995;50:S-41) especially inhibition of orgasm (reversible 3 d after discontinue or responds to Sildenafil (Jama 2003;289:56), pseudoparkinsonism, SIADH, bradycardia with pre-existing arrhythmia. Interaction w β-blockers, IC antiarrhythmics, some benzodiazepines (Am J Psych 1996;153:311); increases bleeding risk w NSAIDs or ASA (J Fam Pract 2006;55:206); SSRI + tramadol (Ultram) or St. John's Wort or sumatriptan can cause serotonin syndrome (Am Fam Phys 2000;61:1745); hypertensive crisis with MAOIs, so 14-d washout before giving MAOI, except 5-wk washout for fluoxetine. Less effective in postmenopausal women than younger women. Withdrawal can occur with SSRIs (Sci Am Med 2000;13:II:9). Mania in 1% general population on SSRIs and more common in bipolar disorder; paranoia, psychosis; extrapyramidal occasionally (Nejm 1994;371:1354).

Preferred SSRIs are citalopram and sertraline due to fewer drug interactions, safer half-life and side effect profiles. Paroxetine also has a favorable half-life and fewer drug interactions, but is associated with a greater risk of extrapyramidal sx.

Table 5.2 Other Antidepressants

Name (Generic Name)	Starting Dose (mg)	Typical Daily Dose (mg)	Max Dose (mg)	Dosing Schedule	Typical Side Effects	Special Considerations/ Dangers	Elimination Half Life
Buproprion SR (Wellbutrin SR) Also called Zyban	100-150	150-300	400 300 for smoking cessation	Bid AM and PM (avoid hs due to insomnia)	Insomnia Headache Nausea Weight loss Worsens HT (Clin Ger 2004; 12:51)	–OK to use with other antidepressants –SR may have less seizure risk –No sexual dysfunction	8-24 hr
Duloxetine (Cymbalta)	20-40	60	60	qd or bid	Anticholinergic and Noradrenergic. Nausea, constipation, dry mouth, fatigue, insomnia; Agitation in elderly	–approved for diabetic peripheral neuropathy –Do NOT use with MAO –avoid use with narrow angle glaucoma	8-17 hr
Mirtazapine (Remeron)	7.5-15	30-45	60	qd hs	Sedation and weight gain, esp. at starting dose	–Agranulocytosis (rare)—check CBC –No sexual dysfunction	20-40 hr

continues

Table 5.2 continued

Name (Generic Name)	Starting Dose (mg)	Typical Daily Dose (mg)	Max Dose (mg)	Dosing Schedule	Typical Side Effects	Special Considerations/ Dangers	Elimination Half Life
Nefazodone (Serzone) (no longer on the market)	25 mg bid	300-600	600	Bid with higher doses hs	Sedating Less sexual dysfunction	3A4 drug interactions: eg, alprazolam, antivirals, cyclosporine –May improve sleep –Black Box Warning –no longer being manufactured	2-4 hr
St John's Wort						May have MAO-like properties, so watch for drug-drug interactions	
Trazodone (desyrel)	25-50	50-200	400	qd hs	Sedating	–Priapism—TO ER STAT –Hypotension –Used for sleep –Prescribe 100 mg and split to save $	4-13 hr
Venlafaxine XR (Effexor XR)	37.5	75-150	225	qd	SSRI-like Anxiety Sweating	–Dose dependent HT –Hits more neurotransmitters at higher dose –increased diastolic BP at higher doses –need to taper off	5-11 hr (XR form slows absorption)

Table 5.3 Tricyclic and Heterocyclic Antidepressants

Name (Generic)	Type	Starting Dose (mg)	Typical Daily Dose (mg)	Max Dose (mg)	Dosing	Typical Side Effects	Special Considerations/ Dangers	Elimination Half Life
Tricyclics in General						Anticholinergic: Dry mouth, constipation, blurry vision, urinary retention Antihistamine: Sedation, weight gain Antiadrenergic: Orthostatic hypotension, Sexual dysfunction	–Fatal in overdose –Use very carefully in elderly –Avoid Tertiary Amines –Never add a TCA to an MAO –OK to use low doses with SSRIs –SIADH –Seizures risk –Switching to mania in bipolar	
Amitriptyline (Elavil)	Tertiary Amine	25-50	125-250	300	qd hs	TCA	–Lower doses for pain –Blood level 50-100 ng/ml	10-22 hr
Clomipramine (Anafranil)	Tertiary Amine	25	125-200	250	qd hs	TCA	–Risk of Seizures –Hyperthermia (rare)	19-37 hr

continues

Table 5.3 continued

Name (Generic)	Type	Starting Dose (mg)	Typical Daily Dose (mg)	Max Dose (mg)	Dosing	Typical Side Effects	Special Considerations/ Dangers	Elimination Half Life
Imipramine (Tofranil)	Tertiary	25-50	125-250	300	qd hs	TCA	–Max dose 100 mg in elderly –Myoclonus –Can precipitate Acute Intermittent Porphyria	11-25 hr
Doxepin (Sinequan)	Tertiary Amine	25-50	125-250	300	qd hs	TCA	–Very sedating and anticholinergic, antihistaminic	11-23 hr
Nortriptyline (Pamelor)	Secondary Amine	10-50	75-100	150	qd hs	TCA	–Less orthostasis –Blood level 50-150 ng/ml	15-39 hr
Desipramine (Norpramin)	Secondary Amine	25-75	125-250	300	qd hs (TID ok)	TCA	–Blood Level > 100 ng/ml –Cocaine abstinence??, less sedating than nortriptyline	12-76 hr
Protriptyline (Vivactil)	Secondary Amine	5	15-30 total	60	TID (qd hs ok)	TCA	–Less weight gain	54-198 hr
Maprotiline (Ludiomil)	Tetracyclic Secondary Amine	140-225					–Not used much –Increased risk of seizures	21-66 hr

TCA = side effects are the same as those of tricyclic antidepressants

Tricylic Antidepressants (TCAs): Tricyclics cause more impotence (while SSRIs cause more anorgasmia), can cause mania (Am J Psych 1995;152:1130); avoid tertiary amine tricyclics (amitriptyline, imipramine, clomipramine, and doxepin) because of increased anticholinergic side effect (Mayo Clin Proc 1995; 70:999), cardiotoxicity (bundle branch block a contraindication) and potent β-blocker activity producing postural hypotension (may not improve w dose reduction).

Most reliable drug levels obtained 12 hr after last dose w the following meds: imipramine (therapeutic level=125 ng/mL), desipramine (therapeutic level=225 ng/mL), nortriptyline (therapeutic level=50-150 ng/mL) (Am J Psych 1985;142:155).

Secondary Amine Tricyclics: For example, nortriptyline and desipramine (BMJ 2002;325:991) (Table 5.3)

Beware of additive effects w other anticholinergic meds (even at therapeutic doses) producing anticholinergic delirium (anxiety, confusion, assaultive behavior, paranoia, hallucinations), which can lead to coma and death. Drugs w anticholinergic side effect include antispasmodics, antidiarrheal agents, low-potency antipsychotics, antiparkinsonian meds, antihistamines, drugs for vertigo, and OTC sleep meds. Tricyclics block effects of clonidine (Catapres) (Am Coll Psychiatrists, 1993; 13:1); quinidine and carbamazepine (Tegretol) increase tricyclic levels.

TCA overdose:

- Prescribe only 1 gm of TCAs at a time to avoid overdose because potentially fatal.
- Rx: recognize anticholinergic side effects of excitation/restlessness w paradoxical progressive sedation, tonic-clonic seizure, flushed-dry skin, pupils dilated, bowel sounds decreased, urinary retention, tachyarrhythmias, hypotension.

- QRS > 0.10 sec predictive of life-threatening ventricular arrhythmia and seizure (Nejm 1985;313:474); R wave in aVR > 3 mm best predictive value for seizure or ventricular arrhythmia (Ann EM 1995;26:196).
- Treat cardiac arrhythmias w propranolol; avoid digoxin, procaine, physostigmine; monitor for several days.
- Initial therapy: pills radiopaque; lavage w charcoal (effective for a prolonged time after overdose because of paralytic ileus due to overdose), alkalinize urine w sodium bicarbonate; can not remove w hemodialysis because protein-bound.

Resistant depression:

- 30% of depressions; increase dose step-wise, and if no response at full therapeutic dosage for 4-6 wks, change drug class. If partial effect seen, augment with lithium (cautiously), bupropion, mirtazapine, methylphenidate, or an atypical antipsychotic at low dose. Pramiprexole (Mirapex) may be useful, but few data yet (Depress Anxiety 2004;20:131). Consider ECT.
- Enhancers: L-Thyroxine 0.025 mg po qd.
- Lithium: Use with extreme caution in geriatric age group; lithium toxicity can occur even on very small doses (Nurs Home Pract 1995;3:17). Trial for 2 wk (Arch Gen Psychiatry 1994;50:387); up to 300 mg po tid (follow 12-hr post dose levels); obtain levels q 5 d (maximum trough 1.0 mEq/L to prevent toxicity). Therapeutic level may be lower (0.4-0.6 mEq/L); in elderly half-life = 36 hr; check TSH, BUN, Cr q 6 mo; withdrawal of caffeine may cause lithium toxicity (Biol Psychiatry 1995;37:348). Carbamazepine increases neurotoxicity of lithium: lethargy, ataxia, muscle weakness, tremors, hyperreflexia.
  - Early toxic effects: flu-type aching joints, sniffles, stiffness, gi distress, disturbance of balance.
  - "Benign" toxic effects: nausea, vomiting, diarrhea, polyuria, polydipsia, fine tremor, wgt gain, edema.

- Acute toxicity: persistent vomiting, uncontrollable diarrhea, hyperactive DTRs, dysarthria, lethargy, somnolence, seizures, coma, and death.
- Chronic toxicity: manifested as goitrogenic hypothyroidism, DI, tubular necrosis; lithium can be lowered by urinary alkalinization; if need diuretic, use amiloride instead of thiazide because lithium competes w sodium reabsorption at the proximal tubule; increased lithium levels from < 2 gm/d sodium diet (a low sodium diet should not be started when pt is on lithium), thiazides, NSAIDs, ACE inhibitors.

MAO Inhibitors: Fourth line due to toxic food and drug interactions causing hypertensive crisis; increase storage of norepinephrine, epinephrine, serotonin; tranylcypromine (Parnate) 10 mg bid and up to 40 mg/d; use tranylcypromine because reversible in 24 hr; used for atypical depression, as well as for hyperphagia, hypersomnia, panic attacks. Safer than tricyclics for heart block, ventricular arrhythmias. Most common side effects are sedation, therefore do not give before 4 PM, and orthostatic hypotension 3-4 wk into rx course because there is an accumulation of dopamine at the sympathetic ganglion. Hypertensive crisis with tyramine-containing foods, such as wine, cheese, aged meats, fermented foods, and with sympathomimetic drugs and catecholamine precursors. Affects all catecholamine precursors: levodopa, pseudoephedrine, OTC cold remedies; interaction with SSRIs causes serotonergic syndrome, consists of rigidity, diaphoresis, hyperthermia, coma, and death. Meperidine (Demerol) increases serotonin release. MAO-B inhibitors have same effects as MAO-A inhibitors when given at higher doses (30 mg).

Electroconvulsive Therapy (Am J Ger Psychiatry 1993;1:30)

Age is not a contradiction to ECT; is preferred treatment with geriatric psychotic depression. Very effective in the elderly (Nejm 1984;311:163), efficacy 80% (Jags 2000;48:560); clear explanation to pt and family because of historical perception of "violence" of rx.

- Indications: drug-resistant or intolerant pts, delusional depression, pts w life-threatening behavior (suicidal, catatonic, stuporous); psychotic depression responds rapidly; usually 6-8 rxs spaced 1-2 d apart; 3/wk more rapid recovery; minimize side effects by using right unilateral lead placement, stimulus intensity at 2.5 × seizure threshold (Am J Psych 1999;156:1865) mortality = 1/10000, relapse rate 10-20% w maintenance drugs.
- Relative contraindications: increased intracranial pressure or mass lesion, MI in last 3 mo, severe osteoporosis; < 1 mo s/p CVA (Jags 2000;48:560; 1987;35:516; Convuls Ther 1989; 5:75); β-blocker for known ischemic heart disease prevents cardiac complications; should also monitor for arrhythmias, bronchospasm, and si of aspiration. Most common side effects are delirium, transient amnesia, and cardiac (Jags 2000;48:560). Pts > 70 yr had no more cognitive impairment post-ECT than younger pts (Am J Psych 1999;156:1865). If delirium occurs early in the course of ECT, do w/u; delirium common in vascular depression (Jags 2000;48:560); dementia not contraindication to ECT (J ECT 2001;17:65; f/u maintenance therapy required, either ECT or antidepressant.

Depression Associated w Parkinson's: SSRIs, buproprion, nortriptyline, ECT transiently improves tremor, rigidity, bradykinesia.

Team Management:

Non-pharmacologic Treatments: Brief, non-pharmacologic interventions may have a bigger effect on subsyndromal or minor depression than antidepressants (Am J Ger Psychiatry 2002;10:256).

Psychotherapy: Talking about clinical basis for disease helps w stigma and improves compliance (Jama 2002;287:1568).

If medication intolerant, psychotherapy alone helps, especially cognitive and behavioral therapy and interpersonal therapy; also good for those with stressful situations and low social support; short-term group therapy (12 wk) utilizing reminiscence therapy, cognitive and behavioral therapy, and limited to small groups (about 6-10 pts) improves self-esteem, insight, social interaction, compliance, and decreases somatization; psychotherapy plus medication more effective in maintaining remission in recurrent depression (Jama 1999;281:39; Nejm 2000;342:1462). Problem solving therapy 4-8 wks (Jama 2002;287:1568); w care manager (Jama 2002;288:2779).

- Model goal setting w family.
- Music therapy: improvement in depression scores even after 9 mo f/u period (J Gerontol 1994;49:P265).
- Nurse-based outreach program reduces psychiatric sx in persons w psychiatric disorders (Jama 2000;283:2809), home based depression rx (Jama 2004;291:1081,1569); Interdisciplinary team (BMJ 2006;332:259).
- Exercise: May act as a long-term antidepressant in the elderly (J Gerontology Med Sci 2001;56A:M497); Improves behavioral management in Alzheimer's Disease (Jama 2003; 290:2015).
- Light: Bright morning light rx (10,000 lux × 30 min/d for min of 5 d) decreased depression scores in institutionalized pts (J Gerontol A Biol Sci Med Sci 2001;56:M356); In Alzheimer's dementia pts with agitated sleep behaviors, bright light therapy × 1 hr/d improved sleep, but not mood (Int J Ger Psych 1999;14:520).

Nursing Home:

- Nurses provide important dx information about non-major depression (Jags 1995;43:1118).
- Individual therapy or group therapy can help in situations involving caregiver stress.

5.2 Anxiety

Int J Ger Psych 1998;13:79; J Clin Psychiatry 1994;55:5; Am J Psych 1994;151:640; N Am Med 1998; 6:2211; Jags 2002;50:18; J Psych 2004;161:1642

Cause: Primary anxiety or mood disorders, medical illness/rx, psychosocial stressors, drug withdrawal.

Epidem: Research is limited. Post-traumatic stress disorder (PTSD) rates are rarely reported in epidemiological studies. DSM-described anxiety disorders less common in elderly, 3.5-5.5% in those > 65 yr old; 6 mo prevalence of all anxiety disorders 20%, lifetime 34%. Anxiety is highly co-morbid with depression in this age group (Int J Ger Psych 2005;20:218). In all age groups, anxiety is also highly co-morbid with substance abuse (Arch Gen Psychiatry 2004;61:807).

Anxiety Disorders and Phobias: GAD most common (5-7%), with phobias also common (5-9%), including simple phobias. Few data exist on PTSD prevalence in this age group, but PTSD persists across one's life, and rates should accumulate over time.

Posttraumatic Stress Disorder: 70% early-onset persisting into old age (Am J Psych 1994;2:239) and symptoms that have been quiescent may recur after retirement (Am J Psych 2001;158:1474). Agoraphobia (without panic) has the highest prevalence of onset late in life; attributed to exaggerated fears of physical illnesses, falls or muggings; < 11% of agoraphobics have coexisting panic disorder; rate of phobias no different in 65-74 yr old than those > 75 yr old in the community.

New-onset Panic Disorder: Uncommon (0.3%) in old age in community samples, may be higher in psychiatric or general hospitals; virtually all are women; associated w CAD, COPD, gi problems.

Obsessive-compulsive Disorder: May occur for the first time in old age in women; obsessive-compulsive and panic disorders more likely to persist in old age than other personality disorders. Hoarding may be a subtype of OCD.

Parkinsonian pts much higher rates of anxiety than pts w arthritis or MS (Neurol 2004;63:293); anxiety in medical pts much less common in old (2-13%) than in young (10-40%).

Pathophys: Serotonin abnormalities resulting in depression, anxiety (J Clin Psychiatry 1994;55:2), medical illnesses (thyroid disease, COPD) or meds/drugs that may induce or exacerbate anxiety (aminophylline, albuterol, levodopa, prednisone, caffeine, OTC decongestants, alcohol or benzodiazepine withdrawal).

Sx: Tachycardia, tremulousness, flushing, restlessness, unsteadiness, light-headedness, and sleep disturbances; somatic and anxiety-related complaints often mask depression.

Si: Hyperventilation, dysphoric mood; subjective feelings of anxiety eg, misinterpreting a tremor as anxiety.

Crs: May persist indefinitely without intervention. May increase risk for mortality males > females (Br J Psychiatry 2004;185:399).

Cmplc: Since new onset is less common than at younger ages, new panic or severe anxiety should prompt a thorough review of systems and screening for medical co-morbidities. Panic disorder: increased mortality, CVD, smoking, drug and alcohol abuse. In some Hispanic/Latin American groups, *ataque de nervios* related to increased suicidality, ER utilization, lower quality of life (J Anxiety Disord 2004;18:841).

Lab

X-Ray: TSH, CBC, lytes, CXR, and EKG for evidence of organic disease; hx, mental status exam, and physical exam (eg, BP) may suggest further studies such as urine metanephrine, 5HIAA or head CT (Mayo Clin Proc 1995;70:1999).

Rx: Identify and eliminate stressors when possible; make sure that abuse is not an issue; provide support and companionship;

PSYCHIATRY

instruction in muscle relaxation techniques; possible cognitive psychotherapy; if pharmacotherapy added, always consider risk of side effects vs benefit of rx; depression is frequently co-morbid, and treatments are very similar.

SSRIs are first-line rx. Less commonly used are the tricyclics due to side effects, eg, nortriptyline and desipramine, are secondary amines with less anticholinergic effects and MAOIs (Tables 5.1, 5.2, 5.3).

- START ANY MED VERY LOW AND GO VERY SLOW to avoid anxiety-related refusal of med.
- β-blockers reduce physical sxs but not necessarily emotional sxs.
- SSRIs have low overdose risk; may either decrease or increase anxiety, insomnia; fluvoxamine (Luvox) approved for OCD symptoms, but has more drug-drug interactions and must be used with caution in this age group; takes higher doses and longer for SSRIs to work for OCD than for depression; down regulation of receptors w chronic use of SSRI causes eventual improvement of sx.
- Risperidone (0.25 mg qd/tid) or quetiapine (12.5-25 mg qd/tid) useful as first-line rx of agitated, anxious pts with dementia or psychosis; antihistamines may induce confusion.
- Buspirone HCl: 6-8-wk trial period may be effective at very low dose 2.5 mg qd to decrease anxiety/agitation in benzodiazepine naïve pts, demented pts.
- Avoid benzodiazepines, if at all possible. If clinically necessary, use lorazepam (available po, im, iv), oxazepam, and temazepam rather than those with long-acting breakdown products, if possible; if pt is on chronic benzodiazepine dosing, wean slowly over several months to avoid acute withdrawal sxs.

Team Management: Discover reversible etiologies; behavioral therapies; short-term cognitive therapy (5 sessions); long-term exposure therapy (exposure to anxiety precipitant); observe carefully for benefits or negative effects of rx.

5.3 Alcohol Misuse

Int J Addict 1995;30:1819; Jama 2000;284:963; Jags 2000;48:985; 2000;48:985; Am Fam Phys 2000;61:1710; Clin Ger Med 2003; 19:743

Cause: Reduced tolerance, lower body water for a given amount of alcohol, resulting in more pronounced effects. Used inappropriately for sleep, pain, loneliness. Health professionals may reinforce denial because of unexamined stereotypes. Atypical presentation delays diagnosis; pain, insomnia, loneliness, depression, death of partner, having a partner who drinks, lack of family and social supports predispose to "late onset" alcohol abuse. Risk factor, family h/o alcohol abuse, in elderly. Coexisting mental illness present in 80% of "lifetime" elderly alcohol abusers (Clin Ger Med 2003;19:743).

Epidem: Prevalence of ETOH abuse in > 65 yr old is 3% in the community, 10:1 M:F (Jama 1993;270:1222), 18% of general medical inpatients and 44% of psychiatric inpatients; Medicare claims data show 1.1% of all hospitalizations in geriatric pts are for alcohol-related diagnoses (Am Fam Phys 2000; 61:1710).

Pathophys:

- Proportion of total body wgt that is fat increases with aging; decreased volume of distribution in elderly increases blood ETOH concentration per unit dose of ETOH; moderate drinking in elderly should be defined as no more than 1 drink qd.
- Increased permeability of blood-brain barrier leads to greater medical morbidity in the elderly alcoholic.
- 66% of elderly alcoholics have had lifelong problems with ETOH ("early onset" defined as onset by 25 yr old); 33% develop habits later in life ("late onset" defined as onset after age 60).

- Reduced GFR, decreased efficacy of hepatic metabolism.
- Gastric alcohol dehydrogenase concentrations decrease, slowing alcohol metabolism.

Sx:

- Drinking 5-6 d/wk, 4-5 drinks per occasion; confusion (10% of dementias are alcohol-related); women no cognitive impairment w one drink/d (Nejm 2005;352:245); self-neglect; self-reported rates of consumption may not accurately indicate impact on elderly lifestyle.
- Traumatic injury (falls, MVA).
- CAGE and MAST screens have decreased sens in the elderly; better when also ask about quantity and frequency (Jama 1996; 276:1964); MAST-G (geriatric version) 95% sens and 78% specif (GRS, 5th ed, 2002; Jags 2000;48:985).
- Sx tend to be nonspecific: "failure to thrive" insomnia, diarrhea, incontinence, repeated falls, loss of libido, increased metabolism of some drugs, eg, tolbutamide (Orinase), phenytoin (Dilantin).
- Have high index of suspicion if hospitalized pt develops new-onset seizures, agitation, confusion, anxiety.
- Can see onset of withdrawal delayed 2-10 d, presenting w confusion.
- Hallucinations; may continue for weeks to months (Drugs Aging 1999;14:405).

Si: Lab abnormalities: nonspecific; high MCV rises w 4-8 wks heavy drinking; abnormal LFTs rise within 4 wks of heavy drinking and fall 4 wks after cessation (Ann IM 1995;155:1907); multiple spider nevi, hypoalbuminemia, fluctuations in INR.

Crs: Improved px w late age of onset of alcoholism, social and family support, absence of dementia.

- Watch for ETOH-med interactions, esp CNS depressants: benzodiazepines, barbiturates, diphenhydramine (Benadryl), psychotropics. ETOH interacts with 50% of most commonly prescribed meds!

- Can precipitate hypoglycemic episodes in DM.
- HT, Afib, stroke, Wernicke's encephalopathy, Korsakoff syndrome, gi bleeding can all result.
- First year after dx of cirrhosis, 50% mortality in individuals > 60 yr old compared to 7% in those < 60 yr old.
- Moderate alcohol consumption (1-6 drinks/wk) may protect against both Alzheimer's type and vascular dementias in some populations and against heart disease thrombotic stroke (Jama 2003;289:1405).

Cmplc:

- Alcoholic women have 4 × risk for CAD.
- Increased cancer risk (liver, esophagus, larynx, nasopharynx, colon, prostate, breast).
- Thrombocytopenia, hyponatremia.

Prevention:

- Pt education to help elderly understand that habitual use of alcohol as aging advances may interfere with achievement of optimal health and functioning in context of increasing chronic disease conditions.
- Avoid trap that the pt has only a few years left, so why not enjoy?
- Emphasize neg effect of alcohol on sleep pattern, nutrition, energy.
- Because of alterations in metabolism of and reaction to drugs, the appropriate number of alcoholic beverages is decreased to 1 drink per d for men, and less for women. Recent studies suggest that moderate alcohol use may protect some women, and to a lesser extent men, from dementia. Alcohol protects against platelet aggregation, raises HDL, improves endothelial function. Wine contains antioxidants.

Therapeutic:

(Clin Ger Med 1993;9:197; Prim Care 1993;20:155)

Treat Withdrawal:

- 10-30% of nondependent problem drinkers cut down to moderate drinking after a brief intervention by a clinician. In older individuals, nonconfrontational, supportive approaches work best.
- Outpatient detoxification from alcohol or psychoactive medications more difficult in older pts. Age is a risk factor for seizures, delirium tremens, other complications. Can be successful if no comorbidities, highly motivated, with social support and willingness to be in daily contact with clinician. Visiting nurses can assess homebound pts.
- Postpone w/u of cognitive loss several weeks.
- Indications for inpatient detox include past h/o complicated withdrawal, polysubstance abuse, use of very high doses of drug or alcohol, suicidality or psychiatric comorbidities, significant medical comorbidities that may be exacerbated by withdrawal, poor social supports for outpatient detox.
    1. Inpatient detox for alcohol involves monitoring symptoms every 1-4 hr, using the CIWA scale. Withdrawal si/sx start within 48-72 hr of last ingestion.
    2. All pts get scheduled thiamine 100 mg po qd for 5 d (protects against Wernicke-Korsakoff), Mg 0.5 to 1 mEq/kg po qd (protects against arrhythmias, seizures). For inpatient detox give first dose as 2-4 mEq iv.
- Keep pts adequately hydrated. Avoid CHF exacerbation.
- Give thiamine before glucose.
- Older pts are more likely to have confusion, sleepiness, weakness (eg, falls), HT as presenting symptoms of withdrawal.
- Several rx options for alcohol withdrawal, including scheduled vs symptom-triggered administration of benzodiazepines, and short vs long acting benzodiazepines.

- Symptom-triggered advantages: shorter hospital stays, less med used.
- Symptom-triggered disadvantages: higher rate of seizures, especially late onset.
- Scheduled med advantages: may protect against "kindling" phenomenon (in which h/o of seizures lowers threshold for future seizures), self tapering, decreased rates of breakthrough sx.
- Scheduled med disadvantages: increased risk of oversedation, with delirium; longer hospital stays. Can have delayed withdrawal from benzodiazepines.
- Pts with acute agitation or illness can be "front-loaded" with hourly doses of short acting benzodiazepines until sx controlled.
- Long- and intermediate-half life benzodiazepines are more likely to accumulate in older pts, leading to a delayed "abstinence syndrome" (withdrawal) occurring days or weeks after alcohol detox.
- Oxazepam and lorazepam are safe to use in those with liver damage.
- Other meds include beta-blockers or clonidine for autonomic hyperactivity. Propranolol can increase delirium. Haldol can be used in addition to benzodiazepines for agitation; lowers seizure threshold, so start low (0.25 to 1 mg).
- Watch for reactive depression and treat w SSRI; when depression co-exists w alcoholism ("dual diagnosis"), both must be treated to achieve success (Int J Addict 1995;30:1819).

Relapse Prevention:

- *DO NOT* PRESCRIBE DISULFIRAM (Antabuse) because elderly susceptible to disulfiram reaction w resultant cardiac complications.
- Naltrexone has been approved for rx of alcoholism by FDA (Am J Med 1997;103:447).

- Ondansetron (Jama 2000;284:963); both naltrexone and ondansetron are indicated for the rx of early onset ETOH abuse, and their role in the rx of older alcoholics is being established.

Team Management:

- Rehab units 1-3 wks; Alcoholics Anonymous (about 33% AA participants > 50 yr old) or social situations that help elderly pursue an abstinent lifestyle.
- Elderly appropriate:
  - Age-specific and proceed at a slower pace
  - Focus on the underlying issues of depression, loneliness, loss
  - Are nonconfrontational and respect privacy
  - Include cognitive behavioral therapy
  - Are linked to medical services
- AA meetings located at senior centers.
- Involve pt's pharmacy to monitor prescription refills; outreach program.
- Pt education: alcohol affects medical conditions (eg, can worsen DM, CHF) and interacts with 50% of meds; informed pts can change behavior.
- Explore family constellation: enablers, scapegoats.

5.4 Substance Misuse

Jags 2000;48:985

Cause: Increased need to treat emotional and physical pain, most commonly for arthritis and sleep; increased risk of drug-drug interaction because of polypharmacy, including OTC.

Epidem: 5% of older adults abuse drugs; vast majority of drug misuse involves benzodiazepines-diazepam (Valium), chlordiazepoxide (librium) and propoxyphene (Darvon); abuse of narcotics is rare among elderly, unless previous h/o abuse at younger age.

Pathophys: Reduction of renal and hepatic function; decreased body water and increased fat proportionally; displacement of one drug from protein-binding site by another makes drug-drug interaction more common and complex to treat.

Sx: "Doctor shopping," "lost pills," anxiety, amnesia, memory loss, depressed mood, agitation, falls, abdominal pain or constipation, personal hygiene deterioration, confusion, obtundation.

Crs: Drug withdrawal longer in older pts; benzodiazepine withdrawal mortality higher; sx (anxiety, hallucinations, tachycardia, nausea, insomnia, tremor, decreased appetite, altered mentation, dizziness) can occur after as little as 2 mo of continuous use, and occur in majority of pts after 4-6 mo of use; up to 30% risk of seizure in untreated withdrawal.

Lab: Drug levels in abuse or w enzyme-competing drugs; LFTs may be elevated.

Rx: Treat drug withdrawal in medically monitored setting due to risk of hyper-autonomic syndrome, delirium or convulsion. Lipid-soluble benzodiazepines cause more difficult withdrawal (diazepam, chlordiazepoxide); may take months. Less lipid-soluble, cut one-half dose for 2 wk, next 1/4 dose for 1 wk, then last 1/4 over 1-2 wk, and monitor vital signs. Sedative hypnotic withdrawal 10-21 d; opioids halved over 5-10 d, then gradual reduction over weeks; treat pain with other meds.

Team Management: Groups specific for older people; chronic pain groups; chemical dependency units, esp important for elderly withdrawal of sedatives/hypnotics; consider NA/AA; psychosocial issues need addressing; abuse/misuse may be self-treatment of stresses or losses of late life; pt education of potential for interaction of complex med regimen and its enhanced effect in elderly.

5.5 Dementias

Cortical Dementia (Dementia, Alzheimer's Type (DAT))

(See Figure 5.2) Ann IM 1991;115:122; Nejm 1986;314:964; 1996;335:330; Clin Ger Med 1994;10:239; Med Clin N Am 1994;78:811; Sultzer DL, Cummings JL. Dementia Dx and Rx Intensive Geriatric Review Course, UCLA, January 1996; Sci Amer 1997;11:xi; Jama 1997;278:1363; 2002;287:2335

Cause: 20-40% genetic transmission.

Early Onset (< 60 yr old):

- Amyloid precussor protein gene on chromosome #21 (Nature 2006;440:284,352)
- Presenillin single gene
- Presenillin two gene type

Late (> 60 yr old):

- Apolipoprotein E gene, E4 allele hetero/homozygotes on chromosome #19 (Nejm 2000;343:450).
- Chromosome #12 autosomal dominant (Jama 1997;278:1237)
  Late onset associated w E4 allele of apolipoprotein E (Jama 1995;273:1274; Nejm 1996;334:752), which facilitates β-amyloid protein deposition in neurofibrillary tangles (Nejm 1995;333:1242), also constricts cerebral blood vessels (Neurol Res 2003;25:642), high concentration of neurofibrillary tangles associated w cognitive decline (Jama 2000;283:1571,1615); higher mortality in pts w dementia and apolipoprotein E phenotype (Jags 1998;46:72); E2 allele protective against the development of Alzheimer's (Jama 1996;275:1612).
- Family hx imparts 3-4 × risk of general population; head trauma imparts 3 × risk of general population; most are acquired and of unclear etiology; toxins, eg, carbon dioxide, carbon monoxide; elevated risk of subsequent strokes in older persons w cognitive impairment, suggesting CVD plays important role in causing cognitive impairment (Jags 1996;44:237);

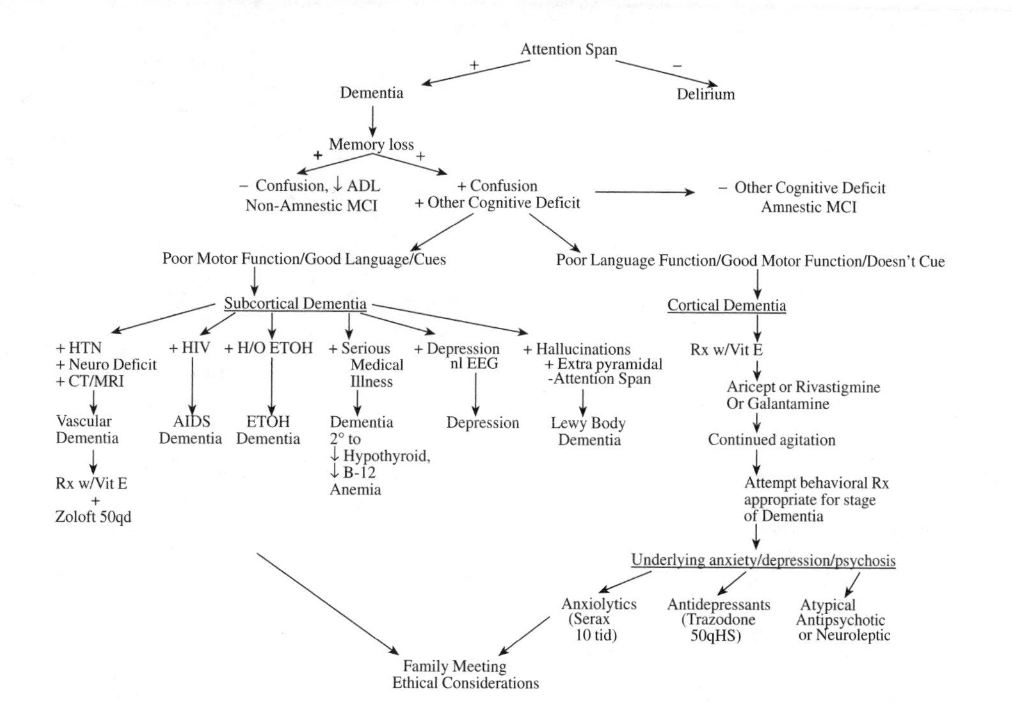

Figure 5.2 Dementia Flow Sheet

Table 5.4 Dementias

	Delirium—Infecting, Metabolic, etc.	AD (60%)	Frontal Lobe Dementia (10%), Pick (1-2%)	Subcortical (2-3%) Huntington's, Wilson's, SNP, NPH, Parkinson	Vascular Dementias (15%) (Multi-infarct, Binswanger's Cortical Infarctions)	Wernicke-Korsakoff
History Onset, duration	Sudden, hours-days (CJD-dementia die within 1 yr)	Insidious, month–years; 8-10 yr AD	2-10 yr	—	Acute, stepwise*	—
Mental status Attention	Fluctuating[a]	—	—	—	—	—
Memory Learning recall, and recognition	Impaired by poor attention	Amnesia early	Amnesia late[a]	Forgetful[a] (retrieval deficit)	—	—
Language Comprehension, repetition, naming	Normal or mild anomia, misnaming, dysgraphia, may be impaired	Aphasia	—	Normal[a]	—	—

Speech	Slurred	Normal	Stereotyped speech, terminal mutism	Abnormal (hypophonic, dysarthric, mute)	—	—
Perception Visual spatial skills, constructional apraxia	Hallucination	Visual spatial	Visual spatial disturbance late	Impaired	—	—
Cognition Calculation, abstraction, judgment	—	Abnormal[a] (acalculia, poor judgment, impaired abstraction)	Calculations spared early	Abnormal (slowed, dilapidated)	—	Confabulation early, antegrade memory loss[a]; can't learn new things
Executive skills Drive, programming response control synthesis	Very poor	—	Impairment of initiation, goal setting, planning	Problems with executive skills	—	—

continues

Table 5.4 continued

	Delirium—Infecting, Metabolic, etc.	AD (60%)	Frontal Lobe Dementia (10%), Pick (1-2%)	Subcortical (2-3%) Huntington's, Wilson's, SNP, NPH, Parkinson	Vascular Dementias (15%) (Multi-infarct, Binswanger's Cortical Infarctions)	Wernicke-Korsakoff
Mood affect	Fear, suspiciousness may often be prominent	Paranoid delusions, 25% disinterested or uninhibited	Personality change early[a] Klüver-Bucy[b] syndrome, apathy, irritability, jocularity, euphoria, loss of fear	Abnormal (apathetic or depressed), blunting, emotional withdrawal	Preservation of personality; emotional lability	Placid, congenial
Motor Posture, tone, movement, gait	Postural tremor, myoclonus, asterixis; AIDS: psychomotor slowing, focal neurologic signs	Normal into final stages (then increased tone and flexed posture)	—	Posture-stooped,[a] SNP (extended or flexed) (Parkinson's) tone, increased, tremor, bradykinesia, chorea, dystonia, abnormal gait	Multifocal defects, in lacunar disease, rigid, EPS, pseudobulbar palsy	Nystagmus, ataxia (detectable in late stages)

AD = Alzheimer; CJD = Creutzfeldt-Jakob disease; AIDS = acquired immunodeficiency syndrome; SNP = supranuclear palsy; EPS = extrapyramidal syndromes.
[a]Most characteristic findings.
[b]Klüver-Bucy—blunted emotional response, hypersex, gluttony.
Modified from tables in Cummings, Benson, and Loverme, 1980. Sultzer/Cummings intensive course in geriatric medicine, 1/96.

low linguistic ability in early life strong predictor of poor cognitive function and Alzheimer's in late life (Jama 1996; 275:582); smoking imparts increased risk (Lancet 1998;351: 1840); nondemented elderly w depressed mood more at risk for developing Alzheimer's dementia (Arch Gen Psychiatry 1996; 53:175).

- Homocysteine a risk factor (Nejm 2002;346:476) vs not a risk factor (Neurol 2004;62:1470).
- Metabolic syndrome and inflamation increase risk cognitive decline (Jama 2004;292:2237).
- Higher antioxidants: ascorbic acid and β-carotene plasma levels are associated w better memory performance (Jags 1997; 45:718).
- Herbal remedies may have heavy metal toxicity/contamination (Jama 2004;292:2868).
- CMV is neurotoxic (Jags 2006;54:1046; 2007;45:131).
- Elevated cholesterol increases risk of MCI (Jags 2007;45:133).

Epidem: Prevalence = 5% at age 70, 20% at 80, 50% at 90 (Jama 1995;273:1354) vs doubles q 5 yr from 1% at age 60 yr to 40% at age 85 yr (Neurol 1998;51:S2; Nejm 1999;341:1670); 50% incidence in family members of late-onset Alzheimer's pts (Geriatrics 2000;55:34); F:M 1.5:1.2 (Arch Gen Psychiatry 1998; 55:809); 100% of Down syndrome pts age > 35 yr (Science 1992; 258:668; Ann IM 1985;103:526).

>40% of elderly dementia is purely Alzheimer's, the rest is vascular multi-infarct type predominantly (Nejm 1993;328:153); 70% of NH pts have Alzheimer's dementia; "mixed dementia" felt to be common.

Pathophys: Structural changes most severe in hippocampus and association cortex of parietal, temporal, frontal lobes; atrophy of corpus callosum differentiates Alzheimer's from healthy elderly and incipient dementia (Jags 1996;44:798); neurofibrillary tangles are paired helical filaments that contain tau and ubiquitin proteins associated w intracellular microtubules (Nejm 1991;325:1849); possible deficiency of acetylcholine vs glutamate (Jama 1999; 281:1401,1433); noradrenergic, serotonergic deficiency (Jama 2002;287:2335; Geriatrics 2000;55:34).

Neuronal dropout; decreased acetylcholine synthesis (Nejm 1985;313:7), hence anticholinergics worsen (Nejm 1985;313:7); plaques a consequence of altered metabolism, primary causative lesions (Neuron 1996;16:921).

Sx: Repetitive behavior predictive (Jags 2003;51:32); Loss of social skills and memory usually unacknowledged by pt unless early stages; depression related to insight into cognitive losses.

Si: (See Table 5.4) Abnormal mental status (Psychiatr Clin N Am 1991; 14:309) w memory loss > 6 mo + 2 other cognitive function impairments for definition of dementia, according to National Institute of Neurological and Communicative Disorders and Stroke-Alzheimer's Disease and Related Disorders (NINCDS-ADRDA). These criteria produce 90-100% accuracy (Neurol 1993;43:250); DSM-IV requires only one cognitive deficit for definition of dementia, producing 80-85% accuracy (Am Psych Association, DSM IV, 1994:142); proper interpretation of MMSE requires knowledge of pt's age and educational level (Jags 1995;43:807).

- Family key to earliest dx if can be encouraged to share information; spousal denial and covering of sx of losses common; retrospective histories suggest 3-4 yr of sxs before presentation to health professional.
- Memory, recent much worse than remote; including orientation to time (d, mo, yr) (day of week is 53% sens, 92% specif) (Ann IM 1991;115:122); recall 3 items associated w medial temporal lobe-hippocampus, mammillary bodies, hypothalamus.
- Perceptive/spatial disorientation (Jags 1998;46:1226), eg, answers to, "How do you get there from here?"; clock face drawing; copy interlocking pentagons associated w parietal, frontal, occipital.

- Language impairments: anomias/paraphasias/aphasias, which often result in neologisms or circumlocutions, fluent aphasia (posterior L brain-Wernicke); use of automatic phrases and clichés; as pt progresses, ask questions that only require short answers to demonstrate comprehension: "Point to the light,"; "Do you put your shoes on before your socks?"; "Is my wife's brother a man or a woman?"; "The lion was killed by the tiger. Which animal is dead?"
- Abstraction impairments: "What does it mean to give someone the cold shoulder?"; categorization; calculations.
- Scoring: < 21 on the MMSE is abnormal for 8th-grade education, < 23 is abnormal for high school education, < 24 abnormal for college education; 18-24 mild cognitive deficit, 10-18 moderate cognitive deficit, < 9 severe cognitive deficit. MMSE insensitive to noncortical dementias; Hachinski scale helps discriminate other dementias from Alzheimer's dementia. If MMSE < 2, ask long-term memory questions because may be mild cognitive impairment, signaling appearance of clear dementia at a later date (Jama 2002;50:1577).
- Executive skills (Lancet 1999;354:1921): motivation, ability to initiate activity, ability to recognize patterns, generate motor programs and the ability to plan and execute a strategy; alternate square and triangle pattern (frontal lobe) (Exp Aging Res 1994;20:73); executive dysfunction highly correlated w the appearance of problem behaviors in Alzheimer's dementia (Exp Aging Res 1994;20:73); executive testing (Am Fam Phys 2006;73:211).
- Affect changes and poor judgment: neuropsychiatric findings with other assessment tests (J Fam Pract 1993;37:599).
- Impairment of verbal memory and category naming associated w incipient dementia (Neurol 1995;45:957).
- Pupillary dilatation not a si of dementia (Arch Neurol 1997;54:55).

- Neuropsychiatric Inventory Questionnaire (Neurol 1994;44:2308) asks about delusions, hallucinations, agitation, disinhibition, apathy, motor disturbance, eating, nighttime behavior (J Neuropsych Clin Neurosci 2000;12:233).

Crs: Slowly progressive; mean survival from first sx = 10 yr, shorter for more severe cases (Ann IM 1990;113:429). Average decline = 3 points per yr on the MMSE; poor prognosis w extrapyramidal si or psychosis (Jama 1997;277:806). Stages (Am J Psych 1982;139:1136) 1 and 2, forget familiar names and places; stage 3, family and coworkers aware; stage 4, difficulty w finances; stage 5, needs assistance dressing; stage 6, incontinence, delusional; stage 7, grunting, nonambulatory.

- Personality changes (from progressive passivity to marked hostility) can develop before cognitive impairments (J Ger Psych Neurol 1990;3:21).
- Delusions in 25% of demented pts; paranoid type most common; accusations of theft, infidelity; hallucinations, usually visual in 25% of pts, early in course predict rapid decline (Jags 2003;57:953; Arch Neurol 1999;56:1388).
- Depression in 50% of demented pts; orbital frontal (irritability), mediofrontal (apathy) early in Alzheimer's dementia; dorsal frontal (aphasia, apraxia, agnosia) occur later (Jags 1997; 45:891).
- Lewy body variant: intraneural inclusion bodies on histopathology, cortical-type cognitive impairment, extrapyramidal si (Arch Neurol 1999;56:1388).
- Clinical characteristics of atypical dementia syndromes (Nejm 1996;335:330): those w language impairment or constructional apraxia out of proportion to memory loss progress less rapidly.
- Agitated behavior occurs sometime during course of disease in 1/3 to 1/2 of pts w Alzheimer's, not predictive of rapid decline.
- Fever common in progressive dementia, most pts recover regardless of antibiotics, question benefit of rx in advanced dementia (Jama 1990;263:3168).

- Rapidly progressing: r/o paraneoplastic limbic encephalopathy. ANN A-1 marker. (Ann Long-Term Care 2006;14:25).

Cmplc:

R/o: *Age-associated memory impairment* (AAMI), also termed *benign*, and if more severe, *malignant, senescent forgetfulness*, may be an early monosymptomatic stage of Alzheimer's dementia; lower N-acetyl-acetate in AAMI and DAT brains than in normal aging brain (Jags 1996;44:133).

R/o: *Mild cognitive impairment* (MCI) (Neurol 2004;63:115; J Neurol Neurosurg Psychiatry 2006;77:714), cognitive deficit greater than normal aging, but does not meet criteria for global cognitive deficit of dementia; memory impairment, do poorly on tests of delayed recall, associated with median temporal lobe atrophy (Neurol 2004;63:94); risk of dementia in MCI 10-15%/yr (Neurol 2006;67:1201; Jags 2006;54:1008). Vit E, does not help delay eventual progression to Alzheimers (Nejm 2005;352:2439); PET can identify MCI (Nejm 2006;355:2632). IADL problems actually signal dementia not MCI (Jags 2006;54:163).

R/o: *Delirium*, if acute, in which attention span is most prominent deficit; test by serial 7's; serial digits up to 7, eg, phone numbers; spell "WORLD" backwards, or repeat days of week backward; associated w increased mortality (Jags 1992;40:759; Jama 1990; 263:1097); if decline on MMSE is > 3-4 pts/yr or score of 15 after only 3 yr h/o dementia, must r/o other problems (Folstein M, Delirium, Bar Harbor, ME, 10/96); rx acute delirium w Haldol 0.5 mg po, iv or im (twice as potent as po) in hospital (Jags 1992; 40:829; Nejm 1999;340:669); sitters, reorienting routines helpful.

- Independent risk factors for developing delirium in hospital include pre-existing dementia, > 80 yr old, fracture on admission, symptomatic infection, male gender, use of antipsychotic or narcotic med, septic encephalopathy (Jama 1996;275:470); other risk factors: comorbid medical conditions, post-operative, immobility, ADL impairment, dehydration, hearing or visual impairment, pain, sleep deprivation, h/o ETOH, fluid and electrolyte abnormalities, hct < 30%, catheters, urinary retention, fecal impaction, use of restraints (Nejm 1999;340:669); severity of Glasgow Coma Score correlates w elevations in BUN, bilirubin, bacteremia.

- Other risk factors include single or multiple drugs; drugs that cause psychiatric sx (Med Lett 2002;44:59); toxins, such as occult solvent/paint exposure, may cause peripheral neuropathy, myopathy, cerebellar signs; elevated blood or urine levels of Pb, As, Hg, manganese, thallium.
- Meds that often cause delirium: anticholinergics (especially diphenhydramine, most common, and scopolamine), TCAs, phenothiazines, NSAIDs, steroids (especially prednisone) H-2 antagonists, digoxin, oral hypoglycemics, diuretics, lithium, many antibiotics, donepezil, β-blockers, SSRIs, anti-convulsants, meperidine (other opioids, less commonly) dopamine agonists, lithium, and many others.

Table 5.5 Dementing Illnesses Arranged by Qualitative Subtypes

Type 1 Dementias	Type 2 Dementias
Alzheimer disease	Frontal types/Pick disease (early)
Atypical AD cases	Alcoholic dementia
Frontal types/Pick disease (late)	B_{12}/Folate deficiency
Creutzfeldt-Jakob	Dementia of depression
Cortical Lewy body disease	Dementia pugilistica
Some vascular dementia	Huntington disease
	Hypothyroidism
	Normal pressure hydrocephalus
	Parkinson dementia
	Polypharmacy
	Vascular dementia (most cases)

Reproduced by permission from Yeager BF, Farnett LE, Ruzicka SA. Management of the behavioral manifestations of dementia. Arch Intern Med 1995;155:250-60.

- Benzopdiazepine and alcohol withdrawal, especially high risk in undiagnosed heavy drinker admitted to hospital for routine procedure.

R/o: *Other Irreversible cortical or Type I dementias* (see Figure 5.2), notable for posterior cortical features (amnesia, aphasia, agnosia, anomia, apraxia) (Jags 1998;46:98).

- *Pick's disease* (1-2% cases, argentophilic inclusion bodies or Pick body on histopathology); if no histopathology, then frontal-temporal dementia (Jags 1997;45:579) similar to Alzheimer's, but much younger onset with less memory impairment and more behavioral change (apathy, irritability, jocularity, euphoria).
- *Klüver-Bucey syndrome* = emotional blunting, loss of fear, oral exploratory behavior, change in eating habits, altered sexual activity); disordered executive function (impairment of initiation goal setting planning); inability to refrain from touching objects-shoplifting; Rx w Risperdal, Zoloft; 2-10 yr duration; no praxis or visuospatial deficit as w Alzheimer's; language-abundant unfocused speech, echolalia, palilalia; is rare, and anatomic changes are isolated to frontal and temporal lobes.
- *Other frontal lobe dementias*, which comprise 10% of dementias (frontal lobe degeneration of the non-Alzheimer's type, progressive subcortical gliosis, amyotrophic lateral sclerosis (ALS)-dementia syndrome); MMSE may be normal w early frontal lobe, Lewy body, Pick's dementias.
- *Primary progressive aphasia* limited to early language findings (Nejm 2004;349:1535).
- *Creutzfeldt-Jakob*, rare, slow virus, prior incubation period several years; no known cure; progresses rapidly once active, death within a year. Cerebellar and extrapyramidal signs, startle myoclonus, asymmetric slowing or periodic polyspike discharges on EEG.

R/o: *Reversible Causes Type II subcortical dementias* (see Figure 5.2), which affect frontal systems (at frontal cortex or subcortical level), while sparing posterior cortical regions. Executive control functions in three main systems are affected: dorsolateral (abstraction and hypothesis generation), orbitofrontal (emotional control), mediofrontal (apathy, impaired goal directed attention). People with executive dysfunction can draw clock, but cannot indicate "1:45" by drawing hands on a clock (eg, the hands point to the 1, the 4 and the 5, instead of the 1 and the 9). Executive function interview screening test for executive dysfunction in mild dementia (Jags 2005;53:1577).

- *Thyroid disorders* (depression, irritability, mental slowing): both hypothyroidism and hyperthyroidism can present w frank psychosis; myxedema; thyrotoxicosis - less common, psychomotor retardation, apathy, less anxiety, tremor, tachycardia than is characteristic of younger pts.
- *Vit B_{12} deficiency:* irritability, psychosis, delirium, amnesia, slowing of thought processes may also occur before peripheral neuropathy (Nejm 1988;318:1720); optic atrophy, older pts symptomatic at higher levels of vit B_{12} (low normal) than younger pts (Jags 1996;44:1355).
- *Subdural hematoma* results from cerebral atrophy and shearing of already stretched bridging veins during trauma.
- *Wernicke-Korsakoff syndrome* w anterograde memory loss, alcohol hx; may recover partially over 1 yr (Nejm 1985;312:16).
- *Pseudodementia of depression:* more "I don't know" answers than the "guesses" of DAT; lack of progression of sxs; preserved awareness of deficits; preserved language skills; cued recall nl; impaired problem solving and word list generation; also often both depression and dementia occur together; more likely to respond to antidepressant if MMSE > 21; rx of apathy responds to stimulant, such as methylphenidate (Ritalin); depression associated w significant memory deficit may be in fact preclinical dementia (Jags 2000;48:479).

- *Syphilitic dementia:* meningovascular (2-10 yr, sometimes 30-40 yr after initial infection); inflammatory arteritis that can result in stroke and vascular dementia; general paresis (7-12 yr after initial infection); delusions, hallucinations, mood disorders often present; pseudobulbar palsy; poor coordination; hyperreflexia or hyporeflexia; pupillary abnormalities; signs of posterior column dysfunction (taboparesis); VDRL and RPR nonreactive in one-fourth of pts w late neurosyphilis; fluorescent treponema antibody (FTA) more sensitive, but remains pos even after rx; not common enough to warrant routine screening (Neurol 2001;56:1143).

Frontal/temporal tumors

R/o: Nonreversible causes type II or subcortical dementias (Ann IM 1984;100:417) which show forgetfulness, executive dysfunction (Jags 1997;45:386) and motor findings early (Arch Neurol 1993; 50:873) unlike the amnesia and early language deficits in DAT.

- *AIDS dementia:* psychomotor slowing, focal neurologic signs, frontal lobe cell loss.
- *Frontal/temporal tumors*
- *Parkinson's dementia* (slowing of cognition), less agnosia and more apathy than w cortical dementias; 40% Parkinson's pts develop dementia; a problem with retrieval, procedural memory; do not do well on interference tasks, visuospatial impairments, verbal fluency (otherwise known as festinating speech or palilalia). Decreased dopamine in the median frontal lobe leads to dementia findings. Psychotic findings may be secondary to executive cognitive deficit, REM sleep disorder, or antiparkinsonian meds. Rx psychotic findings with selegiline, anticholinesterase inhibitor, atypical antipsychotics, ECT; avoid anticholinergics; use clonazepam for REM sleep disorder. More likely dx of *vascular Parkinson's* if no lower body tremor, incontinence, pseudobulbar affect or falls from postural instability, and has h/o HT, stroke, hyperreflexic with upgoing Babinski reflexes, white matter basal ganglia lesion on MRI.

- *Diffuse Lewy body disease (DLBD):* (see Table 5.6) vivid recurrent visual hallucinations that are recognized as unreal occur earlier, and extrapyramidal dysfunction more mild than w Parkinson's and appear w onset of dementia; alteration in alertness, attention resembling confusional states, transient loss of consciousness (Jags 1998;46:1449; Neurol 1996;47:111); sens to antipsychotics, may be life threatening w neuroleptic malignant syndrome, even risperidone; consider olanzapine instead (Nejm 1998;338:6031); minor response with L-dopa (Neurol 1997;48:376); relative serotonergic dominance; ondansetron (Zofran), a 5-HT3 receptor antagonist, used for delusions and hallucinations (Neurol 1995;45:1305).

Table 5.6 Clinical Diagnostic Criteria for Diffuse Lewy Body Disease

1. The central feature is progressive cognitive decline amounting to dementia; deficits on tests of attention, fronto-subcortical skills, and visuospatial ability may be especially significant.
2. Two of the following are required for a probable, and one for a possible diagnosis of DLBD:
   a. Fluctuating cognition with pronounced variations in attention and alertness
   b. Recurrent visual hallucinations that are typically well formed and detailed
   c. Spontaneous motor features of parkinsonism
3. Features supportive of the diagnosis are:
   a. Repeated falls
   b. Syncopes or transient losses of consciousness
   c. Neuroleptic hypersensitivity
   d. Systematized delusions
   e. Hallucinations in other modalities
4. DLBD is less likely in the presence of:
   a. Stroke disease, revealed by focal neurological signs or brain imaging
   b. Evidence of any other physical or brain illness that may account for the clinical picture

- *Progressive supranuclear palsy* (axial rigidity, vertical gaze palsy) may respond to amitriptyline 10-40 mg bid (Jags 1996;44:1072) or zolpidem.
- *Other nonreversible subcortical dementias:* spinocerebellar degeneration, Huntington's, Wilson's, olivopontine degeneration,

systemic diseases: end-stage renal failure, CHF, COPD, DM (subcortical microvascular lesions and hippocampal damage from hypoglycemia).

- *Normal pressure hydrocephalus (NPH)* obstruction of CSF flow around the convexity of the brain, impaired absorption into the sagittal sinus, gait abnormalities initial symptom w small shuffling steps w feet set down at variable force, postural instability, difficulties w fine hand movements, lack of initiative and slowness of thought; best outcomes of shunt done earlier in disease, may be partially reversible, not without substantial morbidity (see NPH).
- *Multi-infarct dementia:* stepwise crs, emotional lability prominent, and h/o HT, CVA, or ASHD; features of mixed cortical/subcortical dementia, see vascular dementias (Arch Neurol 1993;50:873; Am J Psych 1997;154:562).
- *Alcohol-related dementias:* 10-15-yr drinking hx; apathy and noncortical features predominate; irritability; may have normal MMSE; partially reversible w abstinence; direct toxic effect of alcohol has not been established.

R/o: *Paraphrenia:* hallucinations and delusions out of proportion to intellectual dysfunction.

Lab:

- Cost-effectiveness of w/u for reversible dementias questionable (J Neurol 1995;242:446).
- Electrolytes, calcium, kidney and liver function, TSH, CBC, vit B_{12} level w f/u methylmalonic acid level, if < 350 pg/ml, folate, UA, consider VDRL and HIV antibody; dementia occurs in 20% HIV pts.
- Brain histology at postmortem shows neurofibrillary tangles, senile plaques with eosinophilic amyloid.
- EEG occasionally helpful to distinguish Alzheimer's dementia (slow waves) from depression (nl), toxic, metabolic, partial complex seizure or Jakob-Creutzfeldt.
- Consider LP in subacute cases.

- APOE (genotyping for E allele) pos predictive value very high but neg predictive value nil; only recommend in combination w clinical criteria (Nejm 1998;338:506); not for routine clinical dx use; cholinergic markers not present until relatively late in the course of Alzheimer's dementia (Jama 1999;281:1401).
- CSF Tau protein marker (Ann IM 2003;138:400), not yet used clinically.

X-ray: Head CT or brain MRI distinguishes from multi-infarct dementia—periventricular hyperintensities on T2-weighted images w multi-infarct dementia and in deep white matter w Alzheimer's (Neurol 1993;43:250); very low yield of reversible disease, eg, $< 1:250$.

If motor dysfunction, eg, rigidity, reflex asymmetry, abnormal reflexes, then obtain MRI to detect stroke and ischemic changes (Jags 1995;43:138); MRI better than CT for subcortical pathology.

PET, SPECT: Decreased cerebral blood flow and glucose metabolism in parietal, temporal, frontal association cortex bilaterally (Arch Neurol 1995;52:773); mostly a research tool at this point; as early rx evolves, these will become more clinically applicable tests; low sens and specif of SPECT in Alz-heimer's (Jags 1997;45:15; Jama 2003;51:258).

Rx:

Preventive:

- Apolipoprotein E screening not appropriate (Jama 1997; 277:832).
- Pts with extensive social networks may be protected against development of dementia (Lancet 2000;355:1291).
- NSAIDs may decrease risk (Neurol 1997;48:626; Jama 1998; 279:688; Nejm 2001;345:1515,1567) - Large studies only epidemiological, not controlled; not as rx (Jama 2003;289:2819).
- Folic acid slows early cognitive decline in pts w hyperhomocysteinuria (Lancet 2007;369:208).
- Walking associated w better cognitive function (Jama 2004; 292:1447,1494).

- Consider limit or selective screening and preventive care for other diseases based on overall prognosis and life expectancy (Jama 2000;283:3230).

Therapeutic: (Treat GuideL Med Lett 2007;5:9, European J Neurol 2007;14:e1)

- Memory aids (J Fam Pract 1993;37:6): gray matter increased w mental training (Nature 2004;427:311).
- Aricept but not Vit E slows progress of MCI in 1st yr (Nejm 2005;352:23).
- Sertraline for executive dysfunction (Arch Gen Psychiatry 1999;56:713; 2000;57:285; 2002;159:1119).
- Cholinesterase inhibitors: modestly helpful (Jags 2003; 57:5289; Neurol 2007;69:459); improvement in non-cognitive items: cooperation, delusions, pacing (Arch Neurol 1997;54:836; J Ger Psych Neurol 1996;9:1) also decreased behavorial problems (Jama 2003;289:210), increased word finding and memory of important names and events, improved ADLs; 20-30% pts treated demonstrated slowing of decline by 1 yr (Am Fam Phys 2002; 65:2525; Nejm 2003;348:2489, 2508); more likely to have clinically relevant response if mild to moderate dementia w relative preservation of language and praxis; reduces necessity of other psychotropic meds (Ann Long-Term Care 1998;6:92). Se: urge incontinence (Jags 2007; 55:800), wgt loss (Jags 2006;54:1013).
- Rivastigmine may also help w Lewy Body Dementia (Neurol 2000;54:A450). Modest improvement in severe cases (Lancet 2006;367:1031). Parkinsons (Nejm 2004;351:2509).
- Quetiapine, rivastigmine may not help agitation in end stage dementia (BMJ 2005;330:859). May increase agitation (BMJ 2005;330:874).
- Atypical antipsychotics no more likely to increase stroke risk than typical antipsychotics (BMJ 2005;26:3307; CNS Drugs 2005;19:91). Small increased risk of death (RR = 1.65% w all antipsychotics (Jama 2005;294:1934).

- Donepezil (Aricept) 5 mg po (Med Lett 1997;39:53; Neurol 1998;50:135; J Clin Psychiatry 1996;57:30), which may be increased to 10 mg after 4 wk; rivastigmine (Exelon) 1.5-6mg bid; gi side effects, eg, nausea, vomiting, dyspepsia, diarrhea, anorexia; myalgias (Clin Ger Med 2001;43:53); wgt loss, agitation, bradycardia; sick sinus syndrome, advanced pulmonary disease, bladder outflow problems; give in AM to avoid nightmares; helps for 6 mo-2 yr, 8-wk trial suggested helps w Parkinson's, Lewy Body Dementia and AD (Treat GuideL Med Lett 2007;5:9); not cost effective (Lancet 2004;363:2105; Neurol 2004;63:651); drug-drug interactions, CYP isoenzyme interactions (Med Lett 2000;7:28; 2000;42:93) probably not appropriate for NH setting (Jags 2003;50:1431); delay NH placement (Jags 2003;51:937); avoid meds w anticholinergic side effects like ranitidine (Jags 2004;52:2082); (galantamine, see mixed dementia/vascular dementia).
- Memantine (Namenda), NMDA antagonist, for advanced dementia (Nejm 2003;348:1333; Jama 2004;291:317); start with 5 mg qd, increase by 5 mg at weekly intervals to 10 mg bid; side effects dizziness, confusion, expensive (Med Lett 2003;345:73).
- New drug therapies being developed: pharmacologic interventions against the amyloid cascade or inhibitors of β-secretase which liberate β-lipoprotein (Ann IM 2003;138:400; Nejm 2004;351:56), neuroprotective agents, such as glutamate antagonists, antioxidants; huperzine A (a compound first isolated from traditional Chinese herbal medicine), a potent inhibitor acetylcholinesterase, may also protect neurons (Jama 1997; 277:276); injection of neurotrophic agents into ventricular system to retard neural degeneration (Nurs Home Med 1995; 3:3E), brain derived neurotropic factor (Cell 2003; 112:257).
- Vit E, up to 2000 IU qd previously thought to delay death, institutionalization, loss of ADLs, and progression of dementia; decreases cognitive decline (Arch Neurol 2002;59:1125) vs higher all-cause mortality at doses > 400 IU qd (Ann IM

Table 5.7 Medications for Agitated Demented Patients

Insomnia, Anxiety, Fear, Tension	Depressed Mood, Crying	Hostile, Assaultive, Psychotic
Benzodiazepine, oxazepam up to 10 mg qid, or propranolol up to 40 qid plus buspirone	Antidepressant, trazodone 25 mg up to 200 mg/d or SSRIs	Carbamazepine 25 tid mg to 400 mg/d (level = 7), or risperidone 0.5 mg or antipsychotic

Adapted from Royall DR, Polk M. Dementias that present with and without posterior cortical features: an important clinical distinction. J Am Ger Soc 1998;46:98-105.

PSYCHIATRY

2005;142:37) monoamine oxidase-B inhibitors, eg, selegiline 5 mg po bid may have neurotropic effects as well (Nejm 1997; 336:1216,1245; Science 1997;276:675; Neurol 2001;56:1154).

Ginkgo Biloba, modest improvements cognitive function without adverse effects, 6 mo-1 yr (Jama 1997;278:1327), but not a blinded study (Med Lett 1998;40:63); no benefit (Jama 2002;288:836); caution w ASA or anticoagulants.

Treatment of Dementia with Agitated Behavior: Antipsychotic drug uses: anti-aggressive effects of antipsychotics may take up to 8 wk to appear; pts w severe dementia do not respond as well; agitation may result from benzodiazepine withdrawal (Am J Hosp Pharm 1994;51:2917).

OBRA (Omibus Budget Reconciliation Act of 1987), Medicare-approved indications for antipsychotic drug use in NH: agitated psychotic sx=biting, kicking, scratching, or other aggressive behaviors presenting as danger to self or others; functional impairment caused by continuous (24 hr) crying out (Clin Ger 2007;15:12); psychotic sx of hallucinations, paranoia, or delusions; documentation of frequency and duration necessary (Fed Reg 1992; 57:4519).

Table 5.8 Psychotropic Agents Useful for the Treatment of Neuropsychiatric Symptoms and Behavioral Disturbances in Patients with Alzheimer's Disease

Drug	Initial Daily Dose	Final Daily Dose (Range)	Targeted Symptoms
Atypical antipsychotic			Psychosis and agitation
Risperidone	0.5 mg daily	1.0 mg (0.75-1.5 mg daily)	
Olanzapine	2.5 mg daily	5.0 mg (5-10 mg daily)	
Quetiapine	25 mg daily	200 mg (50-150 mg twice day)	
Ziprasidone	20 mg daily	40 mg (20-80 mg twice a day)	
Aripiprazole	10 mg daily	10 mg (10-30 mg daily)	
Neuroleptic			Psychosis and agitation
Haloperidol	0.25 mg daily	2 mg (1-3 mg daily)	
Mood stabilizer			Agitation
Divalproex sodium	125 mg twice a day	500 mg (250-500 mg twice a day)	
Carbamazepine	200 mg twice a day	400 mg (200-500 mg twice a day)	
Selective serotonin-reuptake inhibitor			Depression, anxiety, psychosis, and agitation
Citalopram	10 mg daily	20 mg (20-40 mg daily)	
Escitalopram	5 mg daily	10 mg (10-20 mg daily)	
Paroxetine	10 mg daily	20 mg (10-40 mg daily)	
Sertraline	25 mg daily	75 mg (75-100 mg daily)	
Fluoxetine	5 mg daily	10 mg (10-40 mg daily)	

Tricyclic antidepressant			Depression
Nortriptyline	10 mg daily	50 mg (25-100 mg daily)	
Desipramine	10 mg daily	100 mg (50-200 mg daily)	
Serotonin- and noradrenergic-reuptake inhibitor			Depression and anxiety
Venlafaxine	25 mg twice a day	200 mg (100-150 mg twice a day)	
Noradrenergic and specific serotonergic antidepressant			Depression
Mirtazapine	7.5 mg daily	15 mg (15-30 mg daily)	

Adapted with permission from Nejm 2004;351:56-67.

Table 5.9 Antipsychotic Drugs

Antipsychotic	Side-Effect Profile: Hypotension, Sedation, Anticholinergic	Side-Effect Profile: EPS
Mellaril ("my")	+++++	+
Thorazine ("troubles")	++++	++
Navane ("now")	+++	+++
Haldol ("have")	++	++++
Prolixin ("passed")	+	+++++

EPS = extrapyramidal syndrome.

First Choice Drugs for Dementia with Agitation—Atypical Antipsychotics (Am Fam Phys 2003;67:2335) Serotonin Dopamine Receptor Antagonists:

- *Risperidone* (Risperdal) (J Clin Psychiatry 2003;64:134): decreases neg (depression, social withdrawal, apathy), as well as pos sx (delusions, hallucinations, paranoia) of dementia with agitation and schizophrenia; diminishes depression through its antagonism of 5-HT_2 receptors (American Medical Directors Association 19th Annual Symposium, New Orleans, LA, March 7, 2005); not anticholinergic; less sedation at low doses; starting dose 0.25 mg qd or bid, w slow titration to maximum 1-1.5 mg qd decreases risk of hypotension (J Ger Psych Neurol 1995;8:159); some drug interactions; extrapyramidal side effects (EPS) dose-dependent. Side effects include: orthostatic hypotension, lowered seizure threshold, esophageal dysmotility and aspiration, somnolence, hyperglycemia, elevation of prolactin, weight gain, sexual dysfunction.
- *Olanzapine* (Zyprexa): serotonin-dopamine antagonist w few EPS, but side effect profile otherwise similar, possibly higher risk of hyperglycemia; 2.5-10 mg qd (30-hr half-life); start with

2.5 mg in NH pts (Nurs Home Med 1997;5:7F); double-blind trials support its use (Arch Gen Psychiatry 2000;57:968; 2001; 16:62); IM olanzapine (Neuropsychopharm 2002;26:494).

- *Quetiapine* (Seroquel) 25-400 mg/d, start at 25 bid and titrate gradually to lowest effective dose over several weeks; may be used for sexually inappropriate behavior (Jags 2000;48:707); sedating, orthostasis (Am Fam Phys 2002;65:2525), dyspepsia, weight gain; no EPS; does not induce p-450 enzyme, clearance induced by phenytoin and decreased by ketocoazole.
- *Ziprasidone* (Geodon) (J Psych Pract 2003;9:469).
- Atypical antipsychotics have been known to cause hyperglycemia (Clin Diabetes 2002;20:195).
- Most effective antipsychotics are risperidone and olanzapine (Jama 2005;293:596). All are expensive.
- *Older antipsychotics, phenothiazines:* rarely used since atypicals available, not recommended as first line. In order of increasing extrapyramidal and decreasing sedation/anticholinergic/hypotensive effects (Table 5.9): Mellaril (thioridazine), Thorazine (chlorpromazine), Navane (thiothixene), Haldol (haloperidol), Prolixin (fluphenazine)—mnemonic = "My Troubles Now Have Passed"; 20-25% dose used in younger person.
- Extrapyramidal side effects (EPS): acute dystonic reactions rare in the elderly (Consult Pharm 1992;7:921), treated w diphenhydramine (Benadryl); Parkinsonian signs treated w benztropine mesylate (Cogentin) or anticholinergic or amantadine for 3 mo or switching to lower-potency antipsychotic. Akathisia: 20% prevalence, anticholinergics not as effective at treating as benzodiazepines or β-blockers for effects on GABA (Am J Hosp Pharm 1991;48:1271); also treated w diazepam (Valium); tardive dyskinesia: prevalence as high as 40% and more severe w age (Jags 1987;35:233); 2 × as frequent in blacks as in whites. Increasing antipsychotic dose when this sx

first appears will eliminate it temporarily (supersensitization of dopaminergic receptors after prolonged receptor blockade, abnormal movements can paradoxically worsen when the dosage of the antipsychotic is first decreased). Anticholinergics often exacerbate it. Greatest risk during first 2 yr; adding lithium to antipsychotic may lead to neuroleptic malignant syndrome (NMS) (J Clin Psychopharmacol 1993;54:35); 5-40% tardive dyskinesia eventually remit.

- Orthostatic hypotension: blockade of β_1-receptors more common w low-potency antipsychotics, aliphatic phenothiazines and clozapine; weight gain also w these drugs.
- *Clozapine:* less extrapyramidal sx; no tardive dyskinesia, but causes agranulocytosis in 1-2% pts, which can be fatal; therefore, weekly monitoring and report agranulocytosis to national registry; older pts at greater risk for leukopenia, hypotension, and seizures; can continue med and rx seizures w valproic acid; average dose 37 mg/d; optimal duration of clozapine trial 6 wk-12 mo (J Ger Psych Neurol 1994;7:129; Med Lett Drugs Ther 1994;36:33; 1993;35:16; Drug Topics 1994;138:30; Am J Hlth Syst Pharmacol 1995;52:S9; Am J Ger Psychiatry 1995;3:26; Neurol 1994;44:2247; 1995;45:432; Can J Psychiatry 1995; 40:208) Clozapine significantly reduces gastric acid secretion, resulting in decrease in gastric ulcers (Am J Psych 1995; 152:821).
  - Clozapine overdose: somnolence, tachycardia, aspiration pneumonia, hypotension, seizures; no cases of agranulocytosis reported with overdose; death rare (J Emerg Med 1995; 13:199).
  - Clozapine drug interactions: clozapine and tricyclic antidepressant may produce delirium due to additive anticholinergic effects; cimetidine induced toxicity because of inhibition of cytochrome P-450. Kinetics: cleared mostly through he-

patic enzyme metabolism; start w 6.25 mg to avoid bradycardia (J Clin Psychiatry 1995;56:180).

Second Choice Drugs for Dementia with Agitation:

- *Mood stabilizers/anticonvulsants* (limbic kindling phenomena) (Am J Psych 1998;155:1512): valproic acid (500-1500 mg/d) and carbamazepine (300-600 mg qd); effective in rx of agitation, aggressiveness, impulsivity, and sexually inappropriate behaviors; monitor CBC and LFTs (J Clin Psychiatry 1990; 51:115); and monitor blood levels. Carbamazepine levels decreased by warfarin, theophylline, haloperidol, divalproex sodium, carbamazepine (auto induction); levels increased by macrolides, cimetidine, propoxyphene, INH, fluoxetine, Ca-channel blockers; valproic acid may reduce aggression, temper outbursts, and agitation (Am J Psych 1998;155:54); ASA may increase valproic acid levels, can cause diarrhea. Lamotrigine has fewer se, more effective than toprimate (Neurol 2005;64: 2108); vs mood stabilizers ineffective (Jama 2005;293:596).
- *Buspirone*, when given w antipsychotic drugs, decreases severity of tardive dyskinesia, improves akathisia and parkinsonism. Switching from benzodiazepine to buspirone: change short—or intermediate-acting benzodiazepine, eg, alprazolam (Xanax) to long-acting, eg, clonazepam (Klonopin), add azaperone 5-10 mg 3 × per d up to 30 mg/d; schedule taper of benzodiazepine over 60-90 d; takes 2-3 wk for azaperone to take effect (Am Fam Phys 1996;53:2349).
- *Trazadone* is beneficial in rx of sleep deprivation, aggression, and hostility (J Clin Psychiatry 1995;56:374); give hs because of hypotension.

Other Considerations for Behaviors Associated with Dementia:

- Benzodiazepines for anxiety but not for chronic use, eg, oxazepam (Serax) 10 mg po tid or lorazepam (Ativan) 0.5-2.0 mg/d in 2-3 divided doses; diminished effect after several months. Agitation can be a result of benzodiazepine withdrawal; clonazepam (long half-life) stimulates serotonin production and may lessen aggressive behavior, hyperactivity, social intrusiveness, and impulsivity.

- Propranolol 40-120 mg (Med Clin N Am 1994;78:814).
- Estrogen 0.625-1.25 mg qd for sexual aggression in elderly men (Jags 1991;31:1110); ethics of treatment questionable (Am J Psych 1981;138:5). Rx hypersexuality, paraphilias w SSRI—most safe; atypical antipsychotic or mood stabilizer, then consider antiandrogens or medroxyprogesterone (J Clin Psychiatry 1987;48:368; Ann Long-Term Care 1998;6:248), which causes sleepiness, mild DM, increased appetite and wgt gain, loss of hair, hot flashes, depression, decreased ejaculatory volume; estrogen risk of thromboembolism, vascular risk. GnRH analogues cause hot flashes, erectile dysfunction, decreased libido, and have to use continuously (Jags 99;47:231).

Team Management:

Table 5.10 Alzheimer Disease Assessment Tool

Group	MMSE Mean (±SD)	Characteristic Function and Cognitive Deficit	Approximate Age Function Acquired	Characteristic Function Preserved	Adjuvant Psychological Features	Major Treatment Concerns	Prognosis During 4-yr Follow-up
Forgetfulness (Stage I)	29.6 (±0.7)	None	—	All	None	—	—
Forgetfulness (Stage II)	28.9 (±1.3)	Subjective c/o word finding, forgetting familiar names, normal performance at work	Adult	No objective Memory deficit on clinical interview	Anxiety	Reassurance Treat anxiety	Most will not develop AD but only mild forgetfulness Predicted life expectancy in AD is 8-10 yr
Confusion Stage III	24.6 (±3.5)	Disorientation to time. Clear-cut memory and cognitive deficit Withdrawal from challenging situations (work)	Young adult	Normal ADL and IADL Routine activity well preserved Driving to familiar area	Anxiety Depression	Prevent conditions that increase anxiety Treat depression	80% deterioration in cognitive function Predicted life expectancy 6-8 yr

continues

PSYCHIATRY

Table 5.10 continued

Group	MMSE Mean (±SD)	Characteristic Function and Cognitive Deficit	Approximate Age Function Acquired	Characteristic Function Preserved	Adjuvant Psychological Features	Major Treatment Concerns	Prognosis During 4-yr Follow-up
		Word and name finding deficit					
Dementia Stage IV	20.0 (±3.8)	Disorientation to place Decreased ability to handle finances, perform complex tasks, and remember recent events Decreased driving ability: gets lost, unable to interpret signs	8 yr	Might be oriented ×2 Able to drive to familiar places Able to stay in the community	Denial Paranoid thoughts	Strategy to approach patient with denial Handling finances Use of a notebook as a memory aid Control driving location	25% in nursing home 25% remain in the community Predicted life expectancy 4-6 yr

Dementia Stage V	14.3 (±3.4)	Require assistance choosing attire Forget to bathe Not able to stay in community without assistance	5-7 yr	Able to dress Able to bathe alone	Agitation Reserved sleep patterns	Full home assistance Day care Prepare for long-term care facility	Most in nursing homes Persistent gradual deterioration Predicted life expectancy 3-4 yr
Dementia Stage VI	8.3 (±4.8)	Not remembering names of spouse, child	5 yr	Language impaired Walk with small steps	Violent psychosis, eg, hallucination	24-hr home help Nursing home Treatment for agitation and psychosis	Most will die or be in a nursing home
		Require assistance bathing	4 yr				
		Require assistance dressing	3 yr				
		Require assistance toileting Urinary incontinent Fecal incontinent	2 yr				

continues

PSYCHIATRY

Table 5.10 continued

Group	MMSE Mean (±SD)	Characteristic Function and Cognitive Deficit	Approximate Age Function Acquired	Characteristic Function Preserved	Adjuvant Psychological Features	Major Treatment Concerns	Prognosis During 4-yr Follow-up
Dementia Stage VII	0 (±0)	Dramatic deterioration in:		None	None	Soft food diet NG or PEG tube	14% will die from unknown etiology Possible due to defect in the regulation of vital sign, eg, respiratory function
		Speech activity	15 mo				
		Ambulation	12 mo				
		Sitting	8 mo				
		Smile	4 mo				
		Body posture/head	2 mo				
		Neurologic cortical signs					

MMSE = Mini-Mental State Exam; c/o = complains of; PEG = percutaneous endoscopic gastrostomy; AD = Alzheimer. From Am J Alzheimer Dis Rel Disord Res 1995;10:4.

Table 5.11 Behavior of Demented Patients During Late Stages (Usually in Nursing Home Setting)

Stage V/VII:
Usually placed in NH; aware of surroundings but not aware of their purpose; "all dressed up with nowhere to go"; very unhappy when have to interact w unkempt, aggressive patients; eg, stage VII patients; enjoy opportunity to look after needy cooperative patients (stage VI/VII).

Stage VI/VII:
Not sure where or who they are; need constant reassurance; "Velcro stage"; get along well w stage V/VII patients; like being led around by them; don't mind stage VII/VII patients; not aware enough to be bothered by them.

Stage VII/VII:
If still ambulatory, will follow retreating stimuli; they stop following people when others have stopped moving; tend to follow visitors out of the door of the NH, but are easily redirected.

From lecture by Lucero M, Lewiston, ME, 1994.

- Dementia goals of care: improve pt quality of life, decrease caregiver burden, delay in NH placement, achieve peaceful death (Jags 1998;46:782).
- Can assess caregiver burden w Zarit scale.
- Meeting w the family (Am Fam Phys 1984;29:149): important that pt be included in initial family meeting, may not remember content, but will remember being included and taken seriously.
- Encourage catharsis re (see Table 5.12): family's burden to explain or cover up Alzheimer secret; the family's loss of social roles and identities; violence from pt's catastrophic reactions; being accused of malevolent motives by the pt; guilt regarding reflex anger to physical abuse by pt; blaming themselves for pt's irritability and withdrawal; difficulties w having to constantly supervise pt.
- Facilitate learning of family re: differences between memory loss and attention deficit; stages of dementia; compliment family and pt for recognizing the problem and dispel myths (pt not

lazy, crazy; dementia is not caused by stress, vit deficiency, and not amenable to repetition; pts can still feel embarrassment and shame).

- Encourage caregivers to send letters to family members who are geographically separated, who may not have recognized subtle changes in the pt and who may think the primary caregiver is exaggerating the problem.
- Have family read Alzheimer material and return for a f/u without the pt: identify when guilt has led to self-sacrificing caregiver behaviors; acknowledge their fears for the future and support them in decisions they must make that may be unacceptable to their afflicted parent or spouse, eg, NH placement (explore cultural values and family conflicts).
- Help family draw up a day-to-day care plan for the pt that will provide a predictable environment and repeated reassurance; learn from family as much as possible about the successful approaches and accomplishments to this stage of disease; acknowledge importance of individualized approach for the pt and spouse and assure that care plan will integrate their prior work; create a "team" w family and health professionals; emphasize importance of family's continuing role.
- Encourage family to participate in support group, continue to meet their own individual needs; reinforce that they are developing expertise that is of value to the community at large; support political advocacy when it is suggested by the family.
- Behavioral management: look for precipitants of difficult behavior (what, where, why, when, who); reassurance and redirection effective, do not "reality orient" pts w cortical dementia, may result in "catastrophic reaction"; however, reality orientation and prompting very important techniques in subcortical dementias; otherwise pts may become depressed when caregivers assume pts are less capable than they are.
- Hallucinations, delusions = poor prognosis (Jags 1992;40:768); pts may often conceal so ask subtly: "How are you getting on

with other relatives? Neighbors? Are they annoying in any way? Are they deliberately trying to annoy you? Often when one is elderly, other people are unsympathetic—is that a problem?"

- Sundowning (increased confusion and agitation in the late afternoon secondary to disturbances in circadian rhythm and REM sleep, deterioration of suprachiasmatic nucleus of hypothalamus): restrict daytime sleep, expose to bright light during the day, low-stress activity schedules (J Psychol Nurs 1996;34:40; Acta Psychiatr Scand 1994;89:1), provide routine, be sure pt has glasses and functional hearing aid, avoid sedative hypnotics, place familiar objects on pt's bed or bedside to help ensure safety.
- Wandering: "goal-directed" (disguise exit signs, place stop signs), "aimless wandering" (provide more structure, investigate possible discomfort).
- Repetitive speech: group singing, reminiscing activities.
- Resistance to care: "Good cop, bad cop" intervention in which pt is rescued from purposely overbearing caregiver by gentler caregiver so that the pt will follow the second caregiver and perform a task he or she usually resists.
- Caregivers should be encouraged to recognize their own stress; "36-hr day;" providers may recommend adult day care center.
- In NH, wandering can also be managed by "wandering areas," posted signs, pictures of residents on resident room doors, tape barriers on floors and across doors, half-doors, coded locks.
- Screaming: hearing augmentation devices may prevent hard-of-hearing elderly from yelling (Nurs Home Med 1997;4:515; Jags 2003;52:143).
- Driving: score on MMSE and visual tracking can be used to stratify which cognitively impaired pts can drive safely (Clin Ger Med 1993;9:279; Jama 1995;273:1360; Jags 1997;45:949; 2004;52:143); not at night, not in traffic, but w someone else,

on familiar roads; take driver's test w copilot (Jags 1996;44:815); emphasize family's need to develop clear plan for driving cessation—a necessary eventual goal. Predictive of car accident: visual field testing, falling in past two weeks, poor near vision acuity, limited ROM of neck, visual attention (Jags 1998;46:556,562); mildly cognitively impaired individuals have as many car crashes as controls, but the accidents result in more injury and involve failure to yield (Jags 2000;48:18).

- Ethical considerations: if demented pts unable to carry out decisions and manage the consequences, the presumption in favor of maintaining autonomy may need to be reconsidered (Jags 1995;43:1437); 80% of elderly want to be told about their dx of Alzheimer's disease vs 92% want to be told of a terminal illness of medical origin (Jags 1996;44:404).
- Discussion w pt and family including advance directives (living will, Durable Power of Attorney for Health Care/Health Care Proxy) early on; refer to local Alzheimer's chapter (J Gerontol Nurs 1983;9:93). Discuss "do not resuscitate" (DNR) order; at later stage of disease, hospice; reassure that DNR does not mean "do not treat" (Clin Ger Med 1994;10:91); be certain to establish who is Health Care Proxy and family "communication tree" in crisis. Aim for acute illness care plan that is NH-centered as much as possible, emphasizing risk issues w hospitalization (worsening of cognition, disorientation, lack of understanding by hospital staff); consider orders for "do not hospitalize," "comfort focused care only," "no antibiotics" or "no artificial hydration"; consider goal of "life-enhancing rather than life-prolonging therapies"; tube feeding does not help prevent aspiration, and is risky (Nejm 2000;342:206; Jama 1999;282:1365).

Table 5.12 Phases of Family Adaptation to Alzheimer's Disease

Phase	Issue	Intervention
1. Predx	• Ambiguity, splitting–Mom's ok, I'm not ok • Break down taboos and talk about it to gather info	• Information/education
2. Dx	• Won't seek painful dx until crisis (part of family so may disengage) • Hard to accept dx if process sends them back to predx phase	• Families need to process together (1½ hours) • Keep pt. within family boundary who are going to tell–essential marker of acceptance–starting to organize
3. Role change	• Repeated losses as pt less like himself • Ambiguity about when and how to make major role transformation–eg, driving • Danger = loss of all expectation, pt becomes nonperson	• Change expectations rather than take away role–see the possibility in role–eg, co-driving • Relationship work with demented family member and family (couples work with demented wife and hard-of-hearing husband at age 80)
4. Chronic care giving	• 36-hr day for daughter-in-law while others critique or cheerlead (efficient but overwhelming)–fizzle	• Change boundaries–who can be counted on to help • Change of structure: Roles– Hands-on care Phone calls E-mail • Maintain family vitality normal family life–rituals like Thanksgiving and adolescent fights (conspiracy of happiness = a problem)
5. Shared care giving	• Services not a commodity. Home health means developing new relationships	• New relationships require that culture of caregiver meshes with family's basic values–eg, autonomy vs. safety

continues

Table 5.12 continued

Phase	Issue	Intervention
6. Long-term care	• Almost always traumatic (guilt/failure/marginalized)	• Nurses look so proficient that family may react by checking out or be critical of care • Families need a role + NH expectations of them or else they become a nonentity [Hx and biography providers] • Families need to be partners, not consumers, need collaborative atmosphere (Jama 2004;292:961)
7. End of life	• Ambivalence, relief, guilt, conflict	• Anticipate death early–talk about the good death (pt comfortable, family around, generativity) so family can move along smoothly and with legitimacy • Life review –Feel as though pt that died is still present –Family emerges whole

Adapted from AMDA Lecture, March 5, 1999, Orlando, Florida. Wayne Caron, PhD & James Pattee, MD, CMD.

5.6 Normal-Pressure Hydrocephalus

Nejm 1985;312:1255; Jama 1996;44:445

Cause: Idiopathic, postsurgical, trauma, subarachnoid hemorrhage, infectious meningitis, small-vessel disease.

Pathophys: A "communicating hydrocephalus" (in contrast to foraminal or aqueductal), and obstruction is therefore at cisterna; hence, 4th ventricle may dilate causing cerebellar compression.

Sx: First, trouble walking (ataxia with initiation and spasticity in lower extremity, leading to "magnetic gait," feet grip floor, only lifted with difficulty), progressive dementia and incontinence. Dementia includes psychomotor slowing, impaired ability to concentrate, mild memory difficulties.

Si: Horizontal nystagmus, normal disks, spasticity, frontal lobe signs.

Crs: Progressive dementia.

Lab:

- CSF: transient, but consistent improvement with removal of 50 mL (Acta Neurol Scand 1987;75:566); some neurosurgeons now not doing shunt unless improvement with this first. Miller Fisher test: objective gait assessments before and after removal 30 mL CSF (Acta Neurol Scand 1986;73:566).

X-ray: CT scan shows enlarged ventricles (100%); cisternogram shows delayed or no movement of dye out over hemispheres, but there are false-neg results.

Rx: Surgical shunt, 80% success (Nejm 1985;312:1255).

Cmplc: Infections in 3%-5%; factors associated with pos outcomes from shunting: short duration, known cause (trauma, hemorrhage), gait disturbance before onset of dementia or incontinence, presence of high-amplitude waves on intracranial pressure monitoring (Jama 1996;44:445).

PSYCHIATRY

5.7 Vascular Dementias

Cause:

1. Multiple subcortical (lacunar) or cortical infarctions, multi-infarct dementia (MID).
2. Ischemic demyelinization of subcortical white matter—Binswanger's disease—clinical picture similar to MID.
3. Single infarction; stroke does not always lead to dementia (J Neurol Sci 1968;7:331); generally takes large amount brain tissue destruction (J Neurol Sci 1970;11:205).

Epidem:

Estimates of Prevalence Vary:

- 15% of all postmortem diagnosed dementias are vascular dementias; more common in blacks, Japanese (Neurol 1995; 45:1161); MID overdiagnosed, needs more neuropathic correlation (Neurol 1993;43:243); stroke frequently coexists w Alzheimer's or Parkinson's dementia (Arch Neurol 1989; 46:651); estimated number of vascular dementias inflated when Hachinski index (point system based on presence of neurologic and atherosclerotic disease) used (47-60%) (Nejm 1993;328:153).
- 50% of community-dwelling demented elderly have vascular dementia (Nejm 1993;328:153)

Pathophys: Amyloid deposits in walls of small cerebral blood vessels.

Sx: Subcortical infarctions (basal ganglia, internal capsule, thalamus): slowness, forgetfulness, apathy, executive skill deficit; depression and anxiety more severe in pts w vascular dementia than in Alzheimer's.

Si: Need temporal relationship between stroke and dementia to make dx vascular dementia (Neurol 1992;42:473; 1993;43:250; Nejm 1993;328:153); 10-20% are mixed.

Erkinjuntti criteria for vascular dementia (NINDS-AIREN, Fortschr Neurol Psychiatrie 1994;62:197):

1. Focal neurologic signs + imaging findings: multiple lacunae (multiple motor and sensory deficits, rigidity, extrapyramidal signs, pseudobulbar palsy), extensive white matter lesions, multiple large-vessel infarcts strategically placed (angular gyrus, thalamus, basal forebrain, bilateral infarcts, left hemisphere infarcts).
2. Neurologic deficit and confusion occur within 3 mo of each other.
3. Step-wise progression: unknown dx utility of a h/o "step-wise progression," eg, episodic behavioral complications of

Alzheimer's, eg, UTI may cause deterioration in behavior (Am J Psych 1990;147:435).

Crs: Mortality from vascular dementia is higher; as more older people have strokes and survive, prevalence will increase; decline in ADL in subcortical vascular dementia predicted by age, ETOH, lack of coordination, snout reflex (Jama 2002;50:1969).

Lab:

X-ray: CT: lacunar infarcts 50% of time w MID; MRI: Binswanger's: confluent deep white matter hyper intensities, periventricular white matter lesions (in nl aging, too); central atrophy, 3rd ventricle enlargement marker for vascular dementia (Neurol 1995;45:1456).

Rx: (HMS course *Dementia* 6/5/08: *Vascular Dementia*, Viswanathan, A.)

Preventive: Prevent and postpone atheromatosis and embolization through dietary changes and smoking cessation, ASA, unknown effectiveness of pentoxifylline, ticlopidine. HT control may actually reverse cognitive impairment by treating preexisting HT (Jags 1996;44:411); β-blockers better than Ca-channel blockers and diuretics, resulting in better MMSE score and improved white matter findings on MRI (Jags 1997;45:1423). DM, Afib management (Nejm 1993;328:153), anticoagulants; metabolic enhancing agents have not produced consistent benefits.

Mixed dementias: Galantamine (Lancet 2002;359:1283; Jama 2004;292:2908), Rivastigmine (Eur J Neurol 2000;7:159), Memantine (Nejm 2003;348:1333; Jama 2004;291:317; Stroke 2002;33:1834) modest benefits in functional cognitive outcome.

5.8 Schizophrenia of Old Age (Paraphrenia)

Nurs Home Med 1995;3:248; Jags 1980;8:193; Schizophr Bull 1993;19:701,817

Cause: Sensory impairment debatable.

Epidem: Higher % of new-onset schizophrenia-like psychoses in NH pts; $^{2}/_{3}$ of early-onset schizophrenic pts are left w mild symptoms by old age; M/F = 1:10 in elderly.

Pathophys: Lesions in dorsal lateral prefrontal cortex, superior temporal gyrus, hippocampus, basal ganglia.

Sx: Pos or neg sx lasting for more than 6 mo. Pos: delusions, hallucinations, distorted language and communication patterns, disorganized or catatonic behavior. Neg: restriction in range and intensity of emotional expression, changes in fluency and productivity of thought and speech, changes in initiative. Five categories: paranoid, disorganized, catatonic, undifferentiated, residual type. Risk factors associated with schizoid premorbid personality, few surviving children, deafness, low socioeconomic class, female.

Si: Difficulty focusing attention, formulating concepts, slowing in reaction time; cognitive impairments in memory and construction typical of Alzheimer's dementia not usual w paraphrenia.

Crs: Paranoid delusions w or w/o hallucinations, usually with preservation of personality and affective response; catatonia—may see in schizophrenia as well as bipolar disorder, neurological infections, head trauma, cerebrovascular disease, seizure disorder, hepatic failure, drug abuse (Clin Gerontol 2003;11:26).

Cmplc: R/o dementia, intracranial masses, thyroid disease, infections, liver disease, substance abuse, NPH, delirium, mania, depression.

Lab:

X-ray: CT, MRI: ventricular enlargement, cortical prominence, decreased temporal and hippocampal size, increased basal ganglia size; 5-10% have lesions due to stroke.

Rx:

Therapeutic: Responsiveness to antipsychotics may be more favorable than in younger schizophrenics; risperidone 0.25-1 mg qd, divided bid; quietapine, 25-800 mg qd, divided bid-tid; olanzapine 2.5-10 mg qd.

Team Management:

Nursing Home: Make sure to obtain psychiatric records (should be a requirement for admission); identify antipsychotics taken in past, especially in last month; refer to Alzheimer's management.

PSYCHIATRY

Chapter 6

Infection

6.1 Lung

Pneumonia

Nejm 2001;344:665; 2002;347:2039

Cause: Community acquired: often more than one pathogen; streptococcal pneumonia still most common; tbc in pts > 60 yr old often with co-pathogens: *Streptococcus pneumoniae*, *Staphylococcus aureus*, *Haemophilus influenzae*, aerobic gram-neg bacilli, aerobes and anaerobes (aspiration), *Moraxella catarrhalis*, *Legionella pneumophila*.

NH-acquired organisms of aspiration: *S. pneumoniae*, *Klebsiella pneumoniae*, *S. aureus*, *H. influenzae*, *Escherichia coli*, *M. catarrhalis*, *Mycobacterium tuberculosis*; *Chlamydia pneumoniae* cause of rapid spread of respiratory infection (Jama 1997;277:1214).

Hospital-acquired infection: aerobic gram-neg including periodontal: *Pseudomonas aeruginosa*, *S. pneumonia*, *S. aureus*, *H. influenzae*, *Legionella* (Am Rev Respir Dis 1993;148:14118); *S. aureus* and *S. pneumoniae* most common co-pathogens with influenza.

Epidem: Pneumonia is the leading cause of death from infectious disease in the elderly (Geriatrics 1991;46:25); 11% pneumonia cases, but 85% pneumonia deaths in pts > 65 yr old (Mmwr 1991;40:7); age alone doubles risk of complications and death;

INFECTION

risk increases w each additional comorbid factor, especially CHF, COPD (Am J Med 1990;88:1N; Ann IM 1991;115:428); increase risk w use of gastric acid suppression rx because reduction gastric acid secretion facilitates oral infection (Jama 2004;292:1955).

Pathophys: Age-related changes: decreased immunity, decreased cough and gag reflexes, decreased ciliary activity, increased colonization with resistant gram-neg organisms; comorbid diseases (stroke, etc) affect ability to swallow and increase risk of aspiration pneumonia; 25% of all clinically septic pts (not just from pneumonia) are afebrile due to modified IL-1 response, hypothalamic alterations.

Sx: Shaking chill, fever, cough; decreased function (including cognition), falls, anorexia, 10% no symptoms; < 35% typical presentation (Jags 1989;37:867); 50% of febrile geriatric pts presenting to ER w no other physical si have serious illness, including pneumonia.

Si: Rhonchi, rales, tachypnea; confusion (33% in community-acquired pneumonia vs 53% in NH) (Jags 1986;34:697), tachypnea, dehydration, decreased function, anorexia, worsening of preexisting CHF or COPD (Jama 2006;295:2503).

Crs: Dx may be delayed with "atypical presentation"; this and comorbidity may contribute to longer course of illness, longer hospitalization in the elderly; predictors 30-d mortality in NH: neoplasia, change mental status, RR > 30, syst BP < 90, pH < 7.35, BUN > 10.7, BS < 130.

Cmplc: Delayed resolution, bacteremia (40% mortality), death, mixed infections; r/o other infections, COPD, pulmonary embolus (PE), malignancy, drug reactions, myelodysplastic syndrome.

Lab:

- CBC—important to compare w WBC baseline but be aware 20-40% of all septic pts do not develop leukocytosis (Ger Rv Syllabus 1996;264).

- Electrolytes
- Oxygen saturation (use early and often in NH) to assess severity. If requiring hospital admission, then consider ABGs, blood culture, sputum Gram stain and culture (often impossible to obtain adequate sample; < 50% can produce dx specimen) (Am J Med 1990;88:1N; Jags 1989;37:867).
- Urinary antigen for *legionella;* thoracentesis with stain and culture if significant pleural fluid present (Post Grad Med 1996;99).
- EKG
- Comorbidities predictive: > 85 yr old w Cr > 1.5, < 90 BP, > 110 P (GRS 2002-2004:308).

X-ray: Chest film with infiltrate, though may not be obvious in setting of chronic lung changes.

Rx: Florquinolone if COPD FEV1 < 30% predicted, covers resistant *S. pneumonia*, Gram-neg. *legionella*. Side effects include wide QT, dizziness.

INFECTION

Table 6.1 Treatment of Pneumonia

1. *Route (PO or IM) of Initial Therapy:* Treatment with a parenteral (im) agent Should be considered if: a. there is no response to an oral agent b. vital signs are abnormal c. resident has an acutely altered mental status and is unable to take oral medications (tube feeding not available) 2. *Choice of Parenteral Agent:* Ceftriaxone 500-1000 mg im qd or Cefotaxime 500 mg im q 12 hr In the penicillin allergic pt the type of hypersensitivity (rash, hives) should be considered in making a treatment decision	1. *Choice of Empiric Therapy:* Ceftrixone 500-1000 mg iv qd Cefotaxime 500 mg iv q 8-12 hr Ampicillin/sulbactam 1.5 gm iv q 6-8 hr Cefuroxime 750 mg iv q 8 hr In the penicillin allergic pt the type of hypersensitivity (rash, hives) should be considered in making a treatment decision. An alternative to consider is Levofloxacin 500 mg iv qd *iv erythromycin should be avoided because of the adverse effects such as pain and phlebitis and increasing resistance of pneumococci to macrolides.*	Common organisms Streptococcus pneumonia Haemophilus influenza
3. *Timing of Switch to an Oral Agent:* Residents given im treatment should be switched to an oral agent when they achieve: Clinical stability. In most (75%) residents this will occur on d 3-5 of treatment. Clinical stability is defined as all of the	Antipneumococci florquinolone (Levoquin 500/d) β-Lactam-β lactamase inhibitor plus macrolide Timentin & Zithromax 1.5-3.0 gm q 6 hr 500/d	Atypical pathogens Mycoplasma pneumonia Legionella species Chlamydia pneumonia

following being present: a. improvement in si/sx b. afebrile (< 100.5°F) for ≥ 16 hr c. no acute cardiac or other life-threatening event in the first 3 d of rx d. resident is able to take oral med 4. *Oral Antibiotic Regimens:* Amoxicillin Amoxicillin/clavulanate 2nd or 3rd generation cephalosporin po in the penicillin allergic pt, Levofloxacin 500 mg po qd can be prescribed 5. *Duration of Therapy:* 7-10 d 6. Discontinue when T < 100°F, RR < 24, HR < 100, SPB ≥ 90, Sat ≥ 90%, Baseline COPD × 24°	ICU 3rd gen cephalosporin + antipneumococci florquinolone (Ceftriaxone & Levoquin) –at risk P. aeruginosa antipseudomonal β-lactam-β lactamase inhibitor plus florquinolone piperacillin-tazobactam 3.375 q 6 hr + levoquin –Aspiration Pneumonia: Ceftriaxone 1-2 gm or Levofloxacin 500 –Severe periodontal: ceftriaxone 600 q 8 hr + clinda or flagl 500 q 8 hr 2. *Timing of Switch to an Oral Agent:* When the resident achieves clinical Stability (d 4-6), switch to an oral agent: Amoxicillin Amoxicillin/clavulanate 2nd or 3rd generation oral cephalosporin 3. *Duration of Therapy:* 7-14 d	Same + Staphylococcus aureus, Drug-resistant S. pneumonia Other gram negatives

About 66% will require hospitalization; may be able to avoid hospital with risks of delirium, depression, and nosocomial infection if there is adequate NH or home care and the pt is hemodynamically stable. In some cases, the elderly and their families elect to have no hospital care. Consult advance directives for rx guidance; antibiotics, initially empiric broad-spectrum and then treat appropriate organism if becomes known; oxygen if indicated by decreased O_2 saturation or by clinical respiratory distress.

Prevention: Influenza vaccine annually; pneumonia vaccine q 6 yr, more compliance when pneumonia vaccine given w flu vaccine (Jags 2004;53:25); ginseng (CVT-E002) prevents acute respiratory illness (Jags 2004;52:13), vit E 200 IU prevents URIs in elderly (Jama 2004;292:828).

Therapeutic: See Table 6.1.

- Oral outpatient or NH regimens include erythromycin, azithromycin, clarithromycin, amoxicillin-clavulanic acid, TMP/SMZ, or a 2nd or 3rd generation cephalosporin or TMP/SMZ (up to 24% *S. pneumoniae* resistance).
- If hypoxic, serious underlying illness, or lives alone, cover *S. aureus* and Gram-neg bacilli w iv ceftriaxone or im in NH pts w no iv access, along with oral or iv erythromycin or azithromycin for initial broad coverage. Clindamycin is used when suspicion of anaerobic organisms is high.
- Hospital-acquired infection: iv β-lactam-β-lactamase inhibitor combination, or 3rd generation cephalosporin and clindamycin or piperacillin.
- *S. pneumoniae* sensitivities: 100%: vancomycin; 99.2%: ceftriaxone, doxycycline, levofloxacin; 94%: imipenem; 98.8%: erythromycin; 97.2%: ofloxacin; 96.2%: ciprofloxacin; 95%: cefuroxime; by 1994 increasing resistance developed including against penicillin (14%), ceftazidime (12%), and TMP/SMZ (24%) (Jama 1996;275:194; Nejm 1996;335:1445). If

pseudomonas endemic NH, use ceftazidime; if not, ceftriaxone (Ann Long-Term Care 1998;6:7).

Team Management: Caregiver awareness of baseline to recognize changes; community and institutional efforts to provide appropriate vaccinations and chemoprophylaxis for influenza and pneumonia; use acute crisis to focus future advance directive discussions, particularly w NH pts.

Influenza

Ann Long-Term Care 2003;11:46; Med Lett 2002;44:75; Infections in the Elderly. P. Kamitsuka at Harvard Geriatric Rv Course, April 2004; Am Fam Phys 2001;63:257; Nejm 2001;345:1318; 2000; 343:1778, Jama 2008;299:1127.

Cause: Influenza virus, types A, B, C.

Epidem: Worldwide, 90% of deaths associated with influenza are among those > 65 yr old.

Pathophys: RNA single-stranded viruses spread by respiratory droplets.

Sx: Cough, fever, malaise, sore throat, aches.

Si: Cough; geriatric: exacerbation of cardiopulmonary or chronic illness, changes in behavior/cognition.

Crs: Incubation time only 1-2 d, symptoms usually last 5-6 d, malaise up to 2 wk.

Cmplc: R/o RSV (death less than Influenza A but not more than B (Jama 2003;289:179). Primary influenza pneumonia, secondary bacterial pneumonia, and exacerbation of cardiopulmonary and other chronic illnesses result in increased hospitalization and death.

Lab: Serology on first few cases to establish the type and strain of an outbreak; QuickVue (immunoassay that uses monoclonal antibodies to detect viral nucleoprotein) easiest and fastest test for

INFECTION

rapid diagnosis of influenza A and B; however, neg tests do not exclude influenza (Med Lett 1999;41:121).

X-ray: Chest film if secondary pneumonia suspected (threshold should be low to x-ray).

Rx:

Prevention:

- Influenza vaccine annually for those > 65 and/or working, or living in institutional settings, or in elderly community (Ann IM 1995;123:518; Jama 2004;292:2089); each trivalent influenza vaccine usually includes two inactivated A strains and one B strain chosen each year based on strains from the previous season; new vaccine combination is required each year because of ongoing change (antigenic drift). High dose flu vaccine increases antibody response (Arch IM 2006;106:1121).
- Pneumococcal vaccine should be given every 6 yr to those > 65 yr old and should decrease incidence of secondary bacterial pneumonia; may give pneumococcal vaccine at the same time as influenza vaccine without problems.
- Flu vaccine better at preventing death due to influenza (Arch IM 2007;167:53) in NHs, influenza vaccination prevents an estimated 50-60% of hospitalizations and pneumonia and 80% of deaths; some elderly antibodies fall below protective levels in 4 mo (Med Lett 2002;44:75). Influenza vaccine can decrease the hepatic metabolism of drugs, including theophylline and warfarin by 50% for up to a wk. For those with contraindications to influenza vaccine (allergy to eggs or other vaccine components) use amantadine or rimantadine prophylactically during peak influenza season.
- Start amantadine or rimantadine at first indication of influenza A outbreak in NH, for at least a 2-wk course or until 1 wk after the outbreak is over; this prophylaxis decreases the infection rate of influenza A by 70-80%. Oseltamivir 75 mg qod for elderly w Cr Cl 10-30 ml/min, expensive (Am Fam Phys 2003;67:111).

Therapeutic: Approach to fever in NH: fever > 100° F for all infections, including influenza (Jags 1996;44:74); antiviral resistant strains have emerged and can be shed as soon as the end of one rx course; dosages for those > 65 are the same for prophylaxis and rx:

- Amantadine 100 mg po qd for those with Cr clearance > 50; adjust as per package insert for Cr clearance < 50.
- Rimantadine 200 mg po qd, 100 mg po qd for Cr clearance < 10 or liver disease; observe carefully and decrease dose if CNS side effects noted; may increase seizure activity.
- Neuroaminidase inhibitors: inhaled zanamivir (Jama 1999; 282:31) or oral oseltamivir 75 mg bid × 5 d started within 30 hr after onset of influenza can shorten duration of sx and possibly decrease incidence of complications, Oseltamivir assoc w nausea, vomiting, headache (Med Lett 2002;44:75), but zanamivir associated with bronchospasm in pts with underlying lung disease (Jama 2000;284:2847; Jags 2002;52:608); neither a substitute for vaccination (Med Lett 1999;41:91). Zanamivir better than Rimatidine for control of flu in highly vaccinated NH population (Jamda 2005;6:359).

Pulmonary Tuberculosis

MacLennan WJ, Infection in the Elderly. Boston: Little, Brown 1995; Am Fam Phys 2000;61:2673

Cause: Reactivation, cross-infection in NH.

Epidem: 8% conversion rate in 2.5 yr in NH (Nejm 1985;312:1483); more at risk for reactivation w DM, alcoholism, smoking, cancer, partial gastrectomy, corticosteroids.

Pathophys: Inhaled droplets deposited in alveoli, replicate slowly, spread to regional lymph nodes, then hematogenous spread. May have bronchopneumonia w initial infection, but more often pts develop asx nodule (Gohn complex). Tbc reactivation occurs at sites w high oxygen concentration (upper lobes) because tbc is an obligate aerobe, but mid and lower lobes can be involved in NH pts.

Sx: May not have fever or night sweats; wgt loss, cough, shortness of breath more common; extrapulmonary sx include mental status changes, back, abdominal pain.

Si: Pleural effusion.

Crs: ARDS if miliary spread occurs; segmental atelectasis upper lobe; involvement of lingula or middle lobe can be mistaken for tumor.

Complc: 10% of primary infections may progress to chronic tbc or death (ascribed to antibiotic-unresponsive pneumonia); dissemination bone marrow, liver, gu tract, bone (spine = Pott's disease).

Lab: PPD is negative in active tbc 10-15%; polymorphonuclear leukocytosis, normocytic anemia, elevated ESR; examine 3 sputum samples for AFB, may take up to 12 wk to grow on culture medium (may be inhibited by ciprofloxacin, gentamicin, and amoxicillin-clavulanate, aka Augmentin). Ribosomal DNA/RNA in sputum if have clinical suspicion w negative AFB; pleural effusions may not reveal organisms.

X-ray: Delayed resolution of supposed bacterial infiltrate; classic findings of apical cavitary lesions less common; opacities of middle and upper lobes in isolation or w apical lesions more common; cavitation less common because of decreased cellular immunity.

Rx:

Preventive: See screening Infection Control, Tuberculosis (p 75–76)

Therapeutic: Treat NH residents w INH (300 mg/d) and rifampin (600 mg/d) for 9 mo because no multidrug resistance; drug therapy (INH + rifampin + pyrazinamide) reduces rx duration from 9 to 6 mo:

- INH (300 mg): 5% develop hepatitis; 100 mg pyridoxine to avoid peripheral neuropathy; multiple drug interactions; do not give acetaminophen concurrently.
- Rifampin (450 mg if pt < 50 kg or 600 if pt > 50 kg): 3% hepatitis; 8% hepatitis when taken in combination w INH; skin rash, gi sx; thrombocytopenia (uncommon); optic neuritis; induces hepatic microenzymes.
- Ethambutol (15 mg/kg): modify dosage in renal impairment to avoid retrobulbar neuritis (reduced visual acuity, scotomata, red/green color blindness); good synergistic action w rifampin against resistant mycobacteria.
- Pyrazinamide (1.5 gm if < 50 kg or 2 gm if > 50 kg): 2-6% hepatitis (dose-related), arthralgia, anorexia, nausea, photosensitivity, gout.
- Streptomycin: high toxicity (vestibular, renal).
- Treat in hospital until smear is neg.
- New therapies being developed: compounds that can inactivate enzyme isocitrate lyase, critical in protecting M. *tuberculosis* against macrophage attack (Nature 2000;289:1123; 2000; 406:683).

6.2 Heart

Endocarditis

Jama 1995;274:1706

Cause: Etiology of septicemia found in < 50% of pts; prosthetic valves; pacemakers; S. *aureus* can cause disease in a preexisting healthy valve.

Epidem: More than one-half of pts w endocarditis are elderly because they have more prosthetic valves, hospital-acquired bacteremia, rheumatic valvular lesions.

Pathophys: Alteration in endothelial surface, deposition platelets and fibrin, *vegetation where there is increased turbulence; Streptococcus*

25-70%; *Streptococcus bovis* 25% (associated w gi malignancy, especially colon cancer); *Staphylococcus* 20-30%; *Enterococcus* from gu, 25%; *Streptococcus viridans* less common than in younger pts; culture neg 10-20%.

Sx: Aortic and mitral valve regurgitation most common, heart failure, systemic embolism, cerebral embolism (25% of time presenting as acute confusional state).

Si: Suspect in pts w pyrexia, high ESR, CHF, peripheral emboli, vaguely unwell after recent gi or gu procedure, changing cardiac murmur; still suspect w pos blood cultures despite no heart murmur; may see splenomegaly w *S. viridans;* Janeway's lesions on palms and soles and Roth's spots on fundi indicative of emboli; immune complexes produce Osler's nodes, arthralgias, finger clubbing, petechiae, glomerulonephritis, hematuria.

Crs: 50% mortality.

Cmplc: R/o myocardial abscess if ESR does not normalize w rx, w LBBB, or w progressive lengthening of PR interval.

Lab: Three blood cultures separated in time establish cause in 95% of pts; *S. viridans* (30-45%); assoc w dental procedure, not all penicillin-sens; *Staphylococcus* (10-30%) coagulase-neg associated w prosthetic valves, better px than with *S. aureus;* other streptococci (10-15%) include *Enterococci* (*S. bovis*).

- Associated w colon cancer and diverticulosis, gu manipulation in men, varying resistance.
- ESR > 100 mm/hr, elevated C-reactive protein, 50% positive rheumatoid factor and positive ANA, normochromic normocytic anemia, elevated wbc.

Noninvasive: Echocardiography (transthoracic and transesophageal): vegetations on prosthetic valves, septal or annular abscess; two-dimensional echocardiography allows evaluation of chamber size and serial evaluations can be done if worsening valve dysfunction; if neg and still suspect clinically, recheck echocardiogram.

Rx:

Preventive: For pts w cardiac disorders: highest risk w prosthetic valves, previous infective endocarditis, aortic regurgitation, aortic stenosis, mitral stenosis and regurgitation, s/p intracardiac surgery w residual hemodynamic abnormality (Nejm 1995;332:38; Med Lett 1999;41:75, Am Fam Phys 2008;77:538).

- For procedures involving mouth or respiratory tract: amoxicillin 2-3 gm po 1 hr before procedure (Jama 1997;277:1794; GFT 2005:161).
- Manipulation of gu or gi tract (*Enterococcus*): 1 gm ampicillin and 1.5 mg/kg (not to exceed 120 mg) gentamicin iv 1 hr before procedure and 6 hr later (Jama 1997;277:1794); ampicillin 1 gm im/iv or amoxicillin 1 gm po; if penicillin-allergic, substitute 1 gm vancomycin.
- Prevent hospital-acquired infection.
- Prophylax Prosthetic valves (*Staphylococcus*): use regimen for *Enterococcus*.

Therapeutic (Table 6.2): Require doses that reach bactericidal concentrations; EKG to follow clinical course; surgery may be needed if worsening CHF, embolism, cardiac abscess, vegetations > 10 mm or fungal infection. Valve replacement delayed until residual infection of valve annulus, adjacent structures reduced; anticoagulation not much help.

Table 6.2 Medical Treatment for Endocarditis

Infectious Agent	Drug	Dosage	Duration
PCN-susceptible Strep. viridans or other Strep. (MIC < = 0.1 mu G/ML)	PCN G aqueous (preferred in the elderly)	12-18 million U iv/24 hr continuously or divided q 4 hr	4 wks
	OR		
	Ceftriaxone	2 gm/day iv or im	4 wks
PCN allergic	Vancomycin	30 mg/kg per 24 hr iv in 2 doses (do not exceed 2 gm/24 hr)	4 wks
Strep. Viridans, other strep. (MIC > = 0.1)	PCN G aqueous PLUS	18-30 million U iv/24 hr continuously or divided q 4 hr	4 wks
	Gentamicin* (use w/caution in elderly)	1 mg/kg im or iv q 8 hr	2 wks
β-lactam allergy	Vancomycin	30 mg/kg per 24 hr iv in 2 doses (do not exceed 2 gm/24 hr)	4 wks
Enterococci	PCN G aqueous PLUS	18-30 million U iv/24 hr continuously or divided q 4 hr	4-6 wks
Screen all enterococci endocarditis for antibiotic resistance.	Gentamicin	1 mg/kg im or iv q 8 hr	4-6 wks
	OR		
	Ampicillin PLUS	12 gm iv/24 hr continuously or divided q 4 hr	4-6 wks
	Gentamicin	as above	
B-lactam allergy	Vancomycin PLUS	as above	4-6 wks
	Gentamicin	as above	4-6 wks

Staphylococci, no prosthetic material	Nafcillin or oxacillin PLUS (optional)	2 gm iv q 4 hr	4-6 wks
	Gentamicin	1 mg/kg im or iv q 8 hr	3-5 d
PCN allergy	Vancomycin	30 mg/kg per 24 hr iv in 2 doses (do not exceed 2 gm/24 hr)	4-6 wks
MRSA	Vancomycin	as above	4-6 wks
Staphylococci, with prosthetic material	Nafcillin or oxacillin PLUS	2 gm iv q 4 hr	6-8 wks
(Prosthetic material may need to be removed or replaced)	Rifampin PLUS	300 mg po q 8 hr	6-8 wks
	Gentamicin	1 mg/kg im or iv q 8 hr **(followed by FQ + Rifampin p.o. × 3-6 mo if valve is maintained in place)**	2 wks
MRSA	Vancomycin PLUS	30 mg/kg per 24 hr iv in 2 doses (do not exceed 2 gm/24 hr)	6-8 wks
	Rifampin PLUS	300 mg po q 8 hr	
	Gentamicin	1 mg/kg im or iv q 8 hr	2 wks
HACEK microbes	Ceftriaxone	2 gm iv or im/d	4 wks

*Age over 65 is a relative contraindication for use of gentamicin.
Jama 1995;274:1706; Sci Am Med 1999; 7:XVIII; GRS 2004, p. 312.

6.3 Bones and Joints

Osteomyelitis/Septic Arthritis/Joint Prosthesis Infection

MacLennan WJ, Infection in Elderly Patients. London/Boston: E. Arnold/Little Brown 1994. Little Brown 1995; Nejm 1997;336:999

Cause:

- Septic arthritis: chronic septic arthritis most often caused by *Staphylococcus*.
- Joint prosthesis infection: *Staphylococcus*, Gram-neg, anaerobes.

Epidem:

- Septic arthritis: 25-33% in pts > 60 yr old; impaired immune system; preexisting joint disease, eg, osteoarthritis and RA; *Staphylococcus*, *Streptococcus*, Gram-neg bacteria; hematogenous spread from UTI, cellulitis, endocarditis, *Salmonella* bowel infections; predisposing factors: malnutrition, diabetes, chronic renal failure, hepatic cirrhosis, malignancy, alcoholism, corticosteroids.
- Joint prosthesis infection: 1-2%, hematogenous spread from surgery; sources: gums, gi tract, gu tract.

Sx:

- Septic arthritis: tenderness, redness, warmth; diabetics may not have pain or pyrexia; may only see uncontrolled blood glucose; normocytic normochromic anemia.
- Chronic septic arthritis: may not have pyrexia or tachycardia.

Si: Osteomyelitis: foot: metatarsal heads, proximal phalanges; close to ulcer discharging pus from a sinus; erythema and swelling over infected bone; fluctuant swelling; painful limitation of active and passive movement; usually febrile; difficult to diagnose w preexisting joint disease; masked in sternoclavicular, sacroiliac, hips and shoulder joints.

Cmplc: Septic arthritis: osteomyelitis in adjacent bones, avascular necrosis, septicemia, high mortality; chronic septic arthritis: bacteremia common, giving rise to endocarditis, cholecystitis, cerebral abscess (mortality approaching 50%).

Lab:

- Osteomyelitis: blood cultures pos in 50% pts; culture discharging sinuses w sterile syringe; bone bx; elevated wbc, high ESR may not be present in the elderly.
- Septic arthritis: only 50% elderly have elevated wbc; ESR usually elevated; large-bore needle w heparin to prevent clotting for joint tap: wbc = 100,000, 90% polymorphonuclear leukocytes, elevated lactate, culture pos in 66% pts.

X-ray:

- Osteomyelitis: initial phases show soft tissue swelling over the diaphysis indistinguishable from changes w cellulitis. Two wk after onset: translucency of the cortex of the diaphysis, radiopaque new bone formation under an elevated periosteum; sclerosis anytime after 3 wk.
- In elderly pts, periosteum more likely to be adherent to cortex, so infection does not separate the bone layers; gallium scan to define areas of chronic or subacute infection; CT and MRI to distinguish osteomyelitis from soft tissue infection; MRI less useful in infections related to surgical hardware.
- Osteoporosis may mask areas of lysis; 95% MRI pos in vertebral osteomyelitis.
- Septic arthritis: radionucleotide scan for less accessible joints: hips, sacroiliacs.
- Joint prosthesis infection: translucency of surrounding bone; technetium and gallium scans helpful in late infection; US in detection of abscess.

Rx:

Therapeutic:

- Osteomyelitis: ≥ 3 wk antibiotics to prevent progression to chronic osteomyelitis; oral therapy should be started 24 hr before cessation of iv antibiotics.

- Chronic osteomyelitis: treat for several mo; methicillin-resistant *S. aureus* may respond to clindamycin, erythromycin, rifampin, but vancomycin may be required; Gram-neg, eg, *pseudomonas:* quinolones (especially chronic). Anaerobic osteomyelitis: metronidazole; osteomyelitis difficult to treat in areas w trauma or vascular insufficiency: often requires surgical intervention.
- Septic arthritis: iv antibiotics for at least 6 wks; intra-articular injections of no benefit; benzylpenicillin and aminoglycoside do not achieve adequate levels in joints; surgical debridement and exploration may be needed, especially w hip involvement.
- Joint prosthesis infection: early; 3 wks antibiotics may avoid losing the prosthesis; late; remove prosthesis, pack w antibiotic-impregnated cement and begin parenteral antibiotics 6 wks; persistent in 60% pts, may require joint fusion and new prosthesis.

Preventive: Joint prosthesis infection: 24 hr before surgery use prophylactic antibiotics (J Bone Joint Surg Am 1990;72:1), Amoxacillin 2 gm or clindamycin 600 mg if penicillin allergic 1 hr before procedure (GFT 2005;161); treat mouth, alimentary and gu (including asx UTI) infections prior to surgery.

6.4 Central Nervous System

Meningitis

Symptoms of meningitis in elderly: confusion 57-96%, headache 21-81%; other symptoms include nausea, vomiting, seizures, weakness, and photophobia; fever is inconsistent, and pts can have hypothermia; nuchal rigidity is neither sens nor spec; pos in only 57% cases and can be falsely pos in pts with cervical spondylosis and Parkinson's disease; CSF studies are necessary for a definitive dx.

Table 6.3 Meningitis

Organism	Epidem	Si/sx	Crs/Cmplc	Labs	Rx	Alternate Rx	Prophylaxis
Bacterial Unknown Ethiology	—	—	—	Increased PMNs, glucose > 45 mg/dL, protein < 45 mg/dL	Ampicillin + cefotaxime/ceftriaxone	Add vancomycin if resistant pneumococcus suspected	—
Pneumococcus	17% cases bacterial meningitis Mortality 19-26% Incr. mortality risks: basilar skull fracture, splenectomy, DM, liver disease, ETOH, HIV	Pts often have concomitant/preceding pneumonia, otitis, mastoiditis, sinusitis, or endocarditis Rapid coma, convulsions	Subdural empyema, cerebral vein thrombosis, middle cerebral arteritis causing hemiparesis; permanent memory deficit, NPH	See above	Pending sensitivities: vancomycin + 3rd gen. cephalosporin		Pneumovac-recommended age > 65
					MIC < 0.1 Pen G or ampicillin	Ceftazidime or ceftriaxone	
					MIC = 0.1-1.0 Ceftazidime or ceftriaxone	Meropenem, vancomycin	
					MIC > = 2.0 Vancomycin + ceftazidime/ceftriaxone	Meropenem, substitute rifampin for vancomycin	

continues

INFECTION

Table 6.3 continued

Organism	Epidem	Si/sx	Crs/Cmplc	Labs	Rx	Alternate Rx	Prophylaxis
Meningococcus	5% cases bacterial meningitis peaks late winter/ early spring Mortality 3-13% Incr. mortality risk: age > 60, focal neurological signs at admission, hemorrhagic diathesis	Septicemia, acute confusional state, agitation, aggression	Deafness often permanent, transient paralysis of 6th and 7th CN	See above	Pen G or ampicillin	Ceftriaxone or cefotaxime	Close contacts: rifampin within 24 hr, alt. Ciprofloxacin single 500 mg po

Skin

Young EM Jr, Newcomer VD, Kligman AM, Geriatric Dermatology: Color Atlas and Practitioner's Guide. Philadelphia: Lea and Febiger, 1993

Cause: Thinning epidermis, decreased sebaceous gland secretion compromises barrier between sc tissue and external environment; less effective T-cell immunity.

Pathophys: Sx, Si, Crs, Lab, Rx: see Table 6.4.

Table 6.4 Skin Infections

Disease	Path/Sx/Si/Crs/Lab	Rx
Bacterial		
Cellulitis	Red, tender, warm, swollen, fever, elevated wbc, ESR; distinguish from DVT; often S. aureus or S. pyogenes	Amoxicillin or amoxicillin-clavulanate potassium to cover group A streptococci, *S. aureus;* metronidazole for anaerobes; warm compresses, elevation and drainage of fluctuant areas help expedite healing
Erysipelas	Variant of cellulitis w well-demarcated borders, patches of hemorrhage, exudates and bullous eruption on leg. β-hemolytic strep, *S. aureus;* recur in 2-4 yr; higher risk w peripheral edema	Benzylpenicillin 600 mg im bid 2-3 d, then po penicillin; dicloxacillin or amoxicillin-clavulanate potassium for *S. aureus;* prevent with good hygiene and correct predisposing factors
Furunculosis	Tender red nodule that develops into pustule; abscess in hair follicle; may recur in areas of excessive sweating, restrictive clothing; diabetes risk factor	Drain; antibiotics for *S. aureus;* occasional anaerobes; shampoo and bath w chlorhexidine; if nasal carrier of staph, use bacitracin or mupirocin

continues

Table 6.4 continued

Disease	Path/Sx/Si/Crs/Lab	Rx
Impetigo	Cutaneous inflammation w honey-colored crusts; *S. aureus* or *S. pyogenes*	Topical rx w mupirocin 2% ointment (Bactroban) tid × 7 d; if topical fails, rx w penicillin or anti-staphylococcal agent (dicloxacillin 250 mg qid, e-mycin 250-500 mg qid, cephalexin 250-500 mg qid, clindamycin 150-300 mg qid); recurrent infections rx w mupirocin 2% ointment in calcium base; treat *S. aureus* w dicloxacillin 250 mg qid or topically w mupirocin 2%
Fungal		
Candidiasis	Glazed red skin w satellite lesions; intertriginous; beneath condom catheters, around stomas, fistulas; spread to the fingers by scratching; chronic paronychia w loss of cuticle and brawny swelling	2% miconazole, clotrimazole, ketoconazole, or nystatin; nystatin ointment or imidazole cream in nail fold tid; when topical rx fails, ketoconazole, fluconazole, or triaconazole po
Onychomycosis	Thickening, irregularity and discoloration of toenails and fingernails; increased incidence assoc w aging secondary to slower growth of nail, increased trauma to nail plate, decreased circulation and changes in sizes and width of foot	Treat selectively; podiatry consult for mechanical improvements and to reduce nail mass; terbinafine po 125 mg bid, resolution in 6 mo, mild gi side effects (Lancet 1990;1:636); griseofulvin; rx 4-6 mo for fingernails, 10-18 mo for toenails; ketoconazole 200 mg po qd × 4-6 mo for fingernails, × 10-18 mo for toenails; newer agents w shorter course: itraconazole approved by FDA

Kost and Straus. Nejm 1996;335:1

Elewski and Roderick. Clinical Infectious Disease 1996;23:305-313.

Mathisen. Clinical Infectious Diseases 1998;27:646-648.

Kanj et al. J Am Acad Dermatol 1998;38:517-536.

Ko et al. Med Clin N Amer. 1998;82:5.

6.5 Eye

Conjunctivitis

See Table 6.5.

Table 6.5 Conjunctivitis

	Itching	Tearing	Exudate	Periauricular Adenopathy
Viral	Minimal	+	Minimal (follicle formation) keratoconjunctivitis: subepithelial opacities in epidemics, 3-4 wk	+
Bacterial	Minimal	Moderate	+	Uncommon
Chlamydial	Minimal	Moderate	+	+
Allergic	+	Moderate	Minimal	None

+ = little or few.

6.6 Gastrointestinal Tract

See Table 6.6.

INFECTION

Table 6.6 Gastrointestinal Infections

Disease	Cause	Sx/Si	Crs/Cmplc	Lab	Rx
Oral					
Parotitis	Xerostomia, anticholinergics, malnutrition, DM	Swollen tender parotid gland, red warm overlying skin; pus expressed from Stenson's duct; pt may not complain of pain because sx may be masked by other infections (pneumonia, abdominal abscess)	Cmplc: septicemia, osteomyelitis facial bones, facial nerve palsy, parotid abscess w rupture into pharynx or auditory canal, 10%-50% mortality	Commensal aerobic and anaerobic organisms in the floor of the mouth	Iv cefuroxime w metronidazole or amoxiclavulinic acid until organism identified; hydration; discontinue anticholinergics; may need to drain w external excision
Candidiasis	Anemia, agranulocytosis; CRF; alcoholism; deficiency in riboflavin, nicotinic acid, ascorbic acid; DM, poor oral hygiene (dentures); antibiotics; steroids	Red, raw mucous membrane, w or w/o sheets of whitish pseudomembrane patches	—	Yeast budding cells and pseudohyphae on Gram stain	Nystatin pastilles 100,000 u qid or amphotericin lozenges 10 mg qid, or miconazole gel 10 mL qid pc, retaining near lesion before swallowing;

					fluconazole 100 mg qd systemic therapy; chronic glossitis: coat dentures w nystatin ointment × 2 wk
Stomatitis	Med side effect: furosemide, HCTZ, β-blockers, cholestyramine, desipramine, doxepine, ACE-inhibitors (J Am Ger Soc 1995;43:1414)	—			—
Dental abscess	*Enterococcus* (endocarditis), *S. pyogenes* (glomerulonephritis), actinomycetes (cervicofacial, brain abscess)	—	—	—	—
Gingivitis	*Peptostreptococcus* (lung, brain abscess), gram negative rods	—	—	—	—

continues

INFECTION

Table 6.6 continued

Disease	Cause	Sx/Si	Crs/Cmplc	Lab	Rx
	(pneumonia, endocarditis) (J Am Ger Soc 1995;43:1414), calcium channel blockers				
Peptic ulcer	*H. pylori,* atrophic gastritis, NSAIDs (see gi diseases)	—	—	—	—
Small-bowel overgrowth	Achlorhydria, jejunal diverticular disease; surgery leading to blind loops, overgrowth of bacteria causes more metabolism of vit B_{12} resulting in B_{12} deficiency	Malabsorption, weight loss, diarrhea	Severe overgrowth can lead to protein-energy deficiency; bacteria synthesize folic acid so may see increase in folic acid levels; bacteroides cause deconjugation of bile salts and reduce solubility and absorption of lipids	Macrocytic anemia, ostomalacia, culture jejunal contents	Broad-spectrum antibiotics including metronidazole; surgical intervention

Diarrhea	*C. difficile* PPI's a risk factor (Jama 2005;6:105)	Varying causes of loose watery or frequent stools When severe explosive watery w blood and mucus; pyrexia, dehydration, and shock	R/o noninfectious causes (diverticulosis, inflammatory bowel disease, ischemic colitis, bowel cancer, laxative, theophylline derivatives, NSAIDs, sulfa derivatives, iron supplements, levodopa, cimetadine, ranitidine, allopurinol)	—	Rx *C. difficile:* prevent *C. difficile* w chlorine cleaning fluid, w probiotics (BMJ 2007;335:80); adsorbants don't work. Recurrence 20%; rx *C. difficile* w metronidazole 500 q 6-8 hr and reeval after 6 d switch to Vanco 125 po q 6 hr, if still pos in 4 d add Rifampin 300 mg q 12 hr × 10 d. Then taper w pulse Vanco (Am J Gastroenterol 2002;97:1765); No test of cure except absence of diarrhea.

continues

INFECTION

Table 6.6 continued

Disease	Cause	Sx/Si	Crs/Cmplc	Lab	Rx
					Campylobacter when severe, use erythromycin
	Campylobacter from inadequately prepared poultry *Salmonella* from egg products	Incubation 2-3 d; colicky abdominal pain, diarrhea can be blood-stained Incubation 6-24 hr; vomiting, colic-like pain; watery diarrhea w blood or mucus; sometimes severe dehydration	*Salmonella, Shigella:* may be severe (bacteremia, septicemia) in elderly because of heavy inoculum; lower gi not protected by stomach acidity (achlorhydria); *Salmonella choleraesuis* causes endocarditis		*Salmonella:* always rx w antibiotics: ciprofloxacin 500 mg bid × 7 d or 14 d if bacteremia; or 200 iv bid at first w nausea Rx of *dehydration:* oral (Dextrolyte,

Shigella, fecal oral route direct contact	Incubation 2-4 d, tenesmus; colicky abdominal pain; water, *bloody* or mucus containing stool; elderly may get bacteremia		Glucolyte, Rehidrat) 2-3 Lt; may be difficult in elderly because of impaired thirst and decreased response of renal tubules to ADH; then give 0.9% sodium chloride 3 L/d; avoid D_5 if Na > 160 mmol/L
S. aureus, heat-labile enterotoxin eg, cold meats not recooked	Incubation few hours; vomiting; diarrhea; self-limiting		
Norwalk, rotavirus	Vomiting, mild diarrhea 2-7 d self-limited; except rotavirus in NH can cause fatal dehydration		

6.7 Human Immunodeficiency Virus Infection

Nurs Home Med 1995;3:265; Jags 1995;43:7; 2002;50:605; Arch IM 1994;154:57; 1995;155:184; Geriatrics 1993;48:61; J Comm Hlth 1995;20:383; J Acquir Immun Defic Syndr 1991;4:84; J Gerontol Nurs 1999;25:25; Jags 2007;55:1393

Cause: HIV.

Epidem: 15% of pts w AIDS are > 50 yr old (J Acquir Immun Defic Syndr 1991;4:84); 3% > 60 yr old, expected to reach 10% within decade. Risk factors: homosexual sex 49%, iv drug abuse 17%, heterosexual sex 11%, transfusion/hemophilia 7%, other 16% (J Gerontol Nurs 1999;25:25). 5% of all newly reported cases of HIV infection are in > 50 yr old (J Midwife Women Hlth 2000; 45:176). Older pts represent 10% newly reported cases and 14% of all those living with AIDS nationwide, and expected to incr with the survival benefit of HAART.

Risk Factors: Physicians not considering diagnosis in elderly because elders thought not to be sexually active or assumed to be in monogamous heterosexual relationship; Viagra has increased sexual activity in the over 50 age group; the fastest growing AIDS rate is among the geriatric population.

Increased age risk factors for progression of disease (Int J Epidem 1997;26:1340; J Gerontol Nurs 1998;24:8):

- Pts not perceiving themselves at risk (Oncology 1998;12:749) thus more uninformed regarding risk status and modes of protection: pts age > 50 1/6 as likely to use condoms; 1/5 as likely to get tested as at-risk younger adults.
- Older women becoming infected at greater rate: no risk of pregnancy encourages sexual contact with no protection, atrophy of vaginal wall leads to increased susceptibility to microtears and, hence, viral entry.
- Likewise elderly males may have an increased incidence in anal mucosa tears during homosexual intercourse (J Emerg Med 1996;14:19; J Midwife Women Hlth 2000;45:176).

Pathophys: HIV infection leading to progressive decreased immune function and subsequent opportunistic infection often misdiagnosed as other chronic conditions in older adults. More rapid progression due to inability of older persons to replace functional T cells that are being destroyed (Mech Age Dev 1997;96:137).

Sx and Si:

Early: Viral syndrome; wasting syndrome, candidiasis, HIV encephalopathy occur frequently. Elderly often present with opportunistic infections, five most common opportunisitic infections with associated si/sx are (Jags 1998;46:153, J Gerontol Nurs 1999;25:25):

1. *Pneumocystis carinii* pneumonia (PCP): gradual onset, fever, fatigue, wgt loss, persistent dry cough, shortness of breath and dyspnea on exertion. Median life span 9 mo vs 22 mo for young pts upon dx.
2. *Mycobacterium tuberculosis* (tbc): Fever, bloody sputum with cough, wgt loss, night sweats, and fatigue.
3. *Mycobacterium avium* complex (MAC): Fever, night sweats, wgt loss, nausea, and abdominal pain.
4. Herpes Zoster: Fluid-filled blisters, painful rash skin, fever, fat
5. CMV: Sx based on site of infection
    - Retinitis: floaters, decreased visual acuity and peripheral vision, blindness.
    - Colitis: loss of appetite, dysphagia, substernal and epigastric pain, wgt loss, diarrhea, fever.
    - Neuropathy: tingling and pain in hands or feet late—dementia, AIDS dementia-subcortical type, rapidly progressive as compared to Alzheimer's type; often associated with peripheral neuropathies, myelopathies.

Crs: Faster progression in elderly due to delayed diagnosis and more rapid clinical deterioration (J Gerontol Nurs 1999;25:25), w disease-free period being much less than 11 yr (San Francisco cohort), along with more HIV comorbidity (J Midwife Women

Hlth 2000;45:176). 37% > 80 yr old die within 1 mo of dx vs 12% in younger population (J Emerg Med 1996;14:19).

Cmplc: Specific to opportunistic infection (most common: PCP, tbc, MAC, Herpes zoster, CMV); AIDS dementia complex: mild abnormal on psychometric tests, inability to perform demanding job tasks, can perform ADLs. Progressing to need for cane, then walker, wheelchair, then paraplegia in end stages. Inability to work, upper extremity weakness, progressing to double incontinence, mutism, and vegetative cognitive state in end stages.

Lab: Initial w/u as with other age groups; AIDS dementia often associated w elevated protein levels and relative monocytosis in CSF.

X-ray: Disease-specific (eg, PCP—chest film, serum LDH, ABG).

Rx: Antivirals: nucleoside reverse transcriptase inhibitors, nonnucleoside reverse transcriptase inhibitors, protease inhibitors, entry and fusion inhibitors, microbicides. For rx guidelines refer to Department of Health and Human Services recommendations. Older adults less likely to respond to rx. Drugs provide similar benefits to people over 50, more likely to have their HIV levels under control partly due to better compliance (Jags 2002;50:605). Earlier studies suggesting less likely to respond done before combination therapy. Controversy over aggressiveness of antiviral therapy: aggressive rx because of pts' rapid deterioration (Mech Age Dev 1997;96:137) vs therapy at smaller doses due to increased toxicity; increased se, changes in absorption, distribution, renal clearance, and drug-drug interactions (J Gerontol Nurs 1999;25:25; J Emerg Med 1996;14:19). Zidovudine (AZT) used as 2nd line therapy due to hematological se: anemia, granulocytopenia (J Gerontol Nurs 1999;25:25; Annales de Medicina Interna 1999;16:273).

Prevention: Encourage condom use; health hx forms for older people sensitive to risk factors of AIDS (J Gerontol Nurs 1998;24:8).

Team Management: Multidisciplinary; parenting by grandparents as a result of the AIDS epidemic is increasing.

Chapter 7

Hematology/Oncology

7.1 Hematology

Anemias

Ger Rv Syllabus 2002, 5th ed, p 362; Jags 2003;51:S2

Cause:

- Hypoproliferative is the most common in elderly: Fe deficiency (blood loss), inflammatory diseases, marrow damage or dysfunction, erythropoietin deficiency (renal, thyroid, nutritional).
- Ineffective erythropoiesis: megaloblastic (vit B_{12}, folate), microcytic (thalassemia, sideroblastic), normocytic.
- Hemolytic anemia: immunologic (tumor, drug, collagen vascular, idiopathic), intrinsic (metabolic, abnormal Hgb), extrinsic (mechanical, lytic substance).

Epidem: More than 33% elderly outpatients, after age 85 more common in men (44%) (Mayo Clin Proc 1994;69:730).

Pathophys:

- Sequential changes in Fe deficiency begin w decrease in serum ferritin, followed by low serum Fe and increase in TIBC, then change in rbc indices and decreased hgb.
- Reduced erythropoietin secretion, decreased BP and compensatory increase in heart rate.
- Myelodysplastic syndrome in which hematopoietic precursors abundant, but defective maturation and peripheral cells have

shorter life span; can develop into CML; caused by alkylating agents, RNA virus, somatic mutations, radiation, environmental toxins. Twice as common in men; anemia, thrombocytopenia, leukopenia presenting w fatigue, exercise intolerance, purpura, infection; hepatomegaly 5%, splenomegaly 10%, pallor 50%; find increased Fe stores, hemochromatosis, basophilic stippling, monocytosis in 30%, elevated LDH; average 3-yr mortality, better prognosis if only erythroid dysplasia.

Sx: Fatigue, worsening shortness of breath, angina, peripheral edema related to underlying atherosclerotic heart disease; mental status changes, dizziness, poor balance, pallor may not be noticeable; commonly without sx if slow onset.

Si:

- Fe deficiency causes atrophy of the tongue, buccal mucosa, angular stomatitis; atrophic gastritis which can lead to achlorhydria and vit B_{12} deficiency.
- Megaloblastic: glossitis, mild jaundice, paresthesias and abnormal position and vibratory senses, dementia, depression, mania.

Crs: Megaloblastic stages: first vit $B_{12} < 300$ pg/mL; then hypersegmented neutrophils; then anemia; neurologic damage and dementia seem to occur before hypersegmented phase.

Lab: (Figure 7.1)

- Hgb < 11.
- Check stool guaiac.
- If reticulocyte count high, consider hemolysis (warm-reactive IgG or more commonly cold-reactive IgM).
- Check vit B_{12}, folate if macrocytic, consider methylmalonic acid (MMA) and homocysteine levels to detect subclinical B_{12} (Am J Med 1994;96:239); MMA recommended if vit B_{12} level < 350 pg/ml; previously Schilling test used to identify cause of inadequate absorption but high-dose oral vitamin B_{12} effectively treats deficiency, regardless of cause (Am Fam Phys 2000;62:1565; Blood 1998;92:1191).

- Myelodysplasia: unexplained anemia w macrocytosis & monocytosis (Cancer 2007;109:1536)
- Check transferrin saturation if microcytic or normocytic; if transferrin nl (> 20%), check hgb electrophoresis-fetal and hgbA2 (thalassemia). If transferrin < 20%, check TIBC, ferritin. If TIBC < 250 gm/dL, ferritin > 100 ng/mL, then anemia chronic disease (thyroid, renal). If TIBC > 400 gm/dL, ferritin < 20 ng/mL, then Fe deficiency anemia. If TIBC 250-400 gm/dL, ferritin 15 -100 ng/mL, check for ringed sideroblasts and Fe stores in marrow.

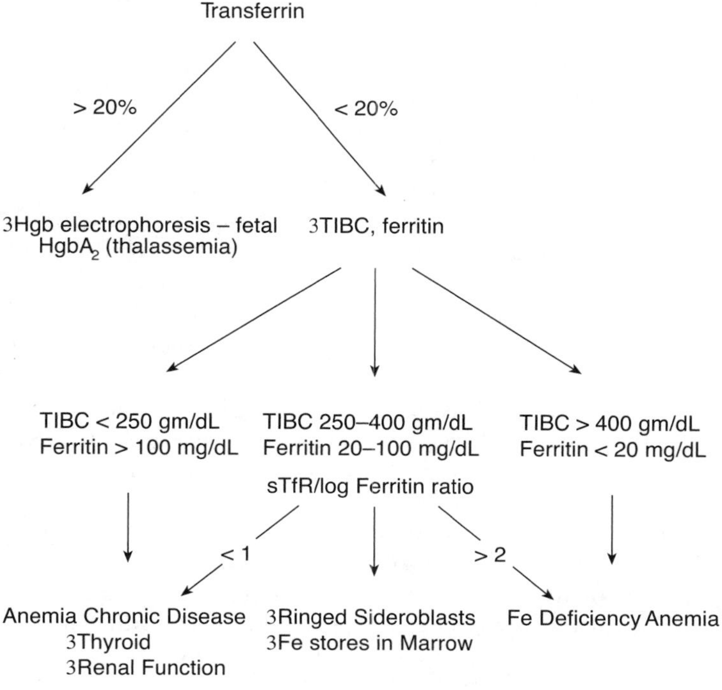

Figure 7.1 Laboratory Tests for Anemia

- Anemias may be "mixed" types in elderly (rbc distribution width elevated).
- If Ferritin > 100 mg/ml, likelihood of Fe deficiency anemia from colonic lesion is low (Am J Gastroenterol 2007;102:82).

Rx:

Preventive: Dietary review routinely.

Therapeutic:

- Chronic disease: erythropoietin 50-100 U/kg weekly, increase dose to 150 U/kg if no response in 2-3 wk (Nejm 1997; 336:933).
- Fe deficiency: ferrous sulfate 325 mg qd; start w 1 tab/d and build up over 2 wk to avoid constipation; 6 mo needed to replenish Fe stores. Less se w low dose Fe rx (Am J Med 2005; 118:1142).
- Fe replacement contraindicated in thalassemia because produces Fe overload.
- Hemolysis: remove offending drug, eg, levodopa, penicillin, doxepin, quinidine, thiazides; rx IgG (warm) w prednisone 60 mg/d, danazol, splenectomy, azathioprine, cyclophosphamide; tfx if unstable; emergency—immunoglobulin 0.4 gm/kg/d 5 d; rx IgM (cold) w transfusion, plasmapheresis.
- Vit B_{12} 1000 μg/d po until serum B_{12} > 300 pg/mL (Nejm 1996;337:1441; Sci Am 1996;III:14; Jama 1991;265:94; Jags 1997;45:124; 1998;46:1125) or parenteral 1,000 μg/d 1st wk then q mo; folic acid 1 mg/d; absorption, cobalamine interfered w by colchicines, neomycin, ethanol, metformin (Nejm 1997;337:1441).
- Myelodysplasia: rx w washed rbc's, granulocyte tfx, blood cell products w hydroxyurea to keep wbcs down.
- Intermittent tfx may be warranted occasionally, particularly in anemia of chronic disease; if pt otherwise stable, will improve quality of life.

7.2 Chronic Lymphocytic Leukemia

Nejm 1995;333:1032; 2005;352:804

Cause: No genes have been identified, while 50% have cytogenetic abnormalities: trisomy 12, chromosome 13 at band q14.

Epidem: Most common form of leukemia in Western countries.

Pathophys: Accumulation of neoplastic B lymphocytes in blood, bone marrow, liver, and spleen; monoclonal proliferation (Leukemia 1994;8:1610).

Sx: Fatigue; malaise; decreased exercise tolerance; exacerbation cardiovascular disease; abdominal pain; early satiety w splenomegaly; > 25% asx.

Si: Enlarged lymph nodes (cervical, axillary, supraclavicular); splenomegaly; hepatomegaly w disease progression; jaundice secondary to hemolysis or biliary obstruction from enlarged periportal lymph nodes (caloris node); ecchymoses; petechiae in late stages secondary to thrombocytopenia; fever in late stages may be secondary to the development of lymphoma.

Crs: 60% diagnosed in asx phase. Findings progress as follows as stage becomes more advanced: lymphocytosis > 50,000/μL, lymph node enlargement, splenomegaly, hgb <11 gm/dL, thrombocytopenia (platelet count < 105/μL); median survival 9 yr.

Cmplc: Hypogammaglobulinemia chief cause of infection (Leuk Lymphoma 1994;13:203).

Lab:

- Criteria: 50-100% of leukocytes are small mature lymphocytes; bone marrow confirms.
- X-ray:

Rx:

Therapeutic:

- Treat constitutional si, bulky lymphadenopathy, splenomegaly causing compression, doubling of wbc in under 1 yr: chlorambucil 0.4-0.8 mg/kg body wgt po q 2 wk for 8-12 mo, yielding response rates of 40-70% vs chlorambucil does not prolong survival (Nejm 1998;338:1506). Addition of prednisone no help; combination therapy does not prolong survival (Ann Oncol 1995;6:219) vs fludarabine cyclophosphamide (Med Lett 2000; 42:83); discontinue rx when response has been achieved and restart w disease progression.
- If no response due to gene mutation, try purine analogue, fludarabine (Blood 1994;84:461a).
- Treat pts w cytopenias w high-dose immunoglobulin, cyclosporine, splenectomy, low-dose radiation of the spleen.
- Hypogammaglobulinemia not helped much by vaccines that produce a suboptimal response.
- Neutropenia from chemotherapy can be treated w hematopoietic growth factors.
- Monoclonal antibodies for minimal residual disease (Ann Oncol 1995;6:219).

7.3 Multiple Myeloma

Jags 1994;42:653; Nejm 1997;336:1657

Cause: Proliferation of plasma cells and plasma cell precursors, usually monoclonal IgG or IgA; translocations 14 q 32 and chromosomes 11, 6, 16, 9, 18, 8; point mutations; monoclonal gammopathy representing 1st oncogenic event leads to multiple myeloma; 2nd oncogenic event may follow (Nejm 1997;336:1657).

Epidem: Mean age at dx = 69.1 yr; black males highest incidence, 9.6/100 000; increased risk w asbestos exposure, farming, atomic bomb survivors, radium dial workers.

Pathophys: First loss of T-cell-mediated control of early B-cell development, then abnormal proliferation of multiple clones, followed by malignant transformation and accumulation of immunoglobulins. Clinical manifestations result from tumor growth, accumulation of immunoglobulin chains, and cytokines released from malignant plasma cells (bone resorption).

Sx: 60-70% of newly diagnosed pts have bone pain (Eur J Cancer 1991;27:1401). Hypercalcemia: anorexia, nausea, vomiting, constipation, weakness, pain, confusion, and lethargy; new onset of DM.

Crs: Prognosis for healthy old people same as for healthy young people (Am J Med 1985;79:316). Px ~ 4 yr if hgb > 10 gm/dL, Ca < 12 mg/dL, nl bones, low M component, IgG < 5 gm/dL, IgA < 3 gm/dL; Px ~ 2 yr if hgb < 8.5 gm/dL, Ca > 12 mg/dL, advanced bone disease, high M component, IgG > 7 gm/dL, IgA > 5 gm/dL and Px ~ 1 yr if Cr > 2.0 mg/dL (Jags 1994;42:653).

Cmplc:

- Renal failure: up to ½ of pts have renal insufficiency at the time of dx; light chains precipitate in renal tubules, leading to obstruction, dilatation, and subsequent atrophy of the nephron. Other mechanisms renal dysfunction: amyloid, infection, hyperuricemia.
- Amyloid and hyperviscosity: results from deposition of immunoglobulin light chains in susceptible organs, eg, kidneys, gi tract, myocardium, peripheral nerves; manifestations of hyperviscosity: mucosal bleeding, retinopathy, CHF; sx may be absent in the setting of anemia, so use caution when deciding to transfuse.
- Hypogammaglobulinemia and infection: major cause of morbidity in multiple myeloma pts, increased risk w encapsulated

organisms: Streptococcus pneumoniae, Haemophilus influenzae, Staphylococcus aureus, gram-neg rods (Semin Oncol 1986;13:282).

Lab:

- 10% atypical plasma cells in bone marrow, monoclonal immunoglobulin in serum, light chains in urine; hgb < 12 gm/dL: normocytic, normochromic w few reticulocytes; rouleaux formation because of excess monoclonal protein; identify in tissue w Congo red stain.
- Prognostic tests: β2-microglobulin < 4 μg/mL better prognosis; plasma cell labeling index is a measure of DNA replication and reflects tumor growth (Blood 1988;72:219); IL-6 levels are higher w severe disease (J Clin Invest 1989;84:2008); follow M protein on SPEP, UPEP; proteinuria; follow recurrence w β2-microglobulin tumor marker.
- X-ray: Multiple osteolytic lesions throughout skeleton, pathologic fractures, and osteopenia on x-ray; scans not sensitive because not enough blastic activity in the lesions; MRI to evaluate cord compression.

Rx:

Therapeutic (Med Clin N Am 1992;76:371):

Initial therapy: melphalan and prednisone (MP); little rationale for using interferon as initial therapy (Semin Oncol 1991;18:18); multi-agent chemotherapy better for those w a poor prognosis (J Clin Oncol 1992;10:334); maintenance therapy: interferon prolongs remission (Semin Oncol 1991;18:37; Nejm 1990;322:1430); resistant disease: vincristine, doxorubicin, dexamethasone, watch for toxicity (Ann IM 1986;105:8); high-dose therapy not recommended for the elderly; pamidronate for pain, to decrease bone turnover, has antitumor effect (Ann IM 2000;132:734).

Supportive Therapy: Hyperviscosity: plasmapheresis; anemia: erythropoietin (Nejm 1990;322:1693; Blood 1996;87:2675), transfusions; hypercalcemia: bisphosphonates; immunization w pneumovax recommended but frequently ineffective because of failure to induce antibodies.

7.4 Lung Cancer

Am Fam Phys monograph 1995;191:26

Cause: 85-90% from smoking; 15 yr must elapse after cessation for risk to approach that of nonsmokers; also from radon, nickel, chromium, asbestos.

Epidem: Most common cause of death due to cancer; greatest prevalence in those < 65 yr old (Jama 1987;258:921); increasing incidence in women because of increased smoking in elderly women (Radiol Clin N Am 1994;32:1; Cancer Pract 1995;3:13).

Crs:

- Elderly have more localized disease at dx than do middle-aged pts; more squamous cell carcinoma and less adenocarcinoma; small-cell lung cancer decreases; therefore, elderly have greater chance of resectable and, hence, curable lung cancer (CA 1987;60:1331).
- 90% of pts w recurrent lung cancer have distant metastases; most recurrences within 2 yr of primary lung cancer.
- Solitary nodule r/o metastasis, carcinoid tumor, granuloma, bronchiogenic cyst; dx of small-cell lung cancer in a nonsmoker should raise the question of misdiagnosis of lymphoma.

Lab:

- Sputum cytology—90% accurate, but not for individual histopathology; fiberoptic bronchoscopy well tolerated by elderly (Chest 1989;95:1043); hgb and hct; pleural effusion: thoracentesis w or w/o pleural biopsy.

X-Ray: Chest film; peripheral lesion needle bx or resection.

- CT: enlarged hilar nodes: bronchoscopy; obtain CT and bone scan to assess for metastasis to liver, brain, bone; if mediastinal nodes enlarged, obtain mediastinoscopy to determine resectability.

Rx:

Therapeutic:

Table 7.1 Non-Small-Cell (Adenocarcinoma, Large-Cell, Squamous Cell) Lung Cancer

Stage	Treatment	Median Survival
Stage I (not involving entire lung, no node involvement or metastases)	Lobectomy	60 mo w small lesion, 27 mo w large lesion
Stage II ipsilateral peri-bronchial or hilar lymph node involvement	Lobectomy or pneumonectomy right lung particularly high risk in elderly (Clin Symp 1993; 45:20); postop chemotherapy may be helpful (cisplatin-based)	17-20 mo
Stage IIIA (entire lung without involvement of the carina, ipsilateral metastases to mediastinal, and subcarinal lymph nodes)	Surgery plus chemotherapy, and radiotherapy (Nejm 1990;323:940)	8-11 mo
Stage IIIB (invading mediastinum, pleural effusion, contralateral lymph nodes)	—	—
Stage IV (distant metastases)	Radiation for pain, obstruction, hemoptysis	6 mo

Table 7.2 Small-Cell Lung Cancer

	Treatment	Survival
Limited	Radiation primary tumor, and mediastinum +/− cranial irradiation (dementia can occur); if aggressive chemo rx cannot be tolerated, try VP-16 (Ger Rv Syllabus 1996; p. 327)	14-18 mo, 15-25% survive 2 yr and considered cured, high association w second primary cancers (Nejm 1992;327:1618)
Extensive	Oral etoposide (Semin Oncol 1990;17:49)	9-11 mo

Chemo Rx: Non-small cell: chemo effectiveness less than for small cell, usually use experimental drugs, paclitaxel + cisplatin; small cell: cyclophosphamide, doxorubicin, vincristine, nitrosurea, etopside, cisplatin (se = nausea, vomiting, renal); newer agents vinorelbine, gemcitabine (Ger Rv Syllabus, 2002, p 372).

Team Management: Determine if pt will tolerate surgery: FEV1 > 2.5 indicates will tolerate pneumonectomy; FEV1 > 1.1: will tolerate lobectomy; controversial whether elderly have higher rate of mortality (J Thorac Cardiovasc Surg 1083;86:654; Jama 1987;258:927); function most predictive of postop outcome; poor prognostic si include advanced disease, wgt loss, nonambulatory for non-small-cell lung cancer; increased age, elevated LDH, alkaline phosphatase, hyponatremia for small-cell lung cancer.

Routine f/u after primary lung cancer rx: H+P examination (pulmonary, abdominal, neurologic sx; cervical, axillary, and supraclavicular lymph nodes; edema of face and neck), and chest x-ray q 4 mo for 2 yr, then q 6-12 mo.

7.5 Breast Cancer

Am Fam Phys 1995;191; Surg Clin N Am 1994;74:145; Jags 2007;55:1636

Cause: Risk factors: breast cancer in 1st-degree relative (Jama 1993;270:1563), age > 30 at birth of first child, late menopause, benign breast disease, heavy radiation exposure, conjugated estrogens, obesity, decreased bone mineral density (Jama 1996; 276:1404), moderate alcohol use: 1-2 × that of healthy age-matched controls (Nejm 1992;327:319); dysplasia in 5-10% of benign bx specimens = 4 × risk; hereditary in 5%, usually younger women.

Epidem: Most common cancer in women; incidence in women < 50 has declined by 13%, but incr in women > 50 by 7%; half of breast cancers occur in women > 65 yr old.

Pathophys: Elderly women more likely to have well-differentiated cancer; both estrogen and progesterone receptors present in 60-70% of elderly pts; biologically less aggressive than in younger women.

Si: Masses more likely malignant in elderly women.

Crs: Overall course more benign, more at risk for subsequent colon cancer (Am J Gastroenterol 1994;84:835).

Compl: Elderly more at risk for emergency complications, eg, hypercalcemia, spinal cord compression, symptomatic brain metastasis.

Lab: CEA, CA27-29.

- X-ray: Palpable lesion may not be detected by mammography 20% of the time; palpable lesion in postmenopausal women requires bx. Bone scans, CT of abdomen, pelvis, chest, and brain not called for in asx pts w normal physical exam findings. Determination of presence of sentinel axillary lymph node reduces requirement for axillary node sampling (Ger Rv Syllabus 2002;5:371).

Rx:

Preventive: See Chapter 2.2, Health Care Maintenance.

Therapeutic:

- Surgical rx w curative intent similar to that adopted in younger pts is appropriate for women > 70 yr old (J Am Soc Ger 1996;44:390).
- Contraindications for breast-conserving surgery: tumor mass > 5 cm, large breast size, subareolar lesion.
- Cancers > 4 cm, preoperative chemotherapy results in substantial tumor shrinkage, allowing for breast-conserving surgery (J Natl Cancer Inst 1991;82:1539).
- Excision alone ("lumpectomy") for tumors < 1 cm.
- Post-operative adjuvant radiation therapy recommended for extensive cancers, eg, > 4 pos lymph nodes; ER-pos more likely to benefit from tamoxifen (Eur J Surg Oncol 1994;20:207). Letrozole (aromatase inhibitor) more disease-free survival than tamoxifen (Nejm 2005;353:2747); exemestrane (aromatase inhibitor) (Lancet 2007;369:559).
- Frail pts w advanced localized lesions respond to tamoxifen (Jama 1996;275:1349) w 40-70% tumor shrinkage, but long-term survival unchanged (Arch Surg 1984;1:548); tamoxifen well tolerated: decreases bone loss, increases HDL levels; increases risk of DVT, endometrial cancer, visual loss.
- Lapatinib (Tykerb): Her-2 and epidermal growth factor receptor (EGFR-1) inhibitor. Decreases tumor cell growth given in combination w capecitabine (Xeloda). Slows progression in women w heavily pre-treated advanced breast cancer.
- Megestrol acetate (Megace), anastrozole fewer side effects (Med Lett Drugs Ther 1996;38:62); decrease recurrence rate w tamoxifen (Br J Cancer 1988;57:612).
- Routine f/u of asx pts after primary breast cancer rx: H+P (skin, chest, breast, abdominal exam) (Am J Clin Oncol 1988; 11:451) q 3 mo × 2 yr, then q 6 mo × 3 yr, then annually after

5 yr; breast self exam q mo for life; mammography q 6 mo × 2 yr, then annually.

- Adjuvant chemotherapy survival benefit for healthy elderly women > 70 yr old (Jama 1992;268:57); responses last 6-12 mo; Paclitaxel (Taxol) for tumors overexpressing HER2 protein (Med Lett 2000;42:83) (see ovarian cancer). Most cytotoxic drugs metabolized in the liver; altered metabolism only with major liver dysfunction. Myelosuppression more common in the elderly; psychosocial adjustments to chemotherapy better in the elderly than in the younger population (Hlth Serv Res 1986;20:961).
- Metastatic breast cancer: median survival 2 yr; palliative therapy for bone, skin, lymph nodes, pleural and pulmonary metastases. Soft tissue and bone metastases will respond to hormonal therapy if they have responded before, eg, progestins, aromatase inhibitors, estrogens (Nejm 2003;348:2431).
- Rx bone mets w clodronate (bisphosphate): decreases bone destruction, decreases tumor burden by inhibiting release of bone-derived tumor growth factors (Nejm 1998;339:357,398).

7.6 Colorectal Cancer

Cancer J 2001;7:213

Epidem: Accounts for 14% of cancers in men and women; 3rd leading cause of cancer death after lung and breast; incidence 4-5 × higher in people > 65 yr old; ⅔ of colon cancers occur in people > 65 yr; increased meat consumption leads to increased risk colon cancer (Jama 2005;293:172).

Pathophys: Minimum of 5 yr for adenomatous polyp to become malignant; if polyp > 2 cm, 40% chance of being malignant; pts w cancers confined to mucosal layers, Dukes stage A (just mucosal involvement), have 80-90% 5-yr survival; Dukes stage B (through bowel wall but no lymph node involvement), 60% 5-yr survival; Dukes stage C (involving lymph nodes), 40% 5-yr survival; Dukes stage D (metastatic), 5% 5-yr survival.

Sx: Anemia, abdominal discomfort; hematochezia, pencil-thin stools, obstruction.

Crs: 5-yr survival for colon cancer worse in geriatric age group (CA 1992;42:9).

Colon Cancer Recurrence: Most likely if tumor penetrated through colon wall; w poorly differentiated histology;

- Presence of obstruction;
- Elevated CEA;
- Increased number of pos lymph nodes.

Rate of Recurrence: 1st yr 50%, 2nd yr 20%, rare after 5 yr; 10% have second primary approximately 11 yr after initial colon cancer.

Pattern of Recurrence: regional lymph nodes, then hematogenous spread to liver; 8% recurrence at site of original surgical anastomosis; local recurrence 25-40%, liver 40%, abdominal peritoneal implants 12-28%; solitary lung nodule has 50% chance metastasis and 50% chance of being primary lung cancer—therefore, need tissue dx.

Sx of Recurrence: abdominal or pelvic pain, lower gi bleeding, change in bowel habits, weight loss, cough, bone pain.

Associated Cancers: breast, ovarian, endometrial (Prim Care 1992;19:607); CEA elevation associated w tumor recurrence in 85-90% of pts and may precede sx by 3-8 mo (Surg Clin N Am 1993;73:85).

Lab:

- CEA good to follow postop for recurrence.
- False-pos: smoking, liver disease, PUD, pancreatitis, diverticulitis, inflammatory bowel disease.

Rx:

Preventive: 10-yr regular ASA use in doses similar to those recommended for prevention of cardiovascular disease substantially reduces risk of colon cancer (Nejm 1995;333:609); COX-2 inhibitors may prevent colon cancer (Jama 1999;282:1254).

Therapeutic:

- Surgical excision only potentially curative intervention; rectal cancer—local resection w "pull-through" procedure to avoid colostomy, use transrectal US to determine depth of lesion and nodular metastasis; rx up to 3 solitary liver nodules w resection.
- Continuous infusion 5-fluorouracil—adjuvant therapy as effective w modulating agents, eg, leucovorin; additional adjuvant therapies cetuximab, irinotecan (Nejm 2004;351:337; J Clin Oncol 2004;22:23).
- Routine f/u: H+P, LFTs, stool guaiac for 2 yr q 3-6 mo, then for 2 yr q 6-12 mo and after yr 4 annually; CEA q 2 mo for 2 yr, then q 4 mo for the next 2 yr, thereafter annually; colonoscopy after surgical resection and 1 yr after, then q 3 yr; chest film q 6-12 mo for 2 yr, then annually (Jama 1989;261:584).

Team Management:

- Refer for hospice.
- Bowel obstruction is an oncologic emergency: preventive: liquid or soft diet, stool softeners, antiemetics (metoclopramide); active conventional "conservative" iv fluids, antiemetics, nasogastric suction may cause resolution; if death imminent, continue symptomatic rx only with pain relief and antiemetics, eg, octreotide (Sandostatin)—dose is 150 mcg-300 mcg sc bid (1 mg/mL multi-use vial); surgical treatment justified only in pt with > 2-3 mo to live, given high morbidity.
- Obstructive uropathy common, may present with retention, dysuria, nocturia, frequency, decreased stream; treated with indwelling catheter or surgery.
- Widespread pelvic metastases can cause difficult-to-manage neuropathic pain.

7.7 Prostate Cancer

Sci Am Med 1995;12:IXA; Am Fam Phys 1995;191:29; Med Clin N Am 1998;83:1423; Urol Clin N Am 1999;25:581

Cause: Hormonal, familial (Prostate 1990;17:337), oncogenic viruses, environmental, not associated w BPH (Lancet 1974;2:115) or vasectomy; incidence decreased by selenium, vit E, decreased soy, decreased tomatoes in diet, increased by high fat diet (Can Med Assoc 1998;159:807).

Epidem:

- 50-70% of men > 70 yr old have histologic evidence of prostate cancer on autopsy and < 3% of them die from prostate cancer; nevertheless prostate cancer is the 2nd most common cause of cancer death in men. As much as 50% of cancers are clinically advanced at the time of discovery; well-differentiated cancer is least likely to spread (10-yr cancer-specific death rate < 10%); most are moderate grade (10-yr cancer-specific death rate 10-20%; poorly differentiated (10-yr cancer-specific death rate 30-60%) (Nejm 1994;330:242).
- Incidence 0.8:100,000 in Asians and 100.2:100,000 in black Americans (Ann IM 1994;120:698); prostate is the most common malignancy in black American males and the 2nd leading cause of cancer death among black American men (CA 1992;42:7; Med Clin N Am 1998;83:1423); men w father or brother w prostate cancer before age 65 yr have a 3-5 × risk of developing prostate cancer (Can Med Assoc 1998;159:807); if they have 2 relatives who developed it before age 65 yr, they have 5-8 × risk.

Pathophys: 95% adenocarcinoma; remainder are squamous, transitional, sarcomas; adenocarcinoma arises in the peripheral portion of the gland (Med Clin N Am 1998;83:1423), while BPH arises from the periurethral area.

Crs: PSA > 20 ng/mL or poorly differentiated, greater likelihood disease not confined to prostate; clinical pattern of recurrence: local pelvic progression; lymph nodes (obturator, iliac, para-aortic); bony metastases to pelvis, spine, and proximal femur; lung, liver, adrenal gland, supraclavicular nodes, brain.

Grading: Gleason score
- 2-4 well differentiated
- 5-7 moderately differentiated
- 8-10 poorly differentiated

Staging:
- (A or T1) extent of tissue involved incidentally on TURP
- (B or T2) detected by DRE confined to prostate
- (C or T3) extend thru prostate capsule
- (D1 or N1-2) lymph node metastases
- (D2 or M) metastases to bone
- (D3) progressive after the initiation of hormone therapy or androgen refractory disease

Lab: Age 60-69 yr: nl PSA range 0.0-4.5 ng/mL; 70-79 yr: nl PSA range 0.0-6.5 ng/mL; U.S. Preventive Services Task Force does not recommend screening w PSA because finding prostate cancer early does not decrease mortality (USPSTF. Guide to Clinical Preventive Services (Jama 2007;298:1533). 1/3 cancers missed w this screening test; false-pos as high as 60%; PSA density > 0.15, more likely cancer and not BPH (Mayo Clin Proc 1994;69:59); best used in men w PSAs < 9 or 10; PSA velocity > 07.5 mg/mL/yr has sensitivity of 72% (Urol Clin N Am 1999;25:581); serial PSA utility unclear (J Urol 1998;158:1243).

- X-ray: Extraperitoneal lymph node sampling via CT-directed needle bx to determine staging and therapy (J Endourol 1992;6:103); bone scan to work up bony metastases; chest film, CT of abdomen and pelvis.

Rx:

Preventive: Large percentage of men w prostate cancer will not die from it; rx causes morbidity; therefore, weigh risks in older people whose life expectancy is limited by other diseases (see HCM p. 70).

Therapeutic: Routine f/u after primary prostate cancer rx:

- H+P (sx of bladder outlet obstruction, pelvic, spine, and long-bone pain, neurologic sx from vertebral collapse, sx of renal failure, fixation of prostate to pelvic wall) q 3 mo × 2 yr, q 6 mo next 3 yr, and annually thereafter.
- PSA q 3 mo × 2 yr, q 6 mo next 3 yr, and annually thereafter; PSA should fall in 2-3 d after surgery; extremely anaplastic tumors are not differentiated enough to produce PSA, so may not be elevated if recurrent.
- Radiation and androgen suppression rx better for localized prostate cancer (Jama 2004;292:864).
- Nerve-sparing radical surgery for moderately differentiated localized prostate cancer in 70 yr old instead of expectant management increased survival time by 6 mo (Jama 1993;269: 2650; 2006;296:2733); improved survival for pts w locally advanced prostate cancer rx w radiotherapy and goserelin (Zoladex) 79% vs 62% 5-yr survival (Nejm 1997;337:295); hormonal (GnRH agonist: leuprolide or goserelin), antiandrogens (flutamide, bicalutamide, nilutamide) (Med Lett 2000;42:83) best for locally advanced mets, relief of bone pain, decrease serum PSA, decrease tumor size, decrease obstruction; may partially reverse anemia, improve appetite (Med Clin N Am 1998;83:1231); watch for osteoporosis; radical prostatectomy is associated w significant erectile dysfunction and some decline in urinary dysfunction (Jama 2000;283:354); nodes can be sampled first, then continue procedure, only if nodes pos.

Team Management:

Conservative management of localized prostate cancer (Jama 2005; 293:2095)

- Pts make decisions based on sx previously experienced, eg, choose expectant management if experience dribbling and radical prostatectomy, if cannot start stream (Jags 1996;44:934).
- Follow PSA rate of rise ≥ 2 ng/mL/cc/yr (Nejm 2004;351: 125,180).

- Pain due to bone mets; megestrol acetate effective for hot flashes in 60% pts.
- Pelvic complications: lower extremity edema from lymphadenopathy, urinary dysfunction, and neurologic impairment.
- Oncologic emergencies: spinal cord compression, obstructive uropathy, SIADH, disseminated intravascular coagulation.

7.8 Ovarian Cancer

Reinke D, Ovarian Cancer, American Academy of Family Practice Board Review Course, Seattle, May 1995; CA 1995;42:69; Semin Oncol 1998;25:281

Cause: Hereditary (5-10%) w early onset; cosmetic talcum to perineum; 80% of ovarian masses are benign; epithelial: 60%, and 5-yr survival = 20-50%; mucinous: 5-yr survival = 60%; stromal sex cord tumors of which 90% are benign, two-thirds occurring in postmenopausal women; metastatic from stomach, colon, breast, uterus.

Epidem: One in 70 women; most common gynecologic cancer-causing death in women; 4th most common cause of cancer death in women; mean age 55-61 yr and incidence of ovarian cancer increases w advancing age into 8th decade; industrialized countries; w ovarian cancer have 4 × the risk breast cancer; w breast cancer have 2 × the risk of ovarian cancer; risk factors: low parity, high-fat diet, no bcp use, sedentary lifestyle.

Pathophys:

- Unregulated cell division/regeneration of ovarian epithelium.
- Pituitary gonadotropin stimulates malignant transformation.

Sx: Nausea, dyspepsia, lower abdominal pain; constipation; early satiety w omental mets; urinary frequency.

Si: Ascites; progressive weakness; wgt loss; ovarian mass.

Crs:

- Three hereditary patterns: ovary alone, ovary w breast, ovary w colon (Lynch syndrome) usually detected in advanced stages;
- Mean survival with residual tumor > 3 cm = 21 mo; < 3 cm = 53 mo; 75% present stage III—5-yr survival rate 10-30%;
- Prognosis: better with young age, good functional status, bcp's, small post-op residual tumor volume, low tumor grade, low tumor ploidy; median time to recurrence 2-4 mo, first detected by CA 125 in asx pts.

Staging:

I = limited to ovary—5-yr survival = 90%
II = pelvic ext—5-yr survival up to 70%
III = intraperitoneal metastasis or pos nodes—5-yr survival = 25%
IV = distant to lung, liver, peritoneal implants occur rapidly—5-yr survival = 10%

Lab: Tumor markers: CEA elevated in 60% epithelial tumors; also pos in cirrhosis, COPD, inflammatory bowel disease, smoking; CA 125—correlates w disease in 93% pts; also pos in endometriosis, miliary tbc, 1% healthy persons.

X-ray:

Noninvasive: US: solid w papillary projections w involvement adjacent visceral, distinguish cyst from ascites, bx metastases; transvaginal US even more effective and should be done if CA 125 > 2× nl; CT: for masses > 2 cm, mets; chest film, IVP, cystoscopy, proctoscopy, BE, UGI, if sx.

Rx:

Therapeutic:

Surgery:

- Laparoscopy discouraged—spill cells
- Debulk primary to < 1 cm = 50% cure, > 1 cm = 20-25% response

- Bx diaphragm, paracolic gutters, pelvic peritoneum, periaortic, pelvic nodes, infra colic omentum
- Peritoneal washings
- TAH/BSOO, omentectomy
- Large-bowel resection required in 20-30% cases
- Bladder or ureteral resection required in 5%
- Diaphragm, liver, spleen resection—rarely need

Chemo-Rx:

- First-line chemo rx = platinum-based combination, response rate = 80%; complete clinical response = 50%.
- Paclitaxel (Taxol) most active agent in ovarian and breast cancer but risk of anaphylaxis requires dexamethasone as well as H1- and H2-antagonist antihistamines, decreasing risk of anaphylaxis from 10% to 1%.
- If creatinine clearance > 45 dL/min and good performance status without comorbid disease—age not a factor (CA 1993; 71:594).
- Only small portion achieve surgical response documented by 2nd look; even then complete surgical responders progress.
- 2nd-line chemo rx = interferon; granulocyte colony-stimulating factor (G-CSF) to prevent neutropenia with chemo rx.

Radiotherapy for small volume tumor, limited by liver and kidney function.

Biological therapy being studied (monoclonal antibodies, gene therapy).

7.9 Treatment of Cancer in the Elderly Hospice/ Palliative Care

Therapeutic: (Tables 7.3, 7.4, and 7.5)

- Adv Studies Med 2004;4:88; CNS Drugs 2003;17:621
- Oldest old tolerate radiotherapy in full doses without serious complications (Jags 1995;43:793; Curr Probl Cancer 1993;

Table 7.3 Dyspnea Control

	Specific Causes and Treatments for Dyspnea
B	**Bronchospasm**—If present, consider nebulized albuterol and/or oral steroids: if not, consider lowering doses of theophylline and adrenergic agents to reduce any tremor and anxiety that often exacerbate dyspnea.
R	**Rales**—If volume overload is present, reduce artificial feeding or stop iv fluids; diuretics are occasionally needed; if pneumonia seems likely, decide whether an antibiotic will rehabilitate the pt or just prolong the dying process; pt and family participation in this decision is essential.
E	**Effusions**—Thoracentesis can be effective, but if the effusion recurs and the pt is ambulatory, consider pleurodesis to prevent recurrent lung collapse; if the pt is close to death, palliate the dyspnea with opioids.
A	**Airway obstruction**—Make sure tracheostomy appliances are cleaned regularly; if aspiration of food is likely, puree solids and thicken liquids with cornstarch or "Thick-it", and instruct the family in positioning the pt during feeding and in suctioning if necessary.
T	**Thick secretions**—If the cough reflex is still strong, loosen secretions with nebulized saline; if the cough is weak, dry secretions with hyoscyamine (Levsin) 0.125 mg po or sl q 8 hr or Transderm Scop 1-3 patches q 3 d, or add glycopyrrolate (Robinul) 0.4-1.0 mg per d to a sc infusion or by sc or iv bolus 0.2 mg q 3 hr prn.
H	**Hemoglobin low**—A blood tfx may add energy and reduce dyspnea for a few weeks; more often, hemorrhage or marrow failure are part of the dying process and are best palliated with opioids and living kindness.
A	**Anxiety**—Sitting upright, using a bedside fan, listening to calming music and practicing relaxation techniques can be extremely effective, as can skillful counseling and the presence of a calming physician; dyspnea exacerbates normal fears and anxiety, so treat with opioids first, then try a benzodiazepine if needed; if the opioid dose is limited by drowsiness, reduce the benzodiazepine and increase the opioid.
I	**Interpersonal issues**—Social and financial problems contribute to dyspnea; counseling and interaction with social workers and other members of the interdisciplinary team may bring relief; when family relationships exacerbate the problem, a few days spent in a peaceful, homelike hospice inpatient unit may help relieve the pt's symptoms.

Table 7.3 continued

	Specific Causes and Treatments for Dyspnea
R	**Religious concerns**—Although faith or an experience of the transcendent can bring profound comfort, some religious beliefs, such as "God is punishing me" or "God will heal me if I have enough faith," can precipitate dyspnea and/or exacerbate its symptoms; take time to listen with full attention and presence; help the pt explore ways to reconnect with God, the cosmos, or the deepest parts of the self; coordinate treatment with the pt's spiritual advisor, chaplain, counselor, other health care professionals, and family members.

Table 7.4 Specific Measures for Treatment of Nausea

Specific Cause	Possible Remedy
Cortical	
• Tumor in CNS or meninges (look for neurologic signs or mental status problems)	• Dexamethasone (consider radiation therapy)
• Increased intracranial pressure (look for projectile vomiting, headache)	• Dexamethasone
• Anxiety and other conditioned responses	• Counseling tranquilizers
• Uncontrolled pain	• Opioids, other pain medications
Vestibular/Middle Ear	
• Vestibular disease (look for vertigo or vomiting after head motion)	• Meclizine and/or ENT consult
• Middle ear infections (look for ear pain or bulging tympanic membrane)	• Antibiotic and/or decongestant
• Motion sickness (travel-related nausea)	• Transderm Scop, meclizine

Table 7.4 continued

Specific Cause	Possible Remedy
Chemoreceptor Trigger Zone	
The most common causes of nausea are mediated by this area in the brain, which senses changes in the blood.	
• Drugs, e.g., opioids, digoxin, chemotherapy, carbamazepine, antibiotics, theophylline	• Decrease drug dose or discontinue drug if possible
• Metabolic, eg, renal or liver failure	• Haloperidol po or sc or ondansetron (Zofran) po or sc
• Hyponatremia	• Salt tablets, demeclocycline
• Hypercalcemia	• Diphosphonate or other therapy
Gastrointestinal Tract	
• Irritation by drugs (eg, NSAIDs, iron, alcohol, antibiotics)	• Stop drug if possible, add H2 blocker or misoprostol
• Tumor infiltration, radiation therapy to the gi tract, or infection (eg, candida esophagitis, colitis)	• Haloperidol sc, possibly with hydroxyzine sc or Transderm Scop
• Distention from constipation or impaction	• Laxative, manual disimpaction
• Obstruction by tumor or poor motility	• Metoclopramide (Reglan)
• Tube feedings	• Reduce feeding volume
• Gag reflex from feeding tube	• Remove it
• Nasopharyngeal bleeding	• Packing, vit K, sedation
• Thick secretions (cough-induced vomiting)	• Nebulized saline if good cough reflex, anticholinergic if poor cough reflex

Table 7.5 Pharmacologic Therapy for Nausea and Vomiting

	Category	Drug	Starting Dosage
vestibular	Antihistamines	Dramamine	50-100 q 4 hr
		Hydroxyzine	10-25 mg qid po, im
	Anticholinergics	Scopolamine	0.3-0.6 mg im, sc, iv, or 1 patch q72 hr
		Hyocyamine	0.125 mg qid po
	Corticosteroids	Dexamethasone	5-10 mg qid po, iv
		Prednisone	5-10 mg qid po
	Benzodiazepines	Lorazepam	0.25 mg qid po, iv, im
		Diazepam	2-5 mg qid po, iv, im, pr
		Compazine PO	5-10 mg 3-4 × per d, 40 max iv 2.5-10
CTZ	Dopamine antagonists	Prochlorperazine	10-25 mg qid po, iv, pr
		Haloperidol	0.25-0.5 mg po, im
		Metoclopramide	1-2 mg po, im, iv (Tardive Dyskinesia)
	Serotonin antagonists		
	Mixed antagonists	Ondansetron	4 mg bid iv, po
		Olanzapoine	2.5 mg q6 hr po

17:145; CA 1993;72:594); used for bone mets, esophageal cancer causing dysphagia—effective in 1-2 wks.

- Fatigue/weakness: rx depending on etiology (Ritalin, transfusion):
  - Hypomagnesemia: magnesium oxide 400 mg 1-2 tab bid-tid.
  - Adrenal insufficiency: hydrocortisone 80 mg iv q 8 hr.
  - Acute bone pain: corticosteroids, bisphosphonates for multiple myeloma.
  - Cord compression: dexamethasone 100 mg iv stat, radiation rx.

- Over-sedation by narcotics: methylphenidate 10 mg at 0800 and 5 mg at 1,200.
- Nausea and vomiting associated w terminal illness: dopamine antagonist, such as phenothiazine; benzodiazepine, antihistamine for anxiety (BMJ 1997;315:1148; 1998;316:286).
- Antiemetics for chemotherapy: start w prochlorperazine (Compazine), promethazine (Phenergan); serotonin-reuptake antagonists granisetron in combination w dexamethasone more effective than either alone (Nejm 1995;332:1); ondansetron (Zofran) 8 mg bid.
- Cachexia: megestrol acetate to rx cachexia, inconsistent results w increasing lean body mass; dronabinol, anabolic androgenic steroid (CNS side effects), psychostimulants to promote appetite—no systemic studies in frail elderly; metoclopramide for gastric stasis, but risk of tardive dyskinesia. ACEI as anti-cachexia drug (Jags 2005;53:2030).
- Daily pain prevention among NH patients w cancer often untreated in older and minority groups (Jama 1998;279:1877); > 33% conscious dying pts have severe pain (Ann IM 1997; 126:97).
- Pain management: analgesic dose in a pt who has become tolerant to a narcotic is not lethal because pt also develops tolerance to the life-threatening side effects of respiratory depression (McCaffery M, Pain Management American Med Dir Assoc Annual Meeting, Phoenix, AZ, 1997); World Health Guidelines for stepwise approach to cancer pain:
  1. Acetaminophen, ASA, OTC NSAID (may be good for neuropathic pain, COX2 fewer gi se, but same renal problems and increased cardiovascular risk), as well as nonpharmacologic interventions (radiation, relaxation, psychotherapy).
  2. Weak opiate (codeine), tramadol less constipation.
  3. Graduated dose of strong narcotic (morphine).

Strong Opioids: (see Table 1.3, Opioid conversion chart, p. 20)

- Can increase long-acting opioid q 24 hr, by 25-50% for moderate pain, and by 50-100% for severe pain.
- When changing from po to iv, there is a large first pass effect so divide by 3 unless converting methadone, then divide by 2.
- Short-lived breakthrough pain can be treated w fentanyl lozenge on a stick via buccal mucosa.
- Opioid rotation if not working; incomplete cross tolerance w second opioid so calculate the equianalgesic dose, then decrease by 25% for severe pain and 50% for moderate pain.
- Spinal cell neurons increase central facilitation leading to allodynia (pain w light touch) from abnormal NMDA pathway. Methadone is an NMDA antagonist, as well as an inhibitor of serotonin and noradrenalin uptake. Relative potency of morphine to methadone varies with dose (see Table 1.3: Opioid conversion chart).

  Avoid meperidine due to accumulation of toxic metabolite normeperidine resulting in dysphoria, myoclonic jerks, seizures (see Geriatric Pharmacology: Pain).
- Constipation from opioids: avoid bulk forming agents like psyllium because may lead to impaction. Give benzodiazepine before manual disimpaction.
- Antiepileptics for neuropathic pain: clonazepam, valproic acid, lamotrigine (Neurol 2001;57:505).

  Alpha 2 blockers act on nociceptive and neuropathic pain, decreasing sympathetic outflow, ie, clonidine.
- Hypercalcemia: iv saline and loop diuretics; pamidronate 60-90 mg iv over 2-24 hr, repeat q 2 wk; or calcitonin 4 μ/kg im or sc q 12 hr; or plicamycin 25 μg/kg iv q 4-6 hr (Drugs 1993; 46:594).
- Pain w terminal delirium: Olanzapine 2.5 mg is both dopamine and serotonin antagonist, so may tx pain, as well w fewer side effects.

Team Management:

- Biofeedback, hypnosis, behavior modification for chronic pain (Ann IM 1980;93:588).
- Formal pt education about pain helpful (CA 1994;74:2139).
- Iv hydration when dying leads to untoward effects such as pulmonary edema (Cancer Nurs 1990;13:62), incr edema, incontinence, dyspnea; endorphins likely released w terminal dehydration.
- Ethical dilemmas in artificially feeding the terminally ill (Jags 1984;32:237; 1984;32:525; Nejm 1988;318:25) (see *Ethics* p. 442).
- Psychological issues: isolation, lack of understanding of dx/px, role changes in family, guilt, financial difficulties, loss of intimacy, anticipatory grief, anger at loss of independence.
- Family meeting w dying pt (simple nonjudgmental listening):
  1. Have pt tell the story of how he/she became ill and the course of the illness; the pt may ask spouse to tell the story, but it is important that the pt do so, regaining confidence and connection w the family this way.
  2. Have pt talk about his/her worries and fears; first, fears for the family:
     A. Spouse—describe how met spouse, evaluate the marriage, voice disillusionments, resentments so they may be let go
     B. "Children"—speak to each, reframe crying not as "breaking down," but as "breaking through"; important for pt to realize that he/she does not have control over how the children will live the rest of their lives and that he/she must let this go; can now only simply give the "gift of love"; grandchildren may have separation and individuation issues (Kübler-Ross E. Children facing death. Presented at the 4th International Seminar on Terminal Care, Montreal, Canada, 1982).

C. "Self"—his/her worries for him/herself: suffering, loneliness, fear, loss of control.

3. Concerning roots: have the pts recount stories about parents and siblings, unmourned deaths.
4. Family tells of the pt: spouse evaluates marriage; secrets may emerge (alcohol, incest) not to inflame guilt, but to keep secrets from being buried only to reappear in future generations (Murphy M. *Hospice Conference*, New York, 1992).
   - Transportation for radiation rx.
   - Caregivers (informal and formal) need to care for themselves (BMJ 1998;316:208).
   - Eligibility hospice care: prognosis < 6 mo; goal of comfort-oriented care; must meet disease specific or general failure to thrive guidelines. Examples:
     - CHF: class IV
     - COPD: O_2 dependent w sx at rest
     - Malnutrition
     - Dementia: bed bound
     - Urinary/fecal incontinence
     - Inability to communicate
     - Comorbid complications

Chapter 8

Cardiology

8.1 Hypertension

Ger Rv Syllabus 2002;5:267; NIH Public No. 93-1088; Arch IM 1993;153:177; 1995;155:563; Clin Ger Med 1999;15:663 www.nhlbi.nih.gov/guidelines/hypertension/jncintro.htm; HT 1994;23:275, Jama 2008;299:1678

Cause: Consider meds, eg, cough and cold preparations, NSAIDs.

Epidem: 50% of pts > 65-74 yr old have HT; 60-70% African American, Hispanic, Native American have HT; > 1/3 have BP > 160 (HT 1995;25:305). Diastolic BP rises until age 55, when it begins to level off; therefore the rise in isolated systolic BP accounts for the overall increase in age-related HT: 10% at age 70, and 20% at age 80 independent of race.

Almost all hypertensive patients older than 75 have sys HT. Lifetime risk of obtaining HT is > 90%; elevated systolic BP or elevated pulse pressure is the single greatest risk for cardiovascular disease in persons older than 65; even isolated sys HT Stage 1. BP 140-159 (Nejm 1993;329:1912); LVH in hypertensives may confer an increased risk for ventricular arrhythmias; ~90% HT primary (essential) assoc w fam hx, DM, obesity, diet, ETOH use, drug/medicine use; ~10% HT secondary: primary renal disease, renovascular causes, pheochromocytoma, Cushing's, Conn's syndrome (Nejm 1992;327:543); it is estimated that less than 20% of elderly hypertensives are contolled at less than sys BP < 140 and dias BP < 90.

Clearly beneficial to treat HT in pts > 80 yr old (Lancet 1999;353:793). Sleep apnea is associated with HT even when adjustment for wgt, ETOH, smoking made; tx of obstructive sleep apnea w BiPAP has been shown to lower BP (Jama 2000; 283:1829); vs > 80 yr, little correlation of BP and mortality (Jags 2007;55:383; 2006;54:912)

Pathophys:

- Increased vascular resistance results from age-related decrease in elastic tissue, as well as the development of atherosclerosis; also a decrease in vasodilatory response to alpha adrenergic stimulation, while adrenergic response remains the same.
- Decreased baroreflex secondary to decreased artery distensibility; requires larger change in BP to activate and then responds w large effects in sympathetic nervous system outflow.
- Renally-secreted prostaglandins protect from HT; renin/aldosterone/angiotensin worsen HT, although not a major cause in the development of HT in the elderly; basal and stimulated levels of renin and aldosterone decline with age; however, older pts respond well to smooth-muscle relaxants and ACE inhibitors.
- Ca and Na intakes modulate BP via PTH and the renin-angiotensin system (Ann IM 1987;107:919).
- "Salt-sensitive" HT depends on Na and Cl together; BP decreases w Na citrate (Nejm 1987;317:1043).

Sx: Usually asymptomatic but long-standing HT may first present with end organ damage, ie, retinal hemorrhage, decreased renal function. Sudden onset (see hypertensive emergency/urgency) or recalcitrant HT suggests secondary HT, particularly occlusive renovascular disease, rarely hyperaldosteronism, hypokalemia, pheochromocytoma.

Si: No proven benefit to treating Stage 1 sys HT, but therapy should not be withheld on the basis of age. Increased risk of rx if dias BP

< 60. Thiazide diuretic or long-acting Ca-channel blocker preferred (Jama 2004;292:1074).

- Sys BP > 140 on three occasions or average dias BP > 90 (consider when stiff arteries cause higher BP readings).
- Systolic BP > 160 mmHg more significant risk factor than diastolic BP > 95 mmHg (Lancet 2000;355:865); ambulatory BP better predictor of risk in elderly (Jama 1999;282:539).
- Auscultate for peripheral arterial bruits, 4th heart sound, displaced PMI; look for retinal changes.
- Palpate during BP measurement to avoid missing an auscultatory gap.

Si of Secondary HT: abdominal bruit (renovascular disease); hyperglycemia, fat distribution (Cushing's); headache, palpitations, diaphoresis and paroxysmal elevations of BP (pheochromocytoma); worsening of BP control or BP that remains uncontrolled on triple rx; malignant HT: abrupt development of diastolic HT (which is unusual in light of the general decrease in diastolic BP in persons > 60 yr old).

Pseudo-HT: presents w rigid arteries that cannot be compressed by sphygmomanometer cuff, giving falsely high readings, but can still palpate radial pulse (Osler's sign, may be unreliable); however, pt often exhibits BP out of proportion to end organ damage (HT 1994;23:275).

Crs: Older pts w HT at higher risk for orthostatic hypotension (> 20 mmHg sys BP drop or > 10 mmHg dias BP drop when changing from supine to standing); pressures should be measured in both sitting and standing position; rx of systolic and diastolic HT up to age 85 yr old (Lancet 1991;338:1281); LVH decreases over 6 mo and function improves in elderly rx'd with verapamil or atenolol (Nejm 1990;322:1350); ace inhibitors best preserve renal function. Increased likelihood of orthostatic hypotension in diabetic patients. Significant correlation between orthostatic hypotension and increased mortality (Circ 1998;98:2290; Am J Med 2000; 108:106).

- Isolated moderate sys HT also associated w increased cardiovascular risks of 1.5 × (Nejm 1993;329:1912).
- Rx of isolated sys HT (> 160 mmHg) in elderly reduces CVAs by 1/3 (NNT − 5 = 33) (Jama 1991;265:3255), stroke mortality by 36%, and cardiac mortality by 25% (Ann IM 1994;121: 355), NNT − 5 = 18 to prevent MI/CVA (Jama 1994; 272:1932).

Cmplc: CVA, hypertensive crisis; chronic renal failure; cardiovascular including Afib and LVH, which increases risk of MI, CVA, Vtach, death and sudden death 3-4 × more than HT alone (Nejm 1992;327:998; 1987;317:787; Ann IM 1986; 105:173).

- Mild cognitive impairment, dementia; antihypertensive therapy may slow progression (Am J Epidem 2001;153:72).

Lab:

- Routine initial w/u:
  Family hx, DM II high likelihood of essential HT, r/o sleep apnea (30%) (Ann IM 1994;120:382; 1985; 103:190).
- Alcohol, sodium (water softeners?), diet (r/o hyperparathyroid, Ca, Mg, K deficiency) and other drug/medicine use, primary renal disease.
- Urinalysis w micro exam, K, BUN/creatinine, EKG (3-8% Sens) or echocardiography (100% Sens, ?specif) for LVH
- For recalcitrant HT or HT emergencies: Renovascular causes (40% have bruits), hypo/hyperthyroidism, pheochromocytoma, Cushing's, Conn's syndrome (Nejm 1992;327:543).
- Elevated CRP has been shown to be related to the future development of HT (Jama 2003;290:2945).

(see specific topics in Chapter 3, Endocrinology)

X-ray: For renovascular HT: renal scan before and after captopril 50 mg po shows decreased flow in affected kidney (90% sens and specif) (Ann IM 1992;117:845; Jama 1992;268:3353).

Rx: Major trials include:

Non-Pharmacologic—The Trials of Hypertension Prevention, DASH, Modification of Diet in Renal Dis, TONE

Pharmacologic—STOP-2, LIFE, SHEP, NHANES III, TOMHS, INDANA, Syst-EUR, SAVE, ELITE, MRFIT, ALLHAT, INVEST, ANBP2, SOLVD, AASK, MRC among others.

Non-Drug Regimens (BMJ 1994;309:436)—reduced sodium intake and wt loss (Jama 1998;279:839); decrease ischemic stroke with leisure time physical activity (Stroke 1998;29:380); reduce ETOH (HT 1992;20:533); avoid or stop NSAIDs (Jama 1994;272:781; Ann IM 1994;121:289).

Pharmacologic Strategies (Ann IM 1994;121:35; NIH Guidelines [2003] www.nhlbi.nih.gov/guidelines/hypertension/jncintro.htm; HT 1994;23:275):

- Guiding principles for drug therapy: start ½ usual adult dose; simple dosing regimens; alternative routes such as patches when needed; lower doses of 2 different agents sometimes better than larger dose of single agent; ½ of elderly controlled w single drug (Jama 1996;277:1577); keep cost in mind.
- Titrate med according to standing BP to avoid orthostatic hypotension.
- Rx goal—gradual reduction of BP as cerebral blood flow to MAP curve is shifted rightward; too rapid decline in BP may precipitate stroke or hypotension, as well as reflex tachycardia/sympathetic activation (esp w α-blockers).
- No more than 10 mmHg decrease per dose increment (over 1 mo) w end goal of 120-140 sys/< 90 diast (lower BP confers added protect for DM); do not lower below 140/85 mmHg [Swedish trial in old persons w HT, STOP-HT (Lancet

CARDIOLOGY

1991;338:1281); Finnish cohort study: lowering BP 5 mmHg from 90 to 86 associated w decreased 5-yr survival (J Hyperten, 1994;7:1183); vs lowering dias BP < 85 did not cause cardiovascular compromise (Lancet 1998;351:1755); BP < 70 a danger (Arch IM 1999;159:2004); when withdraw pts from chronic anti-hypertensives, 40% of pts require restarting them within 1 yr (J Intern Med 1994;235:581)]. Elevated mortality risk secondary to hypotension may be related to underlying illness as opposed to antihypertensive therapy (Ann IM 2002; 136:438). Don't rx oldest old (> 85) (Jags 2007;45:136).

- Treat according to risk stratification: Stage 1 HT (140-159/90-99) w 12 mo lifestyle modification unless risk factors, then treat w 6 mo of lifestyle modification, if target organ damage or clinical cardiovascular disease treat w drugs; Stage 2 HT BP > 160/100 w drugs (> 140 if w DM) (Clin Ger Med 1999;15:663).
- Monitor for hypotension, hypovolemia, kidney function, K esp w diuretics or ACE I or on Digoxin.
- Thiazide diuretics should be first line, careful monitoring for dehydration and electrolyte abnormalities. No benefit if serum potassium < 3.5mg/dL (HT 2000;35:1025). Thiazides reduce Ca excretion, decrease bone Ca loss and hip fractures.
- Second choice should be based on compelling indicators related to comorbidities and risk factors.
- Pts with Stage 2 HT usually require 2 meds.

Diuretics better than β-blockers in decreasing BP and preventing cardiovascular morbidity and mortality (Stroke 1998; 29:380), β-blockers relatively ineffective as monotherapy for older hypertensives (Jama 1998;279:1303); diuretics actually help prevent cardiovascular mortality in hyperlipidemic pts (Jama 1991;265:3255); reduce LV mass (Jama 1998;279:778).

Dyazide (hydrochlorothiazide 12.5-25 mg + triamterene 50 mg) avoids all the MRFIT mortality risks (Ann IM 1995; 122:223; Nejm 1994;330:1852).

Chlorthalidone 2.5 mg qd for isolated sys HT results in 80% risk reduction of CHF in pts w prior MI (Jama 1997;378:212). Chlorthalidone was superior to a Ca-channel blocker and an ace inhibitor in stroke and heart failure protection (Jama 2002; 288:2981).

β-blockers w diuretic also reduce mortality (Jama 1991; 265:3255); atenolol reduced lipid solubility (less depression, lethargy), v.s. only use for compelling indication (J Fam Prac 2008;57:18)

Ca-channel blocker: second choice in elderly after diuretics (Arch IM 1991;151:1954), eg, diltiazem SR 60-180 mg bid, although some studies suggest produces more cognitive impairment than atenolol (Ann IM 1992;116:615); mortality controversy (Jags 1995;43:1309); black men do best with calcium-channel blockers (Med Lett 2007;49:101), long-acting dihydropyridine resulted in 42% reduction in stroke in pts w Isolated Systolic Hypertension (Lancet 1997;350:757). Compelling indications in CAD and DM; avoid Ca-channel blockers in CHF. Ca-channel blocker/ace inhibitor regime no different from β-blocker/thiazide combination in treating hypertensive pts with CAD (Jama 2003;290:2805).

ACE inhibitor may best preserve renal function even w early renal failure, eg, enalapril 5 mg po qd-qid (NNT = 4) (BMJ 1994;309:833); age better predictor of renin response than renin profile (Jama 1998;280:1160); ACE inhibitors more effective than Ca-channel blockers in preventing vascular outcomes in hypertensive Type 2 diabetes (Nejm 1998;338:645; Diab Care 1998;21:597; Lancet 1999;354:1751). ARBs and ACE inhibitors have compelling indications in CHF, DM, and renal insufficiency. More frequent se in blacks. No serum creatinine level in which an ACE inhibitor should not be used.

ACE better than thiazide for all primary endpoints of cardiovascular events and myocardial infarction, despite similar reductions in BP. Results were more significant in men (Nejm 2003; 348:583).

Effects on lipids (Geriatrics 1995;50:13): diuretics increase total cholesterol and triglycerides; sympatholytics decrease total cholesterol and HDL; ACE inhibitors decrease triglycerides; Ca antagonists have no effect on lipids; β-blockers decrease total cholesterol, LDL, triglycerides, and increase HDL; vasodilators decrease total cholesterol, LDL, and increase HDL.

Centrally acting agents are typically not recommended in the elderly. Clonidine patches offer an alternative to the pt not taking oral meds.

HT crisis: rise in BP with imminent risk of organ damage predicated less by BP rise than by the potential vital organ damage; BP must be lowered immediately, but not too low (target BP ~160-170/100-110); make sure pt is euvolemic.

- Assessment: focused physical exam for neuro, cardiovascular, renal, ocular si/sx.
- Hypertensive encephalopathy rx'd w nitroprusside
- LVH and pulmonary edema rx'd w labetolol
- MI or unstable angina rx'd w nitroglycerin ± ACE I
- Dissecting aortic aneurysm rx'd w propranolol
- Adrenergic crisis rx'd w nitroprusside
- Malignant HT rx'd w labetolol captopril
- Acute Renal Failure rx'd w labetolol, minoxidil ± β-blocker
- Perioperative HT rx'd w TNG, nitroprusside (J Am Soc Nephrology 1998;9:133)

Resistant Hypertension: Inability to achieve goal BP while on 2 full dose meds in addition to a full dose diuretic; check BP measurement; attempt ambulatory BP measurement; inadequate diuretic therapy common etiology; loop diuretic better in pts with poor renal function.

Labs: CBC, lytes, BUN/CREAT, UA, CXR, EKG; consider renal US and head CT/MRI, if indicated.

8.2 Coronary Artery Disease

Ger Rv Syllabus 2002;5:253; Jags 1998;46:1157; Am Fam Phys 2002;65:871

Atherosclerosis

Nejm 1996;344:1311; J Am Coll Cardiol 1995;25:1000 (re: women)

Cause: Cholesterol (Nejm 1981;304:65); > 300 independent risk factor in elderly (Jags 1988;36:103, Ann IM 1993;153:1065), vs decreased cholesterol leads to incr death in elders (Jags 2003; 51:991); smoking; HT; lack of estrogen (Ann IM 1976;85:447); genetic (especially in women); not increased by triglyceride elevations alone, although they are markers for other risk factors (Nejm 1993;328:1220); decreased B_6 (Circ 1998;97:437). TFAs increase CAD (Med Lett 2007;49:65; Nejm 2006;354:1601).

Epidem: By age 70 yr, 15% of men and 9% of women have symptomatic CAD; most common cause of death; > 50% of deaths among people > 65 yr (DHHS Pub 97-1789); risk of CHD death from hypercholesterolemia 2.2 × at 60 yr to 11.3 × at 75 yr (Ann IM 1990;1.13:916).

- Incr in diabetes, HT, obesity (Nejm 1990;322:882), homocystinuria (Jama 1992;268:877).
- Low HDL predicts cardiac mortality in pts > 70 yr old; elevated total cholesterol not associated w mortality in men but may be in women (Jama 1995;274:539); decreased in women who take postmenopausal estrogens (Nejm 1991;325:756).

Pathophys: (Nejm 1992;326:242,310)

- Earliest change: lipid-laden cells or fatty streak in intimal layer of artery (Am Hrt J 1994;128:1300); age-related changes: decreases in LDL receptors, cholesterol clearance, bile acid production and estrogen; Insulin resistance syndrome: hyperlipidemia, hyperglycemia, and hyperinsulinemia.

- Wall stress causes fibrous plaques that later infiltrate with cholesterol; impaired fibrinolysis may also play a role in genesis; IL-1, cytokines suggest immunologic mechanism (Basic Res Cardiol 1994;89:41); HDL protective because it stabilizes vasodilator prostaglandin I (Circ 1994;90:1033); HT may induce endothelial dysfunction (HT 1995;25:155); hemorrhage into plaque causes sudden occlusions.

Sx: Claudication, angina, MI, sudden death, TIA/CVA, abdominal angina.

Si: Renal HT; bruits, absent peripheral pulses; CVAs; retinal fundal vessel plaques.

Crs: Reversible with rx (Ann IM 1994;121:348).

Lab: CRP predicts inducible ischemia (Circ 2003;107:245).

Rx: (Jags 1999;47:1458).

NHANES III study (DHHS 97-1789) 50% elderly would benefit from dietary changes; 10-25% qualify for med (NCEP II Guidelines Jama 1993;269:3009):

- Rx of elevated cholesterol, LDL > 130 mg/dL, if two other cardiac risk factors (2002:253), which helps by both decreasing plaques and preventing coronary artery spasm (Nejm 1995; 332;481,488; Circ 1994;89:1329; 1994;90:1056; Lancet 1994; 334:1383; Ann IM 2007;147:1; Jama 2007;297:499); reducing cholesterol may be hazardous (BMJ 1994;308:373); aim to decrease LDL < 100 w 2 or more risk factors, < 160 w 1-2 risk factors (Jama 2111;285:2486); compliance w antilipid rx after age 60 poor in elderly (Jama 2002;288:455,462); statins associated w myopathy (Jama 2003;289:1595).
- Exercise (Jama 1995;273:402) decreases hospitalizations (Jags 1996;44:113); maximum heart rate for men is 220 minus age and for women is 224 minus 0.6 × age because maximal inotropic and chronotropic response to catecholamine and sympathetic nervous system is markedly impaired w age.

- ASA: 85-325 mg qd (Med Lett Drugs Ther 1995;37:14; Arch IM 1995;155:1386).
- Diet that produces LDL < 100 induces plaque regression (Lancet 1994;344:1383); "Mediterranean diet" helps (Lancet 1994;343:1454); Ornish program leads to disease regression, 8% improvement angiogram vs 28% worsening without diet (Jama 1998;280:2001); however, low fat diet may reduce HDL; diet and exercise combined with wt loss may increase HDL; caution dietary changes in pts at risk for malnutrition.

Diet: < 30% fat, < 7% saturated fat, < 200 mg cholesterol/d; Omega-3 FAs more effective than statins w less se (Arch IM 2005;165: 725) then HMG-CoA reductase inhibitor; nicotinic acid 1.5-3.0 gm/d (lowers triglycerides, increases HDL) (Am Fam Phys 1997;55:2250); estrogen replacement decreases ASHD incidents

Table 8.1 Treatments for Elevated Cholesterol

	First Choice	Alternative
ISOLATED ELEVATED LDL	STATIN (in order of most effect on serum lipids): Atorvastatin 10-80 mg qd Simvastatin 5-40 mg qd Pravastatin 10-40 mg qd Lovastatin 10-40 mg qd bid Cerivastatin 0.2-0.3 mg q hs Fluvastatin 20-40 mg qd bid	STATIN + BAS
	BILE ACID SEQUESTRANT (BAS) (eg, Cholestyramine)	BAS + NA
	NICOTINIC ACID (NA)	STATIN + NA*
ELEVATED LDL + LOW HDL	STATIN	STATIN + NA*
ELEVATED LDL + TRIGLYCERIDES (200-400 mg dL)	STATIN	STATIN + GEMFIBROZIL/FENOFIBRATE* STATIN + NA*

*Increased risk of myopathy and hepatitis.

in women by up to 50% (Jama 1995;273:199); alcohol at 2-3 drinks qd decreases mortality by 25% (Am J Pub Hlth 1993; 83:805). Co-enzyme Q10 decreases muscle cramps, decreases HD (Jags 2006;54:4; Ann IM 2000;32:636). Red Yeast Rice decreases cholesterol (Int J Integrative Med 2000;2:9).

- Folate 400 mg/d, B_6 3 mg/d to treat increased homocystinemia, which leads to atherosclerosis (Jama 1998;279:359).
- Estrogen/progesterone reduces risk by 50% (Jama 1995;273: 199,240); perhaps medroxyprogesterone to increase HDL cholesterol in postmenopausal females (Nejm 1981;304:560); in a blinded multicenter trial estrogen did not decrease coronary events in women w preexisting CAD (Jama 1998;280:605).
- Raloxifene 60 mg/d (selective estrogen receptor modulator w estrogen agonist) may have good effects on bone and antagonist effects on breast and uterus and bad effects on LDL-C, fibrinogen, and HDL-C2 (Jama 1998;278:1445).
- Pre-op assessment of cardiac risks:
  - Clinical variables: < 6 mo s/p MI, advanced age, h/o angina, non Q-wave MI, DM, HT, ventricular ectopy requiring rx; asx pts w bradycardia or chronic bifascicular block do not need prophylactic pacing.
  - Pre-op angioplasty in pts w > 3 clinical variables and dipyridamole thallium test that demonstrates either redistribution or EKG changes associated w dipyridamole infusion; if 1-2 clinical variables and pos thallium, risk of having cardiac event (unstable angina, MI, pulmonary edema, cardiac death) increased from 3% to 30% (Nejm 1996;344:1311).
  - Outcome elderly pts w chronic CAD same w invasive vs optimal med rx TIME trial (Jama 2003;289:1117).
- 61% of MIs in 1st wk post-op are silent.

Angina

Mod Concepts Cardiovasc Dis 1988;57:19; Nejm 1984;310:1712; Am Fam Phys 1994;49:1459; Jama 2005;293:350

Cause: Atherosclerotic heart disease; myopathic disorders; mitral valve prolapse; reduced vasodilator reserve in coronary arteries (Nejm 1993;328:1659,1706); mental stress is as good an inducer of angina as exercise (Nejm 1988;318:1005).

Epidem: Silent ischemia: coexistent w angina; potential benefit of β-blockers, Ca-channel blockers, coronary revascularization (Jags 1996;44:83).

Pathophys: Spasm may occur even when there is no fixed lesion; unstable angina usually due to a platelet thrombus (Nejm 1992; 326:287).

Sx: Onset with first exercise after rest; more frequently in unfamiliar settings; worse supine; relieved by TNG (r/o esophageal spasm).

Si: S4; mitral regurgitant murmur during pain.

Crs: Px depends on extent of coronary involvement evidenced by angiography and LV function (Circ 1994;90:2645); C-reactive protein may predict early mortality from acute ischemia (J Am Coll Cardiol 1998;31:4160).

Cmplc: MI

R/o esophageal reflux (mimic PUD) (Ann IM 1992; 117:824), PUD, biliary colic, pleurisy, pancreatitis, pulmonary infarct, pneumothorax (Geriatrics 1995;50:33); consider carbon monoxide induction if onset at home in winter (Nejm 1995; 322:48).

Lab:

Chemistry: CPK-MB may elevate mildly.

Noninvasive: ETT contraindicated in CHF, aortic stenosis, IHSS, unstable angina; can't interpret ST changes in face of LBBB, WPW, digoxin, LVH; submaximal test ($< 85\%$ maximal pulse achieved).

ST depressions (0.5 mm to > 2 mm and start in first 3 min or last ≥ 8 min) (Nejm 1979;301:230) and/or hypotension during ETT:

CARDIOLOGY

this scoring system predicts 5-yr survival and annual mortality (Nejm 1991;325:849). Increased HR > 12 during 1st min of exercise stress test predicts MI cardiac death (Circ 2005;112:1958).

Thallium Scan: at peak exercise and 2-4 hr later a better predictor of long-term outcome than ETT or Holter (Ann IM 1990;113:575); dipyridamole (Persantin) used when pt cannot walk on treadmill.

Echocardiogram w Dobutamine Stress (Am J Cardiol 1993;72:605): about same sens and specif as dipyridamole thallium.

Rx:

- ASA 75-325 mg po qd prevents MIs.
- Antianginal meds (Med Lett Drugs Ther 1994;36:111).
- Nitrates to dilate, reduce spasms, increase collaterals, and decrease platelet adhesion; po, sl, buccal patch, or paste; tolerance develops, so avoid hs or 24-hr rx.
- β-blockers decrease pulse, block action of sympathetic nervous system caused by mental stress (Circ 1994;89:762), lower BP, decrease platelet adhesion; avoid in Prinzmetal type because can increase spasm.
- Ca-channel blockers dilate, reduce spasm but not cardioprotective (Lancet 2004;364:817).
- Ranolazine, fatty acid oxidation inhibitor (Jama 2004; 291:309).
- Imipramine 50 mg po hs helps microvascular.

Surgical:

- Angioplasty (Nejm 1994;331:1037,1044; 1994;330:981) preferred in severely symptomatic pt w 1- or 2-vessel CAD and nl LV EF w multiple medical problems; increased risk for stroke w CABG because of cerebrovascular disease or diffuse aortic disease; increased risk for developing postop cognitive dysfunction or frail physical condition; more complications than medical rx (Nejm 1992;326:10); angioplasty long-term requires more antianginal med and surgical interventions than CABG (Nejm 1994;331:1037).

- Drug-eluding stents reserved for pts at greater risk of restenosis who can receive long-term dual platelet rx (Circ 2007;115:813).
- CABG increases survival significantly (Lancet 1994;344;563; Circ 1994;89:2015); preferred in high-risk symptomatic elderly, even age > 80 yr (Ann IM 1990;113:423) w left main artery disease, in pts w significant 3-vessel disease with EF > 30% (Nejm 1988;319:332; 1987;316:981), in pts w significant 2-vessel disease, decreased LV EF and proximal left anterior descending artery disease, in pts w clinical evidence of heart failure during ischemic episodes w ischemic but viable myocardium w few other medical problems, younger physiologic age and in pts who are prepared for 3-4 mo convalescence; diabetic pts do better w CABG than angioplasty (Nejm 1996;335:1290).
- If unstable angina: ASA 75-325 po qd (Nejm 1992;327:175) in men (Nejm 1983;309:396); heparin alone or better with TNG (Nejm 1988;319:1105).
- If silent ischemia: angioplasty (J Am Coll Cardiol 1994;24:11), atenolol (Circ 1994;90:762).

Myocardial Infarction

Am J Med 1992;43:315; Jags 1998;46:1157,1302

Cause: Atherosclerotic (85%) including spasm; emboli 15% (Ann IM 1978;88:155).

Epidem: Increased incidence with h/o:

- Surgical menopause pts not placed on estrogen, but no sharp increase in natural menopause or BSOO if pts put on estrogen (Nejm 1987;316:1105); increased risk of coronary event in first year on estrogen/progesterone (HERS trial, Jama 1998;280:605), without any significant long-term benefit (HERS II, Jama 2002:288:49).
- Smoking increases risk 3 ×, but risk decreases to nl over 2 yr after stopping (Nejm 1985;313:1511); increases risk 5 × if

> 1 ppd, 2 × if 1-4 cigarettes qd in women (Nejm 1987; 317:1303).

- Elevations of total and/or LDL cholesterol (often with cholecystitis hx) (Nejm 1981;304:1396); low HDL cholesterol (< 35 mg/dL) perhaps more important than high LDL (Am J Cardiol 2000;86:19L).
- Diabetes, by itself, as high a risk as known cardiovascular disease. Diabetic, hypertensive women at higher risk for MI (F = 23%, M = 15%) and mortality rate as high as 46%.
- HT
- Aortic sclerosis a potential marker of coexisting CAD (contribution vs association only) (Clin Cardiol 2004;27:671).
- Myocardium at more risk secondary to comorbidities: decreased heart rate variability, reduced vagal tone makes elderly pt more at risk for sudden death w MI.
- Decreased incidence with exercise> 6 METs > 2 hr/wk divided 3-4 ×/wk (Nejm 1994;330;1549); 2-3 alcoholic drinks qd (Nejm 1993;329:1829; Ann IM 1991;114:967).
- Elderly undertreated and lidocaine overused (Arch IM 1996;156:805): elderly also very under-represented in clinical trials: trial enrollment for 75+ just 9% during 1991-2000, though represents 37% of MI in the U.S. (Jama 2001;286:708).

Pathophys: Platelet aggregations and thrombi (Nejm 1990;322:1549); early morning increase in catecholamine-induced platelet aggregation and decrease in plasminogen activator inhibitor Type 1 contribute to thrombogenesis (J Am Coll Cardiol 1993;22:1228); myocardial damage severe because of long-standing HT, DM, valvular disease associated w LV damage, ongoing electrical instability, multivessel CAD and ischemia, reduced dias compliance, increased vascular resistance increasing cardiac workload.

Sx: Chest pain, substernal, in "distribution of a tree," worse supine; diaphoresis, dyspnea; associated with heavy exertion. 50% > 60 yr old present with CNS sx esp confusion; silent MI more common in the elderly, 15-20% of MIs; DM often the cause; might also be due to increased myocardial collateral circulation from gradual coronary artery narrowing (Jags 1994;42:732).

Si: Elderly may present w flash pulmonary edema, arrhythmia, sudden drop in BP, delirium, sudden weakness. In pts who have dementia or language barrier any pain in torso could be MI; can present w abdominal pain and vertigo, as well; toothache.

- Pericardial rub on day 2+, usually without ST changes (Nejm 1984;311:1211); S4 gallop; fever < 103°; transient S2 paradoxical split (Geriatrics 1995;50:2).
- RV infarct syndrome (Nejm 1994;330:1211) more common in elderly, mortality 75% (Circ 1997;96:436); acute inferior MI, high CVP with low PAPs and PCWPs.
- Rectal exam important for guaiac and detection of BPH so do not omit on admission physical.

CARDIOLOGY

Crs: 42% are "silent" and unrecognized (Ann IM 1995;122:96); non Q wave MI 10% hospital mortality, 36% 1 yr mortality, 23% develop Afib, 53% develop CHF (Am J Cardiol 1995;75:187); TIMI III registry: most severe CAD, least likely to get angiography and most likely to have the most adverse outcomes from their disease both in hospital and at 6 wk (Jama 1996;275:1104). In STEMI, initial Q-wave predicts decreased reperfusion, increased mortality (Lancet 2006;367:2035).

Cmplc: Mortality 4 × higher in elderly, and more in elderly because do not go to the ER as quickly (Circ 1995;92:1133; Ann IM 1997;126:593; Jags 1999;47:151):

- Shock (7.5%) (Nejm 1991;325:1117)
- Arrhythmias
- Rupture of septal wall more frequent in elderly than younger pts.
- Pericardial tamponade (r/o RV infarct)
- Aneurysm, occurs in 40% with anterior MI, develops in first 48 hr, leads to emboli, CHF, and PVCs.

- Mural thrombi without aneurysm in 11% of anterior MIs, 2% of others (J Am Coll Cardial 1993;22:1004).
- Dressler's syndrome.
- Papillary muscle rupture causes CHF.
- Heart block (Mod Concepts Cardiovasc Dis 1976;45:129) occurs in 5% of inferior MIs, 3% of anterior MIs, and in 100% with anterior MI w RBBB causing a 75% mortality.
- Excessive adrenergic tone: analgesia and sedation appropriate, β-blockers should be considered (Am Hrt J 1994;9:1).
- Aflut: if electrical cardioversion unsuccessful, use procainamide; can use sotalol (β-blocker) with no arrhythmic effect.
- CHF: rx systolic dysfunction with dobutamine for positive inotropic effect.

Lab:

Chemistry: Enzymes (Ann IM 1986;105:221):
- Cardiac troponin I and T elevations are specific to myocardium; begin to rise 4-6 hr after MI, usually elevated 6-9 hr afterwards (later than CPK-MB), last 10 d; the preferred markers for evidence of myocardial injury (J Am Coll Cardiol 2000;36:959); troponin I more specific for MI than troponin T (and much more so than CPK and CPK-MB) in renal failure (Nephrol Dial Transplant 1998;13:1709).
- Total CPK and/or fractions up in 12 hr, peak at 2 d, last 4 d; CPK-MB rise during 1st 6 hr after onset of pain has 95% sens and specif and may be used for early r/o MI in ER (Nejm 1994; 331:561,607); total CPK correlates with MI size, but may not be as elevated in the elderly (Mayo Clin Proc 1996;71:184).
- LDH and fractions (isoenzymes 4 and 5) increased; r/o renal and red cell source.
- AST (SGOT) up in 24 hr, peaks at 2-4 d, lasts up to 7 d.
- B-type natriuretic peptide (BNP) levels early in course may assist in risk stratification, though doesn't diagnose MI (Nejm 2001;345:1014; Jama 2005;293:1667).

- Cardiac troponin I elevation is specific to myocardium, useful perioperatively when surgery may increase CPK (Nejm 1994;330:670).

EKG: Non-Q-wave MI more common in the elderly (Mayo Clin Proc 1996;71:184); T-inversions—r/o acute cholecystitis (Ann IM 1992;116:218); in RV infarct, these changes are present in V3-6R, especially V4R w 80+% sens and specif (Nejm 1993; 328:981); new RBBB indicates occlusion of anterior descending proximal to 1st septal branch (Nejm 1993;328:1036); > 10 PVCs/hr associated with a 10+% 1-yr mortality (Nejm 1983; 309:331).

Table 8.2 EKG Changes in MI

Area	Leads	Findings	Artery
Anterior	V_3, V_4	Q, ST elevation, T inversion	Left anterior descending
Anterior septal	V_1, V_2	Q, ST elevation, T inversion	"Watershed"
Anterior lateral	V_4–V_6	Q, ST elevation, T inversion	"Watershed"
Lateral	I, aVL, V_5, V_6	Q, ST elevation, T inversion	L coronary
Inferior	II, III, aVF	Q, ST elevation, T inversion	R coronary
Posterior	V_1, V_2	Tall broad R, ST depression, tall T	Associated w inferior
RV	V_1, V_2	ST elevation	Associated w inferior

ETT: (Nejm 1999;340:340) contraindicated in CHF, aortic stenosis, IHSS, unstable angina; can't interpret ST changes in face of LBBB, WPW, digoxin, LVH, or lack of changes w submaximal test (< 85% maximal pulse achieved).

Nuclear (Sestamibi or Thallium) Scan: at peak exercise and 2-4 hr later better predictor of long-term outcome than ETT or Holter (Jama 1966;277:318).

Non-Exertional Testing: w dipyridamole (Persantine), dobutamine, arbutamine (Med Lett 1998;40:19) as good as ETT- may need in elderly w arthritis, COPD, who may not be able to accomplish ETT; adenosine or dipyridamole better than dobutamine, though contraindicated in hypotension, sick sinus, high-degree AV block (Circ 1990;81:1205), and probably COPD (Chest 1989;95:1345).

Stress Echocardiography: assesses myocardial function and perfusion; used with exercise or dobutamine; increasingly utilized, comparable to nuclear imaging (Heart 2005;91:427).

Angiography Indications: CHF, LV dysfunction (EF < 50%); high-risk noninvasive test results; persistent sx, failure of medical rx; previous angioplasty, CABG, or MI; malignant ventricular arrhythmia (Jama 2005;293:351); contraindications: very elderly; significant risk of bleeding; coexisting medical problems, eg, liver disease, terminal condition; do not need in uncomplicated non-Q-wave MI (Nejm 1999;388:785).

Rx:

Prophylactic Interventions:

- ASA (see Coronary Artery Disease); however, in women, apparent insignificant effect of preventing infarction, except in those over 65 yr old (Nejm 2005;352:1293).
- Stopping smoking decreases risk to baseline in 3 yr (Nejm 1990;322:213).
- Lowering cholesterol helps (meta-analysis) (Nejm 1990; 323:1112), atorvastatin best (J Am Coll Cardial 1998;32:665), as does American Heart Association diet (BMJ 1992; 304:1015).
- 60-70% of coronary deaths due to acute MI before arrival at hospital; pre-hospital thrombolysis important (Am Hrt J

1992;123:181); aggressive rx of acute MI w angiography; angioplasty.

- CABG of minimal benefit (Jama 1994;272:859,891; J Am Coll Cardiol 1995;25:47A) vs CABG beneficial (J Am Coll Cardiol 1994;24:425); 3-yr survival rate 77% with CABG vs 54% with medical therapy alone (Am J Cardiol 1994;74:334).

Coronary Care Unit (CCU):

- O_2 only when objective evidence of desaturation (AHCPR No. 94-0602 1994); ASA 325 mg po stat.
- β-blockers help older post-MI pt (Jags 1995;43:751; Am J Cardiol 1994;4:674); adverse outcome of underuse of β-blockers in elderly survivors of MI (Jama 1997;227:115; Nejm 1998;339:489,551).
- β-blocker rx (metoprolol 5 mg iv q 5 min × 3, then 50 mg po bid × 1 d, then 100 mg bid or atenolol 50-100 mg po qd) if no contraindications help prevent recurrent MIs (Circ 1994; 90:762); mortality reduction 40% in elderly (Am J Med 1992; 93:315).
- Diltiazem for non-Q-wave MI (60-90 mg po qid).
- Captopril 50 mg tid, if ETT is impaired to < 40% (Ann IM 1994;21:750; Nejm 1992;327:669) or acutely × 6 wk for all (Lancet 1994;343:1115) or at least for anterior MI (Nejm 1995;332:80), ages 55-74 yr old (Circ 1998;97:2202).
- TNG rx (iv if volume ok) goal to decrease systolic BP by 10%; excessive reduction in BP may result in extension of infarct (Mayo Clin Proc 1996;71:184); although reduces pain, nitrate therapy (infusion followed by transdermal nitroglycerin) does not improve mortality or LV dysfunction at 6 wk or 6 mo (Lancet 1994;343:1115).
- Heparin does not reduce mortality in old AMI patients (J Am Coll Cardiol 1998;31:964), except if large AMI, where can reduce risk of mural thrombus, emboli, severe CHF, Afib, recurrent ischemia in first few days (Jags 1999;47:271; Lancet 1994;343:311; J Am Coll Cardiol 1996;28:328).

- Lovenox better than Lopurin for non-Q-wave MI (Nejm 1997;337:447).
- Clopidogrel (300 mg loading dose, then 75 mg qd) 1st line tx in UA/NSTEMI if not candidate for early CABG (Circ 2003;108:III-31); benefit in STEMI must be balanced with risk of bleeding in emergent CABG, can be used in place of ASA with severe ASA allergy (ACC/AHA Guidelines 2004).
- Thrombolytics: several studies support the efficacy in pts > 65 yr (ISIS-2, GISSI, ASSET, AIMS), but age distribution skewed in these studies (< 20% in pts > 75 yr old) (Jags 1994; 42:127), benefits in over-75 age group controversial (Am J Ger Cardiol 2003;12:344):
  - Contraindications: prior intracerebral hemorrhage, structural cerebral vascular lesion, intracerebral neoplasm, ischemic stroke within 3 mo (except acute within 3 hr), suspected aortic dissection, active bleeding (excluding menses), significant head trauma within 3 mo.
  - Relative contraindications: poorly controlled HT, severe HT on presentation (SBP > 180, DBP > 110), h/o ischemic stroke greater than 3 mo, traumatic CPR, recent major surgery, recent internal bleeding, pregnancy, active peptic ulcer, current anticoagulant use, prior exposure to streptokinase or anistreplase (ACC/AHA Guidelines 2004); relative contraindications: diabetic retinopathy.
  - Streptokinase preferred over TPA (60% increase risk of cerebral bleeds); ASA+ thrombolytic rx better for survival (ISIS-2), addition of clopidogrel to ASA and thrombolytics improves patency rate and reduces ischemic complications—however, studied in patients 75 yr and younger (Nejm 2005;352:1179); ischemia × 30 min within 6-12 hr w 1-2 mm ST elevation in > 2 leads or presence of LBBB, also w > 12 hr if BP decreased or cardiogenic shock, particularly in elderly who present late; risk/benefit high in IMI (Jags 1998;46:1157).

  - Primary angioplasty comparable if not superior results compared to thrombolytic therapy, if not delayed (Nejm 1999; 341:1413; Jama 2004;291:736).
  - Predictors for thrombolysis: 3 or more risk factors for CAD, > 65 yr, known coronary artery stenosis > 50%, ST-segment deviation on presenting electrocardiogram, 2 or more episodes of angina within last 23 hr, elevated serum cadiac biomarker levels (Jama 2005;293:250).
- Percutaneous coronary intervention (PCI): superior to on site fibrinolysis, provided that transfer takes 2 hr or less (Nejm 2003;349:733); newer recommendations lower "medical contact-to-balloon" time to 90 min, fibrinolysis preferred (ACC/AHA Guidelines 2004); benefit probably greater, in comparison to fibrinolytics, in the elderly (Jama 1999; 282:341); improved benefit when GIIb/IIIa inhibitors given beforehand (Nejm 2001;344:1895), particularly early in rx (Jama 2004;292:362).
- Antagonists of GPIIb/IIIa receptor (the final common pathway in platelet aggregation) (the final common pathway in platelet aggregation) (Jama 1999;281:1407): use in pts w non-ST-elevation acute coronary syndromes w positive troponin (Jama 2000;284:876); IIb/IIIa inhibitors: coronary stenting plus IIb/IIIa (abciximab ReoPro) leads to a greater degree of myocardial salvage and a better clinical outcome than do fibrinolytics w IIb/IIIa inhibitors (abciximab) but antithrombin therapy is still required (Am J Cardiol 2000;85:32C); PURSUIT Trial showed that bleeding more common in IIb/IIIa eptifibatide (Integrilin) group, but no increase in incidence of hemorrhagic stroke (Nejm 1998;339:436); tirofiban (Aggrastat) as part of triple drug rx of unstable angina (Nejm 1998;338:1488,1498,1539); defer use, only selective cases (Jama 2007;297:591).
- ACEIs should generally be started in 24 hr, ideally after fibrinolytic therapy and BP stabilization; increased benefit with

anterior infarction, pulmonary congestion, or LVEF < 40%, though still beneficial; contraindicated in hypotension, renal failure, bilateral renal artery stenosis, or allergy; usually start with po dosing (hypotension with iv); gradually increase dose; ARBs likely beneficial, but less data than ACE-Is (ACC/AHA Guidelines 2004).

- ACE inhibitor (Jama 1995;273:1450; Nejm 1995;332:80) beginning 3 d after MI w EF < 40%, captopril 6.25 q 6-8 hr, stop if hypotensive; diltiazem for non-Q-wave MI if no LVH or CHF.
- Early (24-96 hr) rx of cholesterol with statins recommended, (Jama 2002;287:3087; 2004;292:1307)
- ABCDEs of cardiovascular disease management (Jama 2005;293:350):
  - **A**ntiplatlet rx: ASA, ADP receptor antagonist, except if need for urgent CABG, GpIIb/IIIa inhibitor
  - **A**nticoagulation: LMWH unless Cr Cl < 60 ml/min or early invasive strategy
  - **B**-blockade
  - **B**P control w ACE inhibitors
  - **C**holesterol rx: statin LDL < 70 (Jama 2004;292:1307)
  - **C**igarette cessation
  - **D**iabetes rx: HbA1c < 7%
  - **D**iet: optimal BMI
  - **E**xercise: aerobic 4-5 ×/wk > 30min

Rehab: Depression in CCU s/p MI: 10%, 3-4× increase in mortality rate in 6 mo if persists; return to work part-time in 4-6 wk (Barker LR. Principles of Ambulatory Medicine, Williams and Wilkins 1995;712); if can walk 100 m without angina or dyspnea, can do air travel 10 d after MI (Dardick K. Travel medicine—What the family physician should know. 16th Annual Family Practice Review, St. Petersburg, FL, Bayfront Medical Center, March 1994); lifestyle changes, then thiazides, then β-blockers (Jama 1994;272:842; HT 1994;23:275).

Post MI Rx: (Jags 1998;46:1459):

- β-blocker indefinitely, regardless of whether HT present (Jama 2004;291:1720).
- Cholesterol reduction after MI benefits elderly of both sexes (Circ 1997;96:4211); keep LDL < 100 w simvastatin (Circ 1997;95:1683); new guidelines recommend LDL < 70 (Circ 2004;110:227); rx low HDL with niacin or fibrates.
- ASA 160 mg-325 mg indefinitely (Circ 1996;94:2341).
- Warfarin INR 2.0-3.0 for persistent Afib, LV thrombus.
- Ca-channel blockers, if persistent angina despite nitrates, β-blockers; can be used in place of β-blockers if these are not tolerated.
- Nitrates: increase gradually, isosorbide dinitrate po to 30-40 mg tid or 60 mg dose isosorbide mononitrate sr qd, nitrate free period=12 hr (Nejm 1987;316:1440); β-blocker can be given during nitrate-free period.
- No antiarrhythmics, except β-blocker.
- Implantable cardioverter-defibrillator for VF, VT, high risk sudden cardiac death (Nejm 1996;335:1933; Med Lett 2002; 44:99); also beneficial with LVEF < 30% and h/o MI (Nejm 2002;346:877) vs no benefit in mortality early after MI (Nejm 2004;351:2481).
- Hormone replacement: not as secondary prevention (Nejm 1996;335:453; Jama 1995;273:119; 1998;280:605; Circ 1994; 89:2545).
- CABG 73% success rate vs PTCA 89% success rate.
- Dipyridamole thallium after MI independent predictor of outcome (Jags 1999;47:295).

8.3 Congestive Heart Failure

Clin Ger Med 2000;16:407; Circ 2001;104:2996 (ACC/AHA CHF Practice Guidelines 2004); Jama 2002;287:628; Jags 2003;51:123;

Nejm 2003;348:2007; 2004;351:1097; Chest 2004;125:652; Ann IM 2005;142:132

Cause:

- Systolic: dilated cardiomyopathy (due to ischemia, infarction, HT, MR, chronic ethanol abuse, idiopathic); high output failure (chronic anemia, hyperthyroidism, thiamine deficiency, AV shunting, tachyarrythmia); uncommon (Chagas disease, viral cardiomyopathy, hemochromatosis, sarcoidosis, cardiotoxic meds) (Jags 1997;45:972).
- Diastolic: Hypertrophic cardiomyopathy (CAD and HT) account for > 70% of all heart failure cases, also consider calcific AS, DM, and hypertensive hypertrophic cardiomyopathy; restrictive cardiomyopathy, esp due to senile amyloid deposition (Jags 1997;45:972).
- Precipitating factors: noncompliance with meds and/or diet most common cause, also arrhythmias, excessive fluid intake, (esp iatrogenic), short-acting ca-channel blockers, NSAIDs, estrogen, corticosteroids, clonidine, alcohol, thiazolidinediones (Diab Care 2004;27:256; Jags 1997;45:972).

Table 8.3 Comparing Systolic to Diastolic CHF

Characteristic	Diastolic Heart Failure	Systolic Heart Failure
Age	Frequently elderly	All ages, typically 50-70 yr
Sex	Frequently female	More often male
Left ventricular ejection fraction	Preserved or normal, approximately 40% or higher	Depressed, approximately 40% or lower
Left ventricular cavity size	Usually normal, often with concentric left ventricular hypertrophy	Usually dilated
Left ventricular hypertrophy on electrocardiography	Usually present	Sometimes present
Chest radiography	Congestion with or without cardiomegaly	Congestion and cardiomegaly
Gallop rhythm present	Fourth heart sound	Third heart sound
Coexisting conditions		
Hypertension	+++	++
Diabetes mellitus	+++	++
Previous myocardial infarction	+	+++
Obesity	+++	+
Chronic lung disease	++	0
Sleep apnea	++	++
Long-term dialysis	++	0
Atrial fibrillation	+ (usually paroxysmal)	+ (usually persistent)

*A single plus sign denotes "occasionally associated with," two plus signs "often associated with," three plus signs "usually associated with," and a zero "not associated with."

Reproduced with permission, Nejm 2003;348:2012

CARDIOLOGY

Epidem: See Table 8.3.

- Prevalence of CHF increases two-fold every decade after 45 yr old, so that prevalence in adults > 80 yr old approaches 10% (Jags 1997;45:968); incidence 10 per 1,000 and 20% of all hospital admissions of persons > 65 yr old; most common hospital discharge dx; receives more Medicare dollars than any other dx.
- Diastolic dysfunction much more prevalent in elders, accounts for more than 1/2 of elder pts with heart failure (Ann IM 2002; 137:631; Jags 1997;45:1132). Typically elderly female with HT, obesity, DM. At autopsy, 50% pts with CHF did not have CAD (Mayo Clin Proc 1988;63:552).
- Wide pulse pressure > 67 mmHg, 55% increased risk of CHF (Ann IM 2003;138:10; Jama 1999;281:634), risk of developing HF over 15 yr increases by 5-7% with each increment of 1 of BMI, controlling for other risk factors (Nejm 2002; 347:305); BNP levels independently correlate with risk of developing CHF in asx pts (Jama 2005;293:1609; Nejm 2004; 350:655). Elevated homocysteine and serum insulin-like growth factor 1 levels associated with increased risk of CHF in elderly (Ann IM 2003;139:642; Jama 2003;289:1251).

Pathophys: The heart's ability to respond to stress diminishes normally with age due to four general principles:

1. Reduced responsiveness to beta-adrenergic stimulation → limitations in heart rate, contractility, β2-mediated vasodilation.
2. Increased vascular stiffness → increased afterload.
3. Increased heart stiffness → impaired diastolic filling → increased resting atrial and ventricular pressures → increased preload.
4. Decreased mitochondrial ability to respond to increased demand for ATP (Jags 1997;45:969).
   - Systolic (EF < 40%): Inadequately contracting ventricle resulting from and contributing to several factors (functional,

neurohumoral, and structural), which often are additive in a vicious cycle:

1. Increased afterload: due to increased arterial tone secondary to increased sympathetic tone and increased activation of renin-angiotensin-aldosterone system (RAAS).
2. Increased preload: due to increased venous tone that shifts blood from periphery to central circulation, increasing venous return to heart; also, failing ventricle has decreased cardiac output, causing decreased renal blood flow, causing increased sodium absorption by proximal tubule and increased activation of RAAS.
3. Hypertrophy and dilitation of heart: response to chronic pressure and volume overload or to post-MI remodeling of infarcted area. Hypertrophied muscle operates at lower inotropic state than normal muscle. Remodeling may also lead to arrythmia or to altered flow, causing further damage (eg, mitral regurgitation). Angiotensin II, aldosterone, and catecholamines are all directly involved in adverse remodeling process—possibly directly cardiotoxic.
4. Natriuretic peptides: released in response to atrial (ANP) and ventricular (BNP, ANP) stretch and filling pressure. Increases GFR, natriuresis, and diuresis. Counteracts effects of aldosterone, renin, norepinephrine, and endothelin; causes vasodilation.

- Diastolic (EF 50% or greater): impaired capacity of ventricle to fill due to impaired ventricular relaxation, increased myocardial stiffness (Nejm 2004;350:1953); leads to increased end-dias pressures, decreased stroke volume, decreased lung compliance; heart less able to accommodate small hemodynamic changes, resulting in exercise intolerance.

Sx: Most common presenting sx are of decreased exercise tolerance or fluid retention. However, elderly may present with atypical sxs–eg, cough, mental status change, or self-limitation of IADLs.

Must distinguish sys from dias dysfunction, as this will determine therapy; however si/sx are often similar (J Am Coll Cardiol 2003;41:1519):

- Systolic: fatigue, sx of prerenal azotemia, cool skin, mental obtundation, anxiety, insomnia, nightmares, anorexia, nausea; orthopnea, PND may not occur due to compensatory pulmonary vasculature changes (Jags 1997;45:1129).
- Diastolic: increased filling pressures causing congestion, exercise intolerance.

Si: JVD most reliable sign in the elderly (98% specific) (Am Fam Phys 2004;70:2145); Pulmonary and peripheral edema occur late in disease, and are neither sens nor spec in elderly (Jags 1997; 45:1129); resting tachycardia uncommon; S_4 very non-spec in elderly, and may simply reflect age-related diastolic dysfunction; pulse contour abnormalities obscure due to stiff vessels (Jags 1997;45:1129); daily weights helpful early sign of fluid retention once dx has been made.

Course:

- 1-yr mortality for symptomatic heart failure is 45%, rate of sudden death is 6-9 × higher than the general population; mortality rate directly related to age and presence of CAD; mortality in pts with Class I-II NYHA sxs most often sudden cardiac death; in Class III-IV, most often due to progressive heart failure (Ann IM 2004;141:381).
- Fewer than 30% elderly persons survive 6 yr after first hospitalization for CHF (Clin Ger Med 2000;16:407). Average 5-yr mortality from time of dx–55% in men, 45% in women (Nejm 2002;347:1397; Jama 2004;292:344).
- Elderly pts with sys dysfunction have higher mortality than pts with dias dysfunction (Jags 1995;43:1038). Annual mortality 5-8% dias, 10-15% sys (Circ 2002;105:1387).

- Single marital status correlated w death from CHF (Am J Cardiol 1997;78:1640). Atrial natriuretic hormone and BNP levels predictive of mortality from CHF, sudden death (Jags 1998;46:453; Circ 2003;107:1278; 2002;105:2392). LBBB is predictor of sudden death.
- Elevated JVP and third heart sound: increased risk of CHF hospitalization and death (Nejm 2001;345:574). Shift in differential wbc (decreased lymphocytes) correlates with poor px in pts with CHF (activation of sympathetic nervous system) (Circ 1998;97:19) 6-min walk test provides independent prognostic data in pts w LV dysfunction (Jama 1993;270:1702). AHA/ACC Classification 2002:

  Useful for progressively staging CHF, unlike NYHA (a functional assessment, allows movement between classes)
  Stage A – high risk, but no structural or functional heart abnormality
  Stage B – structural abnormality, but no past or current symptoms of heart failure
  Stage C – structural abnormality with current or previous symptoms of heart failure
  Stage D – end stage symptoms refractory to standard treatment, requiring special interventions

Lab: CBC, UA, lytes, BUN, Cr, glucose, Ca, magnesium, phosphorus, albumin, liver function, TSH; consider HIV, ferritin, ANA, Rh in select pts.

BNP: Not yet recommended by ACC/AHA as part of routine outpatient evaluation. Increases with age, LV thickness, and in women (Circ 2004;109:984); cannot distinguish between sys and dias HF. In pts with acute dyspnea, very useful in ruling out CHF – BNP < 50 pg/ml = NPV 96% (Nejm 2002;347:161); elevated BNP >100 may suggest either stable or decompensated CHF or other causes of BNP elevation (PE, cor pulmonale),

CARDIOLOGY

depending on the clinical setting. BNP elevation also of Px value (BMJ 2005;330:625; Jama 2005;294:2866).

Noninvasive Studies:

- Echocardiography in all cases to assess ventricle size and function, atrial size, diastolic filling, valvular function, pericardium; normal EF in elderly is 50-60% (Curr Probl Cardiol 1987; 12:1).
- EKG for evidence of LV dysfunction due to CAD (eg, Q waves) or LVH.
- CXR, though cardiomegaly need not be present and pulmonary congestion may be subtle or absent in elderly pts (Cardiol Clin 1999;17:125).
- Noninvasive stress testing to detect ischemic myocardium in pts without angina but with high probability of CAD who would be candidates for revascularization (J Am Coll Cardiol 1995;26:1376).
- Functional capacity, including physical capacity, emotional status, social function and cognitive factors (J Am Coll Cardiol 1995:1376).

Invasive Studies: Coronary revascularization has been shown to be beneficial in pts with combination of ischemia and left ventricular systolic dysfunction, therefore coronary arteriography is recommended in pts with angina and heart failure who have no contraindications to coronary revascularization.

Rx: Majority of trials still do not include representative proportions of minorities or women. Very few include persons > 75 yr old (Arch IM 2002;162:1682).

For recommended doses: Captopril 6.25 tid up to 50 tid; enalapril 2.5 mg qd to 20 mg qd; Lisiropril 2.5 qd up to 20 qd; Losartan 50 mg qd maintenance, Isosorbide dinitrate 120 mg qd maintenance, Carvedilol 3.125 mg bid up to 25 mg bid. Metoprolol CR/XL 12.5 mg qd to 250 mg qd, spironolactone

25 mg qd maintenance cautions use ACEI if BP < 90, K > 5.5, Cr > 3.0 (Jags 1998;46:545)

Systolic:

Stage A – high risk, but no structural or functional heart abnormality

** Risk factor reduction and pt education. Consider ACEI.

- Treat HT, hyperlipidemia, DM aggressively – goal dias BP < 80
- Lifestyle modification – stop smoking, illicit drugs, decrease alcohol
- ACEI in high risk pts (PVD or DM) without CHF sxs or low EF reduced risk of CHF at 5 yr by 77% – NNT = 40 (Ramipril, HOPE – Nejm 2000;342:145)
- ARB reduces first CHF hospitalization in type II diabetics with nephropathy by 32% – NNT = 21 (Losartan, RENAAL – Nejm 2001;345:861)

Stage B – Structural abnormality, but no past or current sxs of heart failure.

** Minimize disease progression, prevent new injury. Use ACEI and β-blockade in all pts.

- Asymptomatic pts with EF < 35%: ACEI reduces risk of developing symptomatic CHF over 3 yr by 37% – NNT = 11 (Enalapril, SOLVD-P - Nejm 1992;327:685)
- Claudications also helped by ACEI (Ann IM 2006;144:660)
- Pts s/p MI with low EF but no overt HF: ACEI reduces 3-yr risk of severe CHF by 29-37%, mortality by 19-22% – NNT = 20 (Captopril, SAVE - Nejm 1992;327:669; Trandolapril, TRACE - Nejm 1995;333:1670)
- Pts s/p MI with low EF, receiving ACEI: β-blocker reduced mortality by 23% at 16 mo – NNT = 33 (Carvedilol, CAPRICORN - Lancet 2001;357:1385)
- Lifestyle modification and risk factor reduction as in Stage A

Stage C—structural abnormality with current or previous sxs of heart failure

CARDIOLOGY

** Alleviate symptoms, slow disease progression. ACEI, certain β-blockers in all pts.

** Diuretics and sodium restriction for volume overload. Add digoxin if needed for symptom control.

** Consider aldosterone antagonist, hydralazine + isosorbide or ARB as second line.

** Interdisciplinary interventions are very effective and underutilized (see below).

- ACE inhibitors: help all pts with symptomatic heart failure; meta-analysis showed 35% relative risk reduction in rate of death or hospitalization. Pts with lowest EF have the greatest benefit. (Enalapril, CONSENSUS - Nejm 1987;316:1429; Enalapril, SOLVD - Nejm 1991;325:293; Enalapril, V-HeFT II - Nejm 1991;325:303; Ramipiril, AIRE - Lancet 1993;342:821; Jama 1995;273:1450).
- β Blockers: Carvedilol, Metoprolol, Bisoprolol only in class with proven benefit to reduce death, sxs, and hospitalizations in CHF; in addition to ACE, diuretic, digoxin, tx decreased all-cause 1-yr mortality by 32-65% in Class II-III heart failure pts - NNT=21-27 (Carvedilol, Nejm 1996;334:1349; Bisoprolol, CIBIS-II - Lancet 1999;353:9; Metoprolol CR/XL, MERIT-HF- Lancet 1999;353:2001; Jama 2002;287:883).
- Other β-blockers have not shown comparable effects: Bucindolol in moderate CHF patients showed no significant difference in mortality (BEST – Nejm 2001;344:1651).
- Diuretics: reduce volume overload in symptomatic pts; should not be used in isolation. Meta-analysis showed reduction in mortality, improved exercise capacity (Int J Cardiol 2002; 82:149); follow closely for electrolyte abnormalities, intravascular volume depletion.
- Moderate salt restriction: 2-3 gm/d recommended, but not well-studied (Jags 1998;46:525).

- Avoid meds that exacerbate CHF sxs, including NSAIDs and COX 2 inhibitors (Lancet 2004;363:1751; Arch IM 2002; 162:265), thiazolodinediones & metformin (Diab Care 2004; 27:256), certain anti-arrhythmics: quinidine, sotalol (Arch IM 2004;164:711).
- Digoxin: decreases hospitalizations for heart failure by 23% over 3 yr in pts in NSR – NNT=13, with greatest effect in patients with EF < 25%; no difference in overall mortality (dig - Nejm 1997;336:525); Serum concentration does not correlate with efficacy, lower concentrations (< 0/9 ng/ml) preferable due to toxicity (J Am Coll Cardiol 2002;39:946; Jama 2003; 289:871). Suggestion of increased mortality in women on digoxin–may be related to gender differences in drug pharmacokinectics (Nejm 2002;347:1394,1403).
- Aldosterone antagonists: spironolactone reduced 2 yr hospitalization for CHF by 35% and overall mortality by 30% in NYHA Class III or IV pts on ACEI and loop diuretic– NNT= 9 (RALES - Nejm 1999;341:709). Eplerenone reduced mortality by 25% in pts with CHF s/p MI – NNT= 43 (EPHESUS - Nejm 2003;348:1309); Both drugs are significantly associated with hyperkalemia; use low doses and follow renal function, electrolytes closely (Nejm 2004;351:585).
- Angiotensin II receptor blockers: effective and safe alternative to ACEI, if unable to tolerate due to cough or angioedema; ARB reduces 3 yr CV death or hospitalization by 18% in pts with low EF compared to placebo, NNT= 14 (Candesartan, CHARM-Alt—Lancet 2003;362:772). ARB not inferior to ACEI in pts s/p MI with CHF, but no overall mortality benefit for combination ACEI and ARB (Valsartan vs Captopril, VALIANT—Nejm 2003;349:1893; CHARM-Added—Lancet 2003;362:767, Ann IM 2004;141:693)
- Nitrates and Hydralazine: Recommended for pts on β-blocker, dig, and diuretics, who cannot tolerate ACE/ARB or aldosterone antagonists due to renal insufficiency (Nejm 1991;

325:303). Hydralazine helpful if pt has low cardiac output and pre-renal azotemia (Sci Am 1998;II:12); combination reduced 3-yr mortality by 36% in pts on digoxin and diuretic (V-HeFT - Nejm 1986;314:1547), similar effect seen in African American pts–43% mortality reduction, 33% reduction in CHF hospitalization (A-HeFT - Nejm 2004; 351:2049).

- Ca-Channel Blockers: Short-acting negative inotropes (nifedipine, diltiazem, verapamil) not recommended in CHF due to increased risk of hospitalization (Circ 1990;82:1954). Felodipine and amlodipine have a neutral effect on survival in CHF, therefore use only if needed to control HT or angina (Felodipine, V-HeFT III - Circ 1997;96:856; Cardiol Clin 1999;17:128; Amlodipine, PRAISE-2 – Cardiol Clin 2000; 23:457).

Stage D—end stage symptoms refractory to standard rx, requiring special interventions.

** Primary goal is relief of symptoms – requires meticulous monitoring, control of volume status.

** All medical rx, as above. Consider referrals for surgical intervention and/or palliative care.

- Carvedilol beneficial even in symptomatic pts with EF $< 25\%$ − reduced mortality by 35% − NNT=15 (COPERNICUS, Nejm 2001;334:1651)
- In acute decompensation: Assess perfusion (warm or cold?) and congestion; Address low perfusion first with vasodilators (nitroprusside, nitroglycerin, morphine, nesiritide) then address persistent congestion with diuretics (loop + metolazone); inotropes (milrinone, dobutamine) may not be necessary and often are detrimental, causing arrythmia and ischemia (Jama 2002;287:628; Nesiritide, VMAC—Jama 2002;287:153; milrinone, OPTIME—Jama 2002;287:1541).
- Ventricular assist device: reduced 1-yr mortality of Class IV pts by 48%, compared to medical rx − NNT= 4, also improved

quality of life but increased adverse events (Nejm 2001; 345:1435).

- Consider referral for transplantation; however elderly pts should be informed of increased risks of post-op NH placement, change in quality of life (Am Hrt J 2004;147:347).
- Palliation: 1-yr mortality = 40-50% for Class IV pts receiving optimal therapy. Important to discuss px with pts to help set treatment goals, complete advance directives. Criteria for hospice referral include: intractable or recurrent symptoms of CHF despite optimal rx as tolerated, impaired nutritional status, pt aware of px, and elects primarily palliative rx goals. Multidisciplinary approach of hospice may also improve sxs and prognosis (Jama 2004;291:2476).

Special Clinical Situations:

- Valvular dx: pts should be evaluated early (Stage B) for valve replacement or repair.
- Symptoms of ischemia: revascularize if absence of comorbid disease (renal failure, pulmonary disease, EF < 20%, life expectance < 1 yr); potential benefit highest if severe of limiting angina or anginal equivalent (Jags 1998;46:545).
- Intraventricular conduction delay: resynchronization (biventricular pacemaker) reduces mortality by 20% in pts with Class III or IV sxs, low EF, prolonged QRS, and optimal medical rx; also reduces hospitalization and improves 6 min walk distance (Ann IM 2004;141:381; Circ 2003;108:2596).
- Afib: anticoagulation and rate control—amiodarone or dig if β-blockade not effective (see Chapter 8.6); catheter ablation with preliminary success in improving LV function and symptoms of CHF in pts with Afib and low EF (Nejm 2004; 351:2373).
- Ventricular arrhythmia or h/o cardiac arrest: ICD (implantable cardioverter-defibrillator) recommended to reduce risk of sudden death; in Class II-III pts without past h/o arrhythmia,

ICD placement reduced death at 4 yrs by 23%, as compared to placebo (SCD-HeFT—Nejm 2005;352:225).

- Renal insufficiency: calculate creatinine clearance to assess severity. Review med list, diet closely for nephrotoxic drugs (NSAIDs) or sources of extra potassium. Clear evidence to suggest benefit from ACEI with GFR > 30, possible benefit for GFR < 30, but monitor closely (Ann IM 2003;138:917). Pts with initial rise in creatinine after starting ACEI may have greater cardiac benefit long-term; tolerate creatinine rise as long as normal potassium can be maintained (Jags 2002; 50:1297). Spironolactone dose should not exceed 25 mg daily, if given with ACEI; avoid combination if GFR < 30 (Nejm 2004;351:585).

Dx: Paucity of large-scale randomized controlled trials in pharmacologic rx of dias heart failure; current rx recommendations are theoretical, consensus-based (Circ 2002;105:1503). Reduce cardiac risk factors; manage volume status; encourage lifestyle modification. Improve ventricular relaxation with rate control; prevent further LVH with blood pressure control.

- Diuretics, nitrates: effective in managing sxs of volume overload, but be cautious with preload reduction; use diuretics and vasodilators judiciously and in low doses (Jags 1997;45:1252; BMJ 2004;328:1114).
- ACE-Inhibitors: ACEI promotes filling by reduction of venous and arterial tone, regression of LVH and interstitial fibrosis, attenuation of coronary vasoconstriction (Jags 1995;42:1040); benefits of ACEI in blocking effects of RAAS activation are assumed to apply to pts with CHF.
- Angiotensin receptor blockers: candesartan reduced CHF hospitalization, but not mortality in pts with symptomatic CHF (Lancet 2003;362:777); 2-week trial of Losartan improved exercise capacity in pts with dias dysfunction and marked hyper-

tensive response to exercise (J Am Coll Cardiol 1999; 33:1567).

- Ca-channel blockers: (non-dihydropyridine only) decrease afterload, regress LVH, enhance ventricular relaxation, and give improved exercise tolerance in pts with hypertrophic cardiomyopathy (Jags 1995;43:1039; Am J Cardiol 1990;66:981).
- β-blockers: slow rate and promote ventricular filling, therefore increasing stroke volume and reducing symptoms (Cardiol Clin 1999;17:129); β-blockers also effective anti-ischemic agents and reduce LVH (Am J Cardiol 1997;80:207); propanolol + ACE + diuretic decreased mortality and increased LVEF in pts > 80 yr old with CHF, normal sys function, and prior MI (Am J Cardiol 1997;80:207).
- Digoxin: not recommended as first-line therapy due to inotropic effects; May be beneficial in pts with Afib; Subgroup analysis of pts with EF > 45% suggested reduction in hospitalizations and deaths due to heart failure (dig—Nejm 1997; 336:525).

Prescribing Principles:

- Get to target doses: start low, go slow, but benefits seen in trials will be achieved only when pts are taking target doses. Majority of pts in primary care practice and in NHs are not receiving optimal therapy (Lancet 2002;360:1631; Jags 2002; 50:1831).
- Start two drugs together: standard practice to start both β-blocker and ACEI (and diuretic, if needed) w initial diagnosis of heart failure; small doses of both will give greater benefit than max dose of only one. If symptomatic hypotension develops, lower diuretic dose before lowering ACEI or β-blocker.
- Contraindications to ACEI: not necessarily renal insufficiency or hyperkalemia! True contraindication is angioedema, intolerable cough. Significant survival benefit is seen from use of

ACEI even in pts with "perceived contraindications" of Creatine > 3.0 or hyperkalemia > 5.5 (Jags 2002;50:1659).

- Contraindications to β-blockade: Not necessarily advanced heart failure! True contraindications are severe bronchospasm, advanced heart block, or frequent hypoglycemia. Use caution in starting during acute CHF exacerbation or volume overload, but do start as soon as stable. Transient worsening in sxs may be expected, followed by improvement over 6-12 wk.

Team Management:

- Team management and group visits to address pt education, sx management (daily weights, support stockings), and dietary and med compliance resulted in significantly decreased hospitalization rates; may improve quality of life (Jama 1994; 272:1442; 2004;291:1358; Jags 2004;50:1590). Benefit is greater in higher-risk populations and if contact is direct, rather than by telephone (Ann IM 2004;141:644).
- Dietary supplementation in elderly heart failure pts (see table in Clin Ger Med 2000;16:480).
- Scheduled exercise program: supervised aerobic exercise for 30 min 3×/wk × 6 mo was safe and resulted in improved exercise tolerance (Ann IM 1996;124:1051). Benefit and safety have yet to be established in frail elderly, but they are likely to benefit the most (Jags 2003;51:699); meta-analysis of exercise training in pts with low EF showed decreased hospitalization and mortality rates (BMJ 2004 online, doi:10.1136/bmj.37938.6452200.EE).
- Cardiac rehab activity should address duration, and not intensity of activity. Supervision of activity initially recommended for those with Class III-IV failure (Cardiol Clin 1999;17:130).
- Community Nurse Management improves quality of care (Ann IM 2006;145:273).

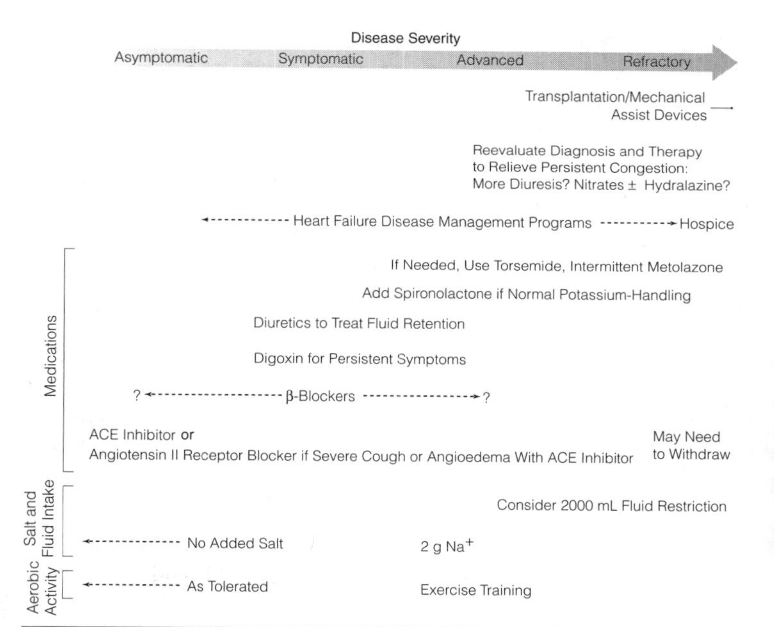

The step diagram demonstrates addition of therapies in relation to the clinical severity of heart failure with reduced left ventricular ejection fraction. Angiotensin-converting enzyme (ACE) inhibitors are prescribed at every level of disease severity, but they may have to be withdrawn for symptomatic hypotension or progressive renal dysfunction in 10% to 30% of patients approaching end-stage disease. Angiotensin receptor–blocking agents (ARBs) are a reasonable alternative for patients who cannot tolerate ACE inhibitors due to angioedema or severe cough but they are not appropriate for patients intolerant to ACE inhibitors due to symptomatic hypotension, renal failure, or hyperkalemia. β-Adrenergic blocking agents are prescribed for patients with mild to moderate symptoms of heart failure, but they are not initiated in patients with severe symptoms of heart failure unresponsive to stabilization with other therapies. Diuretics are prescribed to maintain fluid balance, with spironolactone added in patients with severely symptomatic disease when renal function and potassium handling are preserved. Fluid retention persisting despite high-dose loop diuretic therapy may be better managed with torsemide, a loop diuretic with better absorption. Metolazone effectively potentiates loop diuretic effects, but regular use should be avoided due to severe electrolyte depletion. When severe symptoms persist, patients should be reevaluated to diagnose and treat persistent congestion. Some patients may benefit from addition of nitrates with or without hydralazine. Transplantation and mechanical assist devices are relevant to only a very small population with advanced heart failure. Restriction of sodium and fluid intake is increasingly required as heart failure becomes more severe. Exercise is recommended for all patients except those with severe resting dyspnea. Heart failure management programs are most cost-effective in patients at high risk for repeated heart failure hospitalizations, but they may be useful at every stage of disease.

Figure 8.1 Stepped Therapy for Heart Failure (Jama 2002;287:631).

8.4 Syncope

Cardiol Clin 1997;15:295; Ger Rv Syllabus 2002:165; Eur Hrt J 2001;22:1256; Ann IM 1997;126:989; Nejm 2000; 343;1856; Geriatrics 2004;59:22; Jama 2004;292:1221

Cause: Unlike in younger pts, syncope is usually multifactorial: occurs usually in the setting of multiple medical problems, meds, and age-related physiological impairments.

Cardiac: (associated w 18-33% 1 yr mortality rates vs. 6% for non-cardiac syncope)

- Electrical: Vtach, Afib, tachy or bradyarrhythmias ie, Stokes-Adams-Morgagni
- Mechanical: aortic stenosis (most common, lesion is severe or critical when sx of syncope ensues) with decreased preload or arrhythmia, hypertrophic cardiomyopathy: pts > 60 yr old represent 33% of cases.
- MI: approximately 1% present as syncopy; rare: aortic dissection, pericardial tamponade, PE, pulmonary HT, billowing mitral valve.

Medications: antihypertensives, nitrates, diuretics, phenothiazines, tricyclics; acepromazine, haloperidol, L-dopa (J Clin Epidem 1999;50:313).

Hypotension

- Orthostatic: decreased baroreceptor sensitivity, volume depletion, venous pooling. Orthostatic hypotension occurs in 14.6% of community-dwelling older adults and 52% of NH residents (Geriatrics 2004;59:22). Primary cause of 16% of falls, contributes to 26% (Ann IM 1990;113:308).
- Postprandial: pts w HT more at risk for postprandial hypotension (Circ 1993;89:391; Ann IM 1995;122:286).
- Addison's disease: chronic adrenal suppression.

Reflex-Mediated (all compensatory mechanisms less responsive in aging):

- Vasovagal: pain, fatigue, fear, venipuncture, heat exposure.
- Situational: cough, defecation, micturition: 3+ voidings per night in men associated with 1.9 × mortality rate over 54 mo. Carotid sinus hypersensitivity R > L; commonly in M > 60 yr old (found in 23% of unexplained or recurrent fallers).

Autonomic Insufficiency:

- Diabetes: autonomic instability, osmotic diuresis with dehydration
- Parkinson's disease
- Shy-Drager syndrome

Other:

- Neurologic: vertebrobasilar insufficiency (rare, usually causes dizziness), migraine with basilar artery component, carotid-basilar artery steal, subclavian steal) (Ann IM;1997;126;989); subarachnoid hemorrhage (CVA/TIA, rare cause of syncope, would expect to find other neuro deficits, would require all four neck arteries—2 carotids, 2 vertebrals—to be occluded). Psychiatric (rare): panic, MDD
- Septic shock.
- Deconditioning, starvation.
- Positional (eg, turning over in bed—assoc with atrial myxoma or thrombus).

Conditions Frequently Misdiagnosed as Syncope: hypoglycemia, epilepsy, cataplexy, alteration in mental status (eg, from ETOH).

Epidem: Annual incidence 6% in the elderly.

Sx:

Cardiac: premonitory sxs are usually absent; possible palpitations, dyspnea, angina. May be related to effort/exertion. If arrhythmia, occurs in any position, sx clear quickly after event.

Vasovagal: nausea, fatigue, dimming vision, diaphoresis, dizziness upon wakening. Usually standing, aborted if person lies flat. Continued sx and fatigue common after event.

Carotid Sinus Hypersensitivity: turning head, shaving, taking carotid pulse.

TIA: diplopia, dysphagia, confusion after episode.

Sxs are not useful for risk stratifying pts w unexplained syncope (Arch IM 1999;159:375).

Si: Orthostatic BP from lying or sitting to standing after 1 min; pos if P increases > 30 mmHg, and/or sys BP decreases > 20 mmHg (Jama 1999;281:1022). Hypotension following position change with min change in heart rate indicates baroreceptor reflex impairment, hypotension with tachycardia indicates volume depletion (Geriatrics 2004;59:22).

Aortic stenosis: murmur delay of carotid artery impulse.

- Observe for signs of trauma.
- Check stool for occult blood.

Cmplc:

- R/o seizures (tonic-clonic movements and rigid tone—arrhythmias and vasovagal usually flaccid), bowel/bladder incontinence, aura, tongue biting.
- Fall-related injuries and fractures; r/o dizziness from vestibular etiology, in which case vestibular rehab of help (Neurol 2004;63:150).

Lab: H+P reveal 56-85% of ultimately identifiable causes (Ann IM 1992;268:2553); laboratory tests are generally low yield, although CBC w differential, electrolytes, blood glucose, BUN, creatinine, and drug levels can be helpful; Dx infection with CXR, UA.

Noninvasive (Cardiol Clin 1997;15:195): EKG indicated in all pts presenting with syncope (establishes dx in 5% but 50% will have abnormal EKG). Features suggesting a cardiac cause of syncope: Afib/Aflut, MAT, paced rhythm, frequent PVCs, ventricular arrhythmias, BBB, LVH, q waves indicative of prior myocardial infarction, Mobitz 2 or higher AVB, WPW, prolonged QT interval.

- Cardiogenic (arrhythmic): monitor 24 hr; Holter monitoring not that helpful because complex ventricular arrhythmias recur despite treatment and 50% of pts without significant findings on Holter have recurrence of arrhythmias; poor correlation of sxs with Holter recorded arrhythmias (Chest 1980;78:456); telemetry rarely diagnostic, as most arrhythmias are brief and not associated w sxs.
- Pt-activated memory loop recorders: useful and cost effective in pts with infrequent episodic syncope with previously negative w/u; records several min before event; continuous implantable loop recorders also available for use up to 18 mo.
- Ambulatory BP monitoring: may help detect orthostatic, postprandial, or medication-induced hypotension.
- Electrophysiologic studies (EPS): 3-4 yr mortality = 60% w abnormal EPS vs 15% w normal EPS; EF > 40% correlates highly w neg EPS (Jama 1992;268:2553). Poor sens and specif for bradyarrhythmias (Nejm 1989;321:1703).
- Cardiogenic (nonarrhythmic): echocardiogram indicated to w/u aortic stenosis/HCM. Stress test helpful to look for exertionally-induced hypotension reflective of left ventricular dysfunction or myocardial ischemia (Jama 2004;292:1221); efficient to perform stress echo as a single procedure.
- Cerebrovascular: carotid US not useful, as presence of stenotic lesions does not establish cause of syncope (useful if planning to do carotid sinus massage on elderly pt) (Nejm 2000; 343:1856). CT/EEG not indicated, unless focal findings or sxs of neurologic disease. Carotid sinus massage can establish CSH as source of syncope (contraindicated with acute MI, recent stroke or TIA, h/o VF/VT): pt should be supine/monitored

with EKG. Defibrillator/cardiac drugs present. Gently/firmly touch carotid sinus for 5 sec. If no response, massage carotid sinus for 5 sec, no more than 10 sec. Pos response is 3 sec asystole or drop in sys BP of 50 mmHg (Jama 2004;292:1221).

- Electroencephalogram: minimal value, unless pt exhibits focal neurological abnormalities or si/sx of seizures.
- Tilt table: helpful for evaluation of recurrent, unexplained syncope in pts without underlying heart disease; pos endpoints are vasovagal sxs; common protocol is 60° for 45 min; sens 67-83% and specif 75-100% for vasovagal mechanism of syncope (Am J Med Sci 1999;317:110); variable reproducibility (Am J Cardiol 1997;80:1492); probably should not be used to assess therapeutic efficacy (Eur Hrt J 2001;22:1256).

Neurally-mediated hypotension (Jama 2000;343:1856): strong ventricular contractions may cause via C-fiber-induced peripheral dilatation (Ann IM 1991;115:871); brought out w tilt table and isoproterenol infusion; if bradycardia and hypotension occur quickly on tilt alone, may be more sure of dx (Nejm 1993; 328:1117).

Rx:

Therapeutic:

- Although most syncope in the elderly is multi-factorial, therapy should be aimed at reducing specific contributory diseases and processes:
  - Cardiac
  - Cardiac (nonarrhythmic): valve replacement for aortic stenosis.
  - Neurocardiogenic: rx by avoiding diuretics, vasodilators and tricyclics; increase salt intake; try fludrocortisone (Florinef) if no HT, hypokalemia or heart failure. β-blockers and anticholinergics like disopyramide (Norpace) (Jama 1995; 274:961) or SSRI, like paroxetine 20 mg qd (J Am Coll

Cardiol 1999;33:1227). Consider pacing if drug rx not effective (Circ 2002;106:2145).

- Orthostatic hypotension: elastic stockings, fludrocortisone 0.1 mg/d increasing to as much as 1.0 mg/d, perform dorsiflexsion of feet or handgrip exercises before standing. Adequate control of BP reduces incidence of orthostatic hypotension. β-blockers, ACE inhibitors and CCBs assoc with lower frequence of orthostatic hypotension than diuretics, α-blockers and central α-agonists. Avoid ETOH.

Post-prandial: Avoid ETOH and large carbo meals. Caffeine. Remain recumbent after meal.

Carotid-Sinus Hypersensitivity: avoid triggers. Consider pacemakers (falls reduced by 2/3 in CSH pts who receive pacemakers)

- Medication-induced: document and review pt meds; consider alternatives or discontinuation.
- Address driving in elderly with syncope.

Valvular Disease

Ger Rv Syllabus 1991, 1994, 1996, 2004; Nejm 1997;337:32 (See Table 8.4)

Table 8.4 Valvular Heart Disease

	Aortic Stenosis	Aortic Insufficiency	Mitral Stenosis	Mitral Regurgitation
Cause	Degenerative valve disease > rheumatic disease; associated w DM, hyperlipidemia; calcific AS age 50-60 yr (50% associated w CAD)	Rheumatic heart disease (mitral disease may also be present); cystic medial necrosis of the aortic root associated w aneurysm of the ascending aorta; HT and renal disease can lead to fenestrations of the valve	Rheumatic heart disease, 1/3 of mitral valve disease in the elderly	Rheumatic fever rare; CAD w papillary muscle dysfunction, ventricular dilatation, prolapse mitral valve, rupture chordae tendineae, CHF may be presenting sx
Pathophys	Leaflet calcification in the elderly rather than fusion of the commissures as w younger pts	—	Commissural fusion fibrosis and calcification of leaflets and chordae	Calcium posterior cusp leaflets lifting them toward L atrium resulting in MR
Sx	Exertional chest pain, dyspnea, syncope; sedentary elderly: low-output state: weight loss, pleural effusions, hepatic and renal failure; afib can lead to CHF in low-output state	CHF; more problems at rest than when they maintain exercise	Afib precipitates clinical deterioration	If dyspnea, orthopnea, edema, or fatigue present, valve replacement indicated; associated w afib
Si	Low-output state: murmur not very loud; late peaking systolic ejection murmur as opposed to early peaking in AS; may be confused w MR;	W aortic root dilatation high-pitched blowing diastolic murmur heard best at the right rather than the left sternal	In older pts calcified leaflets less mobile, therefore first heart sound at apex is diminished, no	May be difficult to differentiate from AS in elderly because increased AP diameter results in diminished

	S_4, decreased carotid upstroke, associated AI murmur w calcific AS	border; wide pulse pressure; LVH	opening snap; diastolic murmur heard best w bell at apex w pt in left lateral position; often associated w murmur of mitral insufficiency	AS murmur MR if not crescendo-decrescendo, and radiates axilla or left sternal border
Test	Doppler gradient > 40; hemodynamic studies needed for low-output state; aortic area < 0.75 cm² or peak systolic valve gradient of 70 mmHg, > 50 severe	Pts where end-systolic dimension exceeds 5 cm² may be approaching LV dysfunction—indication for valve replacement before irreversible damage takes place	LAE on EKG; echo for severity	End-diastolic valve dimension > 4.5 cm², refer cardiologist, once EF < 60 px worsens
Prognosis	W onset sx: mortality rate = 30-50%, aortic valve surgery (Circ 1993;8:17): encouraging results w human homographs; treat porcine and human homographs w warfarin for 3 mo at INR of 2-3, then D/C warfarin; mechanical heart valves: use warfarin long-term (INR at 2.5-3.5); ASA 160 mg/d may provide added protection;	Nifedipine delays need for valve replacement (Nejm 1994;331:689); replace valve w exercise intolerance and before LV dysfunction (Ann Thorac Surg 1992;53:191); presence of coronary disease worsens postop outcome; may see associated rheumatic MS al-	Anticoagulate if afib present, valve replacement for progressive, severe sx; malfunction of bioprosthesis if high-frequency holosystolic murmur (Nejm 1996; 335:407); good outcome w valvotomy if class I or II (New	If CAD present, operative mortality = 25% (Ann Thorac Surg 1993;55:333); then manage medically w diuresis, afterload reduction; afib: rx w anticoagulation, embolus less likely w MR than MS; good prognosis w valve

continues

Table 8.4 continued

	Aortic Stenosis	Aortic Insufficiency	Mitral Stenosis	Mitral Regurgitation
	favorable results of CABG +/− valve replacement in pts >80 yr old (Cardiovasc Surg 1993;1:68); may eventually restore contractility in CHF (Nejm 1997); malfunction of aortic bioprosthesis if aortic diastolic murmur (Nejm 1996;335:407); surgery if LVH dysfunction at rest, hypertensive hypertrophic cardiomyopathy, ventricular ectopy, pts may be denying their sx. Postop tx fluids rather than pressors for (Nejm 1997)	though less common in older people but when seen is more often accompanied by afib than in younger pts; afib worsens sx of fatigue and CHF, and embolization may occur resulting in stroke	York Heart Association) or class III, IV in octogenarians (J Am Ger Soc 2000;48:971)	repair of mitral valve prolapse

D/C = discontinue; LAE = left atrial enlargement.

8.5 Arrhythmias

Supraventricular Tachyarrhythmias

Ger Rv Syllabus 1996;222; Am Fam Phys 1994;49:823,1805; 1994; 50:959; Nejm 2004;351:2404; 1995; 332:162; J Am Coll Cardiol 1994;23:916; Clin Ger Med 1999;15:645; Jags 2000;48:224; Ann IM 2004;141:745

Cause:

- Afib: associated w HT in 70% of pts; associated w mitral stenosis, atrial septal defect; also associated with hyperthyroidism or subclinical hyperthyroidism especially in the elderly (Nejm 1994;331:1252); toxic multinodular goiter present in 20% of the elderly with Afib associated w hyperthyroidism (Med Aud Dig 1983;30:18); alcoholic myocardiomyopathy; COPD; CAD; fever; pericarditis; Aflut; WPW, and multifocal atrial tachcardia often (60%) from pulmonary disease including pulmonary emboli. The term "lone afib" describes Afib in the absence of demonstrable underlying cardiac disease or h/o HT.
- Supraventricular arrhythmias: hypokalemia, low serum magnesium; concomitant administration of dig and quinidine has 6.5% complication rate in older population.

Pathophys: Afib: age-associated loss of sinoatrial node fibers, atrial myocardial fibers, amyloid deposition; atrial dilatation from decreased ventricular compliance; SVT reentrant pathways; a rapidly firing focus (or foci), usually located in or near the pulmonary vein, which may mimic the appearance of Afib on the surface EKG (Circ 1997;95:572). Lone Afib is due to fibrotic areas in the atrium that predispose pts to arrythmia, to increased susceptibility to autonomic neural stimuli to the heart (J Am Coll Cardiol 1998;32:695), or to localized atrial myocarditis (Circ 1997;96:1180).

Epidem: Afib: 6% of pts > 65 yr old; 50% of pts w Afib > 75 yr old.

Sx: Polyuria, palpitations, faintness, neck pounding in AV reentrant types, but not accessory pathway SVT (Nejm 1992;327:772); CHF and stroke in Afib.

Some pts with afib have minimal sxs or none, whereas others may have severe sxs, particularly at the onset of the arrhythmia. Sxs may range from palpitations to acute pulmonary edema, but fatigue and other nonspecific sxs are probably the most common (Eur Hrt J 1996;17:48). The cognitive function of elderly pts with persistent arrhythmia may be impaired as compared with that of aged-matched controls in the sinus rhythm (Jags 2000;48:387).

Crs: Afib: unfavorable markers for successful conversion: > 1-yr duration or markedly dilated LA (5 cm) or recurrent after previous conversion.

Cmplc: Elderly more dependent on atrial kick, thus Afib may lead to CHF; 7-fold risk of stroke in non-rheumatic Afib and a 17% risk in mitral stenosis; post-PAT T-wave inversions may last days to wks (Nejm 1995;332:161); chronic Afib causes embolic CVA in 20% if recent CHF, chronic HT or previous embolus (Ann IM 1992;116:1); pts older than 61 yr who have lone Afib have an increased risk of stroke and death (Arch IM 1999;159:1118; Eur Heart J 1999;20:896); increased cognitive disorders (Jags 2000;48:387).

Lab:

Chemistry: TSH.

Noninvasive: EKG; sick sinus syndrome is diagnosed by SVTs alternating w some heart block; suggested by P < 90 after 1-2 mg atropine or asystole > 3 sec after carotid sinus massage; supraventricular arrhythmias: normal QRS, regular tachycardia without visible P waves = AV nodal re-entrant arrhythmia: controlled w digoxin or verapamil.

Multifocal atrial tachycardia: P > 100 and 3 or more different PR intervals and P-wave morphologies; looks superficially like Afib, but dig will not help.

Rx:

Therapeutic: Current guidelines recommend a ventricular rate during Afib of 60-80 bpm at rest and 90-115 bpm during exercise (J Am Coll Cardiol 2001;38:1231); all but β-blockers may prolong or cause ventricular arrhythmias (Ann IM 1992;117:141); need to lower dig dose by one-half in the presence of quinidine to avoid digitalis toxicity (Nejm 1992;326:1264).

Acutely: Iv verapamil, diltiazem, β-blockers like esmolol, metoprolol, sotalol (Ann EM 2000;36:1), which is a nonselective β-adrenergic blocker, also helps decrease CHF, sudden cardiac death (J Am Coll Cardiol 1999;34:1522); for VT implantable cardioverter-defibrillator (J Am Coll Cardiol 1999;34:1090); dig to slow; useful in combination with other agents (J Am Coll Cardiol 1999;33:304); conversion with dig alone no better than placebo (Ann IM 1987;106:503); rate easily overridden by catechol/exercise stimulation (Ann IM 1991;114:573); if recalcitrant, may need quinidine po (holds in NSR better, but death rate 3 × placebo) (Circ 1990;82:1106) or procainamide or amiodarone (Ann IM 2003;139:1009; 1992;116:1017) or clonidine (0.075 mg po, repeat in 2 hrs, decreases sympathetic tone (Ann IM 1992;116:388).

- If LA size is < 50 mm, use cardioversion (Jags 1999;47:740); use heart-rate control with iv diltiazem, iv β-blocker, dig or some combination. If pt remains in Afib, then give unfractionated or sc LMW heparin. Further treatment depends on the duration of the Afib. If duration of Afib ≤ 48 hr and no clinically significant LV dysfunction, mitral valve disease, or previous embolism: iv ibutilide; or oral propafenone (600 mg) or flecainide (300 mg); or oral quinidine (400-600 mg); or direct current shock. If duration of Afib > 48 hr, unknown duration, or high risk of embolism: TEE-guided cardioversion; or adequate anticoagulation for 3 wks, followed by direct-current cardioversion, with or without concomitant antiarrhythmic drugs (Nejm 2001;334:14).

- Chronic/paroxysmal (failed conversion): With coumadin, 50-70% reduction of stroke risk (Nejm 1995;332:238). Valvular: if no contraindications, heparinize and coumadinize, rate control; non-valvular: controversial, depends on risk of bleeding versus risk of embolic disease in particular pt; increased risk of stroke if age > 65: diabetes, high BP, h/o stroke/TIA, CHF, LV dysfunction, mitral stenosis or if age is > 75. Increased risk of bleeding if stroke, gi bleed, severe recent illness, Afib, high INR, age > 80 (debated). Special case: "lone Afib," meaning no comorbidities and age < 65, then no rx or ASA. Any age with one or more risk factors for stroke: coumadin (unless clear contraindication); unless contraindications exists, adjusted-dose coumadin with INR of 2-3 (J Am Ger Soc 2000;48:224; Nejm 1995;333:5); yields 64% risk reduction vs placebo and 40% vs ASA (Nejm 1995;332:238). Similar guidelines found in Clin Ger Med 1999.
- ASA for those who cannot take coumadin.
- Warfarin is underused in at-risk populations with Afib (Nejm 2002;347:84; 2002;347:1825; Jama 2002;288:2441; Ann IM 1999;131:927, 159:1322; Jags 2000;48:224; 1998;46:1423; Arch IM 1998;158:2093; Lancet 1998;352:1167).
- Bleeding risk cited among reasons not to anticoagulate (Jags 1997;45:1060); 9 studies show no age-related risk of bleeding; 10 studies show age-related risk of bleeding (Ann IM 1996; 124:970). Appears that risk is balanced best with effectiveness if INR maintained at 2-3 (Lancet 1996;348:633). A high rate of intracranial hemorrhage complicated the use of warfarin in elderly pts in one trial (Lancet 1994;343:687), but analysis of the degree of anticoagulation at the time of bleeding indicated that virtually all episodes occurred at an INR greater than 3.0

(Arch IM 1996;156:409); increased intracerebral bleeds in pts > 80 yr (Neurol 2007;68:118).

- PAT and Aflut: carotid sinus pressure; then, for PAT only, adenosine 6-12 mg iv, metabolized in 10 sec, potentiated by dipyridamole and carbamazepine, inhibited by theophyllines (Med Lett Drugs Ther 1990;32:63) or verapamil 5-10 mg iv; perhaps propranolol 1-5 mg iv, then either dig + quinidine or electrical cardioversion with syncope; OK to do even if dig on board, as long as levels therapeutic and not toxic and K+ OK (Ann IM 1981;95:676).
- Multifocal atrial tachycardia: verapamil iv with pretreatment with iv CaCl2 (Ann IM 1987;107:623) or po for chronic; MgH iv, especially if low; β-blockers if no COPD.

8.6 Bradyarrhythmias and Heart Blocks

Cause: ASHD, dig.

Epidem: Idiopathic 3rd degree heart block fairly common in the elderly.

Sx:

- 1st degree heart block usually causes no sx.
- 2nd degree may cause dizziness or dyspnea.
- 3rd degree may cause syncope, especially during standing.

Si:

- 1st degree heart block = PR > 0.22 sec
- 2nd degree = some unconducted P waves
- 3rd degree = no relationship between P waves and QRS intervals
- Sick sinus syndrome (sinoatrial node dysfunction due to CAD or sclerodegenerative process) presenting w chest pain, palpitations or sinus pause; treat brady part of the bradycardia-tachycardia syndrome w permanent pacer.

Crs: 5-yr mortality 50%; not significantly reduced by pacing, but pacer improves sx.

Lab: Noninvasive: EKG; Holter monitor may still miss a majority of intermittent heart blocks (Nejm 1989;321:1703); event monitor.

Rx:

- 2nd and 3rd degree: isoproterenol iv or sl, atropine iv or external pacer until can get transvenous pacer; symptomatic pts w sinus pause > 3 sec with sx or pause > 2 sec with sx, as well as Mobitz type II block should be considered for pacemaker; pts w Mobitz type I should avoid digitalis, β-blockers, Ca-channel blockers, and antidepressants.
- Sick sinus syndrome: lower incidence of Afib w dual-chamber pacing (Lancet 1994;344:1523; Nejm 1998;338:1097).
- Transvenous pacemaker: temporary first, then permanent, unless inferior MI, when block will usually reverse spontaneously.
- Permanent pacemaker (Nejm 1996;344:89; Mod Concepts Cardiovasc Dis 1991;60:31): dual-chamber types more expensive; use only when need atrial kick (Ann IM 1986;105:264).

Table 8.5 Indications for Permanent Pacer

A. Acquired Atrioventricular Block in Adults

1. Third-degree AV block at any anatomic level association with any one of the following conditions:
    a. Bradycardia with symptoms presumed to be due to AV block.
    b. Arrhythmias and other medical conditions that require drugs that result in symptomatic bradycardia.
    c. Documented periods of asystole ≥ 3.0 seconds or any escape rate < 40 beats per minute (bpm) in awake symptom-free patients.
    d. After catheter ablation of the AV junction. There are not trials to assess outcome without pacing, and pacing is virtually always planned in this situation unless the operative procedure is AV junction modification.
    e. Postoperative AV block that is not expected to resolve.
    f. Neuromuscular disease with AV block such as myotonic muscular dystrophy, Kearns-Sayre syndrome, Erb's dystrophy (limb-girdle), and peroneal muscular atrophy.

Table 8.5 continued

2. Second-degree AV block regardless of type or site of block, with associated symptomatic bradycardia.
3. Asymptomatic third-degree AV block at any anatomic site with average awake ventricular rates of 40 bpm or faster.
4. Asymptomatic type II second-degree AV block.
5. Asymptomatic type I second-degree AV block at intra- or infra-His levels found incidentally at electrophysiological study for other indications.
6. First-degree AV block with symptoms of pacemaker syndrome and documented alleviation of symptoms with temporary AV pacing.

B. Chronic Bifascicular and Trifascicular Block

1. Intermittent third-degree AV block.
2. Type II second-degree AV block.
3. Syncope not proved to be due to AV block when other likely causes have been excluded, specifically ventricular tachycardia (VT).
4. Incidental finding at electrophysiological study of markedly prolonged HV interval (≥100 milliseconds) in asymptomatic patients.
5. Incidental finding at electrophysiological study of pacing-induced infra-His block that is not physiological.

C. Sinus Node Dysfunction

1. Sinus node dysfunction with documented symptomatic bradycardia, including frequent sinus pauses that produce symptoms. In some patients, bradycardia is iatrogenic and will occur as a consequence of essential long-term drug therapy of type and dose for which there are no acceptable alternatives.
2. Symptomatic chronotropic incompetence.
3. Sinus node dysfunction occurring spontaneously or as a result of necessary drug therapy with heart rate < 40 bpm when a clear association between significant symptoms consistent with bradycardia and the actual presence of bradycardia has not been documented.

D. To Prevent Tachycardia

1. Sustained pause-dependent VT, with or without prolonged QT, in which the efficacy of pacing is thoroughly documented.
2. High-risk patients with congenital long QT syndrome.

continues

Table 8.5 continued

E. Hypersensitive Carotid Sinus Syndrome and Neurally Mediated Syncope

1. Recurrent syncope caused by carotid sinus stimulation; minimal carotid sinus pressure induces ventricular asystole of > 3 seconds' duration in the absence of any medication that depresses the sinus node or AV conduction.
2. Recurrent syncope without clear, provocative events and with a hypersensitive cardioinhibitory response.
3. Syncope of unexplained origin when major abnormalities of sinus node function or AV conduction are discovered or provoked in electrophysiological studies.

F. After the Acute Phase of Myocardial Infarction

1. Persistent second-degree AV block in the His-Purkinje system with bilateral bundle branch block or third-degree AV block within or below the His-Purkinje system after AMI.
2. Transient advanced (second- or third-degree) infranodal AV block and associated bundle branch block. If the site of block is uncertain, an electrophysiological study may be necessary.
3. Persistent and symptomatic second- or third-degree AV block.

Based on evidence and favorable opinion about efficiency by American College of Cardiology/American Heart Association practice guidelines (ACC/AHA)

Cause: Venous stasis from incompetent valves; increased hct leads to greater blood viscosity and clotting.

Epidem: Occult cancers; extended sedentary periods (illness, travel); obesity; hip fracture; estrogen.

Pathophys: Decreased levels of antithrombin III can lead to venous dilatation and stasis.

Sx: None or calf pain; unilateral edema.

Si: None or increased calf diameter/tenderness/elevated skin temperature; Homan's sign not sens/specif.

Cmplc: Chronic postphlebitic syndrome: occurring after thrombosis involving destruction of the deep and communicating valves of the leg and obliteration of thrombosed veins. Rarely painful. Chronic edema (enlarged and hard leg because of trapped fluid from lymphedema due to scarring); hypopigmentation; stasis dermatitis; hyperemic ulcers; varicose veins; rx w 30 mmHg pressure stocking toe to knee; legs 3-4 inches above heart level at night, if significant swelling persists; elevate legs intermittently, but ambulation should not be limited.

Lab: Neg d-dimer excludes DVT (Ann IM 2004;141:1839).

Noninvasive: Duplex US: in pts w sx, better than IPG (Nejm 1993;329:1365); in high-risk asx pts only 38% sens (Lancet 1994;343:1142); in pts w sxs of recurrence, it is difficult to distinguish on US up to 1 yr after initial DVT (Acta Radiol 1992; 33:297); use serial IPG if had normal IPG before; venograms may be indeterminate, therefore use degree of clinical suspicion in deciding anticoagulation (Geriatrics 1995;50:29).

Rx:

Preventive:

- In hip replacement initiating low-molecular-weight heparin treatment 1 mo prior to elective surgery results in fewer DVTs (Nejm 1993;329:1370; 1996;335:696).
- Enoxaparin plus pneumatic compression prevents DVT orthopedic surgery (J Bone Joint Surg Br 2004;86:809).

Therapeutic: Heparin iv × 5 d + coumadin started on day 1 (Nejm 1992;327:1485); continue coumadin × 6 mo (Nejm 1995; 332:1661); 1-2 mo only if transient spec cause; lifelong if recurrent idiopathic (Nejm 1995;332:1710); low-molecular-weight heparin as good as heparin for DVT (Arch IM 1995;155:601) (see Hip Fracture re: hiradin, p 365).

8.7 Anticoagulation

Treatment Guidelines 2008;6:29

Anticoagulants:

- ASA (Nejm 1994;330:1287) 75-325 mg po qd (Med Lett Drugs Ther 1995;37:14) inhibits platelet aggregation; can be used safely w coumadin (Nejm 1993;329:530). Adverse effects: gastric intolerance (Ann IM 1994;120:184), asthma, increased bleeding time for 2 d, platelet dysfunction for 7-10 d. Cheap.

- Enoxaparin (Lovenox) 30 mg sc bid, low-molecular-weight heparin (Med Lett Drugs Ther 1993;35:75) are clearly better with less bleeding (Ann IM 1994;121:81) and better DVT/PE prevention over 6 d (Nejm 1992;326:975); $23/d as rx for DVT (Nejm 1996;334:677,682; 1996;335:1816); after 24 hr, Lovenox may start warfarin and may discontinue heparin after 4 d if INR 2.0 for 2 consecutive d (Nejm 1996;335:1821; 1997; 337:657,663,688; Arch IM 1998;158:1809); not for recurrent pulmonary embolus (Geriatrics 1998;53:40; Clin Ger Med 2001;15:15).
- Heparin: also inhibits activated prothrombin-platelet interaction; renal excretion, half-life = 105 min (Nejm 1991; 324:1565); prophylactic regimen = 5,000 U iv q 12 hr; therapeutic regimen = 5,000-U load, then 1,200 U IV/hr; measuring q 6 hr PTT until stable at 1.5-2.0 × control.
  - Ticlopidine (Ticlid): stoke prevention after cardiac stenting, may cause neutropenia, thrombocytopenia, cholestasis, TTP, therefore only use 2-4 wks (Ann IM 1998;128:541).

Prophylaxis of thromboembolism for surgical or orthopedic procedure, where short term need (< 1 mo): qd evening doses of 5.0-7.5 mg; lower doses should be used in elderly pts; during initiation of therapy, PT INR should be monitored qd, response to a given dose may not be accurately measured for up to 36 hr, doses should not be changed for 3-5 d; 3 wk before procedure: hct, PT, APTT, and platelet count; overlap prolonged PT 2-5 d with heparin as switch over (Nejm 1984;311:645) because it inhibits liver synthesis of factors X (3-d half-life), IX (1.25 d), VII (7 h), and II (4 d); INR of 2-3 for routine anticoagulation, 3.0-4.5 for artificial valves (Am Coll Phys J Club 1994;120:52).

Pre-op and on coumadin: withhold 4 d prior to surgery and use heparin; discontinue antiplatelet rx 5 d prior to surgery and restart 48-72 hr after surgery (Chest 1995;108:312S).

Coumadin Protocol: If INR < 1.5, increase total dose/wk by 10%; INR > 3.4, decrease total weekly dose by 10% after one dose is held; INR 5.0-9.0 w increased risk of bleeding, coumadin may be omitted and vit K (1.0-2.5 mg) given po w additional dose in 24 hr if INR remains high; > 9.0 without serious risk of bleeding may give vit K 3-5 mg po; significant elevation of INR w severe bleeding, give vit K (10 mg) slow iv infusion q 12 hr prn w FFP and tfx, if needed.

For minor surgery w pts at low risk for thromboembolic event, stop coumadin several days pre-operatively and perform surgery when INR < 1.5; for pts w significant risk for thrombolic event, admit for heparin infusion when INR reaches 2.0; stop infusion 4 hr prior to surgery, resuming as soon as possible postoperatively (Jags 2000;48:226).

Adverse effects: bleeding, especially when given with probenecid or if renal failure; risk of serious bleeding > 10%/yr in therapeutic range; correlates w higher PTs and 1st 3 mo of rx, not age or gender (Ann IM 1993;118:511); risk of intracranial bleed = 2%/yr w PT 2 × control, risk much higher if PT higher (Ann IM 1994;120:897); blue toe syndrome (cholesterol emboli) rare complication (South Med J 1992;85:210; Surgery 1989;105:737).

Potentiated by foods and drugs (Ann IM 1994;121:676) that either displace from carrier protein or compete for degradation enzyme; includes allopurinol (Nejm 1970;283:1484), amiodarone, Antabuse, ASA, cimetidine (Ann IM 1979;90:993); or by decreased warfarin metabolism (cimetidine, erythromycin, tricyclics, TMP/SMZ); vit K deficiency (inadequate diet, fat malabsorption, mineral oil, broad-spectrum antibiotics); unknown mechanisms: clofibrate, quinine, phenothiazines, acetaminophen (Jags 1998;279:657).

Decreased w increased coumadin metabolism (barbiturates, carbamazepine); excess vit K (dietary supplements); impaired coumadin absorption (malabsorption syndromes, mineral oil, cholestyramine).

Chapter 9

Pulmonology

9.1 Chronic Obstructive Pulmonary Disease

Jama 2003;290:17; Clin Ger Med 2003;19:1; Geriatrics 1995;50:24; Ger Rv Syllabus 1996;278

Cause: Smoking in 90% of pts (Nejm 2004;350:26), α one antitrypsin deficiency, airway hyperesponsiveness; asthma may "reappear" late in life and can be provoked by URI, GERD, cardiac, and glaucoma meds.

Epidem: COPD 4th leading cause of death, develops only in 10-20% of smokers.

Asthma (increased bronchial and bronchiolar responsiveness to various stimuli resulting in airway narrowing): 1-3% of new cases in the elderly; prevalence 3.8% in men and 7.1% in women; increased mortality in elderly.

Pathophys: Normal changes in lung w aging: decreased elastic recoil resulting in collapsed airways during respiratory cycle, especially in lower part of lung leading to V/Q mismatch; chest wall compliance, number of alveoli, vital capacity, maximum voluntary ventilation, FEV1, maximum expiratory flow rate all decreased by 25-30 mL/yr and if smoker 60-70 mL/yr:

- Increase in residual volume and functional residual capacity; all changes accentuated by pulmonary disease.
- Limitation of expiratory flow, usually combination of emphysema and chronic bronchitis.

PULMONOLOGY

- Emphysema: destruction of air spaces distal to terminal bronchioles.
- Chronic bronchitis: Remodeling due to chronic exposure and infiltration of walls by inflammatory cells leads to narrowing of the small airways (Nejm 2004;350:2689); daily production of sputum for 3 mo during 2 consecutive yr.
- Asthma: relatively few new cases in elderly and may have collagen-vascular etiology.

Sx: Cough, sputum production, dyspnea, fear of shortness of breath may lead to blunting of emotional response in interpersonal interactions (Heart Lung 1973;2:389).

Si: Final stages: cor pulmonale—barrel chest, prolongation of expiration, wheezing, pulmonary HT, elevated jugular venous pressure, pronounced pulmonic closure sound (P2), hepatic congestion, peripheral edema, cyanosis.

Asthma: indicators of acuity: difficulty walking 100 feet or more; speech fragmented by rapid breath; syncope; pulsus paradoxus > 12 mmHg; inability to lie supine; accessory muscle use; respiratory rate > 30; heart rate > 120; FEV1 or peak expiratory flow rate $< 30\%$ predicted value.

Cmplc: R/o lung cancer, CHF, GE reflux, recurrent aspiration, thromboembolic disease (pleuritic pain, hemoptysis, unexplained right-sided heart failure, hypoxemia), cough secondary to β-blockers, ACE inhibitors.

Lab: (Jama 2003;290:17) Normal PaO_2 for pt > 65 yr old = 80-85 mmHg (Eur Respir J 1994;7:856); PaO_2 decreased approximately 3 mmHg/decade or $pO_2 = 100-(age/3)$; FEV1/FVC < 0.70; FEV1 falls 30 mL/yr and 75-80 mL/yr in smokers.

Asthma: Reversible w bronchodilators; FEV1 improves by 15% or 200 mL.

X-ray: Chronic bronchitis: increased bronchiolar markings, increased heart size; emphysema: elongated heart, hyperinflation of lungs, bullae.

Rx: (Figure 9.1)

Therapeutic: Bronchodilator therapy: symptomatic improvement, but does not change survival; 40% pts use metered-dose inhalers (MDIs) inappropriately, spacers help (re correct use see: National Asthma Education Program, National Heart, Lung, and Blood Institute 1991;57); reasons for noncompliance include expense, memory lapse, denial, anxiety; all pts; cause tremor, tachycardia, arrhythmia; need instruction:

- Exhale slowly w pacer in mouth
- Press down on canister when begin to inhale slowly and deeply
- Hold breath 10 sec or 5 sec, if can't do 10 sec.
- Exhale through nose and pursed lips.
- Wait 30-60 sec.
- Repeat same instructions for second puff (Can CME 2000; 12:207).

β2-adrenergic agonists most effective for acute episodes of asthma and prevention of exercise-induced asthma; long-acting β2-adrenergic agonists prevent nocturnal asthma and should be prescribed only at regular intervals (never prn); Arformoterol nebulizer a long-acting β2 agonist (Clin Ther 2007;29:261; Med Lett 2007;49:53); elderly asthmatics have diminished receptor response and may not respond as well to β-adrenergic agonists (Geriatrics 1995;50:24; Nejm 2004;350:2689);

Anticholinergic—ipratropium bromide best as chronic therapy in addition to β2-adrenergic receptor agonists; Tiotropium—has a duration of effect of more than 24 hrs; not advantageous to use both in the acute setting (Ann Pharmacother 1994;28:1379); precipitates glaucoma if sprayed in eye.

Corticosteroids: COPD: do not appreciably alter the rate of decline in lung function by themselves but rather reduce the

PULMONOLOGY

number of exacerbations and thus the progression of the disease (Beclomethasone, Triamcinolone, Flunisolide, Fluticasone), but do not alter decline in NH (Jama 2004;5:31). Steroids for rhinitis (J Allergy Clin Immunol 2005; 116:1289).

First-line therapy for asthma; loss of bone density if given systemically; rinsing mouth after inhaler avoids oral candidiasis, cataracts.

Cromolyn anti-inflammatory blocks mast cell degranulation, 1-2 puffs qid; nedocromil anti-inflammatory w sometimes unpleasant taste, nausea, vomiting, rhinitis occasionally.

Theophylline (Chest 1995;107:206S) (Table 9.1): in older pts w emphysema may be of value initially for airflow obstruction that is irreversible; may reduce the work of breathing, augmenting diaphragmatic breathing and acting centrally to increase respiratory drive; may also work as a mild diuretic; high serum levels may be more helpful to pts w asthma, but toxicity (nausea, cardiac arrhythmias, confusion, seizures) 17× more frequent in the elderly, therefore has limited role in COPD (Nurs Home Pract 1995;3:17); erythromycin and cimetidine inhibit cytochrome P-450 metabolism of theophylline; liver disease and CHF reduce clearance; decrease theophylline by 50% if giving ciprofloxacin at the same time; measure levels after 2-5 d of therapy; therapeutic trough = 5-15 μg/mL.

<table>
<tr><td rowspan="5">Stage 0
At Risk

Chronic Symptoms
(Cough and Sputum
Production)</td><td rowspan="4">Stage 1
Mild $FEV_1 \geq 80\%$ Predicted</td><td rowspan="3">Stage 2
Moderate
FEV_1 5-% to 79%
Predicted
Often asx
Dyspnea w/mild exertion
Cough slightly purulent
sputum</td><td rowspan="2">Stage 3
Severe
FEV_1 30% to 49%
Predicted
Occurs asx
Same as mild
Wheezing on forced exp
and
hyperinflation</td><td>Stage 4
Very Severe
$FEV_1 < 30\%$ Predicted Dyspnea
Or
Chronic Respiratory Failure
Or
Right-Sided Heart Failure</td></tr>
<tr><td>Digoxin judicious HcTz
Consider transplantation or other
asurgical treatment</td></tr>
<tr><td colspan="2">Add pulmonary rehabilitation
Add long-term oxygen to correct arterial hypoxemia</td></tr>
<tr><td colspan="3">Add long-acting bronchodilator(s) for relief of persistent dyspnea
Add inhaled corticosteroids for persistent dyspnea or bronchodilator(s) or repeated exacerbations
[combined steroid β-2 agonist (Lancet 2003;361:449) v.s. Not helpful COPD just asthma (GRS 5th edition)]
Consider pulmonary rehabilitation for patients who are persistently dyspneic despite therapy with long-acting bronchodilators and inhaled corticosteroids</td></tr>
<tr><td colspan="4">Add short-acting bronchodilator for relief of intermittent dyspnea Ipatropium bromide</td></tr>
<tr><td colspan="5">Smoking cessation for all smokers
Vaccinations against influenza and pneumoccocal infection for those older than 65 years</td></tr>
</table>

Figure 9.1 Stages of Disease Severity and Recommended Treatments

Table 9.1 Theophylline Levels

Increased Levels	Decreased Levels
Caffeine	β-Blockers
Erythromycin	Barbiturates
Clarithromycin (Biaxin)	Phenytoin
Ciprofloxacin (Cipro)	Rifampin
Pentoxifylline (Trental)	Felodipine (Plendil)
Cimetidine	High protein
Ranitidine (Zantac)	Low carbohydrate
Enoxacin (Penetrex)	Carbamazepine (Tegretol)
Disulfiram (Antabuse)	Smoking
Mexiletine (Mexitil)	
Ticlopidine (Ticlid)	
Estrogen/progestin	
Isoproterenol (Isuprel)	
Propranolol	
Flu shot	
Untreated hypothyroid, CHF	
Thiabendazole (Mintezol)	

Indication for long-term oxygen therapy at home: O_2:PO_2 < 55 mmHg or cor pulmonale or polycythemia w PO_2 < 60 mmHg; goal is to increase PO_2 > 60 mmHg; after 1, 6, 12 mo, ABGs should be measured to determine ongoing need for and appropriate dose of oxygen; long-term oxygen therapy: increased survival (Nejm 1995;333:710); COPD pts on oxygen need to increase oxygen flow rate by 2 L per min during air travel.

Team Management:

- Avoid irritants: smoking, dust, air pollution, humidity; pts > 65 yr gain 4 yr of life expectancy if they quit smoking; MAO inhibitors may help w the addiction, counteracting nicotine stimulation of dopamine release (Jama 1995;275:1217).

- For substantial sputum production: percussion and postural drainage given by a family member; flutter valve device pts can use alone.
- Severe dyspnea: conscious slowing of respirations, purse-lipped breathing, relaxation techniques.
- Arm movement exercise controversial.
- Daily 15-min periods of exercise-induced hyperpnea increase ventilatory capacity in pts 65-75 yr/old; 8-wk training program produces significant reduction in breathlessness (Geriatrics 1993;48:59); pulmonary rehabilitation program improves exercise capacity in older pts w COPD (Chest 1995;107:730).
- Nutrition: high ratio of fat to carbohydrate; fat metabolism generates the least amount of carbon dioxide, carbohydrates the most; very hot and very cold foods stimulate coughing; in NH more frequent small meals, minimize chewing-soft foods, fluids not during meals, avoid foods that cause bloating (Clin Prac Guidelines AMDA 2004).
- Psychosocial support: family education, eg, care and crisis.
- Asthma: color-coded peak expiratory flow meters may make it easier for older pts to monitor asthma in outpatient setting (Am Fam Phys monograph 1995;2); stepwise approach to asthma management (Med Lett 1999;41:5; Geriatrics at Your Fingertips, Reuben, David B et al. 7th ed, AGS 2005;171):
  1. Intermittent (sx $<$ 2/wk nocturnal $<$ 2/mo, FEV1$>$ 80% peak flow rate $<$ 20%): prn inhaled β2-agonist less than twice a week. Inhaled β2-agonist or cromolyn or nedocromil before exposure to trigger.
  2. Mildly persistent (sx 2 ×/wk, nocturnal $>$ 2/mo, FEV1 $<$ 80%, PFR 30%): daily inhaled corticosteroid (200-500 mcg) w β2-agonist prn less than once a week.
  3. Moderately persistent (FEV1 60-80% PF $>$ 30%): daily inhaled corticosteroid (800-2000 mcg) plus long-acting β2-agonist plus prn β2-agonist not exceeding 3-4 d/wk.

PULMONOLOGY

4. Severely persistent (FEV1 < 60%, PF > 30%): inhaled corticosteroid (800-2000 mcg) plus long-acting β2-agonist plus sustained-release theophylline and or ipratropium plus prn β2-agonist (NIH, Geriatrics at Your Fingertips, 7th ed AGS, 2005;171).

Always heed "subjective" responses to empiric rx trials as well as "objective" (eg, peak flow responses), since perception of breathlessness important to pt, reducing anxiety component.

Pre-op Assessment: Only absolute indication for preop PFTs, even in COPD pts, is to measure lung volume before lung resection; consider local vs general anesthesia to avoid a 30-50% fall in tidal volume; preop postural drainage w chest percussion to avoid complications post-op; bronchial secretions increase for 6 wk after cessation of smoking, increasing risk for post-op infection (Ger Rv Syllabus, 5th ed., 2002; p81)

9.2 Pulmonary Embolus

Cause: Hypercoagulability, immobilization, trauma (up to 1 mo post-op) (Nejm 1998;339:93)

Epidem: 15% of cancer pts will have one within 2 yr (Ann IM 1982; 303:1509). Common in COPD exacerbation (Ann IM 2006; 144:390)

Pathophys: Thrombophlebitis causes thrombus migrating to lungs; recurrent small emboli more common than single large one; mostly thigh and pelvis veins (Ann IM 1981;94:439); no si or sxs in 50%.

Sx: Dyspnea may be sudden, intermittent, or chronic; pleuritic chest pain w infarct; hemoptysis; fever; syncope w large emboli; common to have minimal sxs.

Si: 33% pleural effusion of which 67% bloody (rbc > 100 000/dL); unexplained arrhythmias; resistant heart failure; tachycardia.

Crs: Resolves over 10-30 d (Nejm 1969;280:1194); 60% survival without rx, 90% w rx 3 d heparin.

Cmplc: Chronic leg edema, chronic pulmonary HT.

Lab: nl a-a = < 10-15 mmHg, and is abnormal if there is intrinsic lung problem.

Negative D-dimer rules out PE w near certainty; false positive results appear to be less likely in nonsurgical pts or without underlying cancer or liver disease (Am J Resp Care Med 1999;159:1445).

EKG: Partial RBBB (S1S2S3), right axis deviation 20%, S1Q3T3.

X-ray: V/Q scan mismatch (PIO-PED-Jama 1990;262:2753); B-mode duplex US; arteriogram false-neg rate w 1-5% complication rate, 1-4/1000 mortality rate; spiral CT.

Rx:

Preventive: Mild to moderate alcohol consumption decreases risk of DVT and pulmonary embolus (Jags 1996;44:1030). Complete leg US adequate to r/o DVT (Radiology 2005;237:348).

Therapeutic: Heparin PTT 1.5-2.5 × control for 5-10 d; overlap coumadin 5 d and continue 6 mo at INR 2-3 (Nejm 1995;332:166).

If major bleeding, stop heparin and allow anticoagulation effect to dissipate over hours; if cannot tolerate coumadin long term, give heparin sc 10,000 units q 12 hr; vena cava filter for pts w persistent contraindication to anticoagulation; adverse effects include chronic leg edema, thrombus formation above the filter, recurrent embolization through collateral veins, perforation of vena cava, migration of filter.

Aim of prophylaxis is to prolong quality of life; if pt terminally ill, eg, w cancer, anticoagulation may only prolong suffering. ? subcutaneous unfractionated vs low-molecular-wt heparin in venous thromboembolism (Jama 2006;296:935).

9.3 Pulmonary Hypertension

Cause: LVH, valvular heart disease, COPD, chronic recurrent thromboembolic disease.

Epidem: F > M

Pathophys: Excess platelet thromboxane A, deficient endothelial cell prostaglandin (Nejm 1993;328:1732).

Sx: Dyspnea, chest pain, pedal edema, fatigue.

Si: Right-sided S_3, pulmonary systolic and diastolic murmurs, tricuspid insufficiency, enlarged RV.

Crs: If PA pressure > 85 mmHg, then median survival time 2.8 yr.

Lab: ABG: low PCO2.

Rx:

Therapeutic: Selective use of oxygen; low-dose diuretics; phlebotomy for hct exceeding 50%; Ca-channel blockers; coumadin anticoagulation (Nejm 1992;327:76); epoprostenol (Prostacyclin) infused or inhaled has some hemodynamic and sx benefit (Ann IM 2000; 132:425), may be no long-term benefit (Nejm 2000;342:1866); Iloprost (Ventavis) not yet studied in elderly (Respiration 2007; 74:498); Boseatan (Tracleer) po, treprostinil (Remodulin) sq (Med Lett 2002;44:79). Sildenafil (Viagra): phosphodiesterase-5 inhibitor significantly improves long-term function in pulmonary HT secondary to chronic thromboembolic disease (Eur Respir J 2007;e-pub).

Chapter 10

Orthopedics/Rheumatology

10.1 Osteoporosis

Nejm 1992;327:620; Bull Rheum Dis 1988;38:1; Ann IM 1995;123:452; American Medical Director Association 23rd Annual Symposium March 16-19, 2000, San Francisco, CA, S Cummings, MD, Update on Osteoporosis Mar 18, 2000.

Causes: Causes are listed in Table 10.1.

Epidem: More common in female smokers from changes in estrogen metabolism (Nejm 1994;330:387; 1985;313:973); less frequent in blacks and Polynesians who have higher adolescent bone densities (Nejm 1991;325:1597); 7% of U.S. women over the age 50 have osteoporosis (Jama 2001;286:2815).

Pathophys: Simple estrogen deficiency postmenopausally (Nejm 1980;303:1571).

Sx: Fx usually of vertebrae, distal forearm bones, proximal femur; bone pain, especially vertebral, although many w/o sx.

Si: Decreased height/kyphosis from vertebral compression fractures; if incidental vertebral fracture of T7 or 8, pt has osteoporosis by definition (Cummings 2000); kyphotic pt stands with back to wall, and heels touching wall, wall-occiput distance > 0 cm= thoracic vertebral compression fracture, inferior rib to superior pelvis distance anteriorly < 2 finger breadths = lumbar vertebral compression fracture (Jama 2004;292:2890); hip fx, other than due to severe trauma means dx of osteoporosis.

Table 10.1 Causes of Osteoporosis

Acromegaly
Alcoholism
Chronic Liver disease
COPD
Cushing's disease/syndrome (even 10 mg prednisone qd enough), including chronic steroid use in asthmatics (Nejm1983;309:265) and rheumatoid arthritis (Ann IM 1993;119:963)
Diabetes, type I
Estrogen deficiency in postmenopausal women or amenorrheic athletes (Nejm 1984;311:277); hypogonadotrophic hypogonadism in men
Gastric surgery
Heparin
Homocystinuria
Hyperprolactinemia
Hyperparathyroidism
Hyperthyroidism
Idiopathic, at least some of which is genetic in structure of bone matrix protein (Nejm 1998;338:1016)
Malabsorption
Myeloma
Porphyria
RA
Renal calcium leak (rx'd w thiazides)
Soda intake excessive ($\uparrow PO_4$)
Thalassemia
Vit A, chronic excessive intake (Ann IM 1998;129:770)
Vit D, winter time deficiency (Jama 1995;274:1683; Jags 2007;55:752)
Vit D antagonist meds like phenytoin

Vit D deficiency an explanation for nonspecific aches and pains and fatigue (Mayo Clin Proc 2003;78:1457,1463).

Crs: Chronic, slowly progressive.

Cmplc: Rib and vertebral fractures (Nejm 1983;309:265), hip fractures.

Lab: Chemistry: TSH, calcium, phosphorus, BUN, Cr as initial labs; PTH if indicated to r/o hyperparathyroidism.

X-ray: Osteopenic bones and fractures; bone mineral densitometry (BMD) screening controversial, much debated (Ann IM 1990;112:516; 1990;113:565; Nejm 1991;324:1105; 1987; 316:212); BMD test if will affect rx; screen high-risk pts (chronic steroid use, renal disease, hyperparathyroidism, Graves' disease, malabsorption); value in repeating BMD once on rx is uncertain: dual-energy x-ray absorptiometry (DEXA) most precise and lowest cost (Am Fam Phys 1996;1:1; Med Lett 1996;38:103); T score (standard deviation from mean density of younger normals) > 2.5 has a 5 × incr risk of fracture; Z score compares to same age group; scores may take 2 yr to change w rx (Jama 2000; 283:1318); femoral neck measurement most accurate because does not pick up calcification of aorta that a spine measurement might; vs FIT trial data suggests that yr to yr variation makes it difficult to use DEXA to follow therapy.

Rx:

- All rx is preventive or instituted to slow progression (Med Lett Drugs Ther 1992;34:101) including progression of steroid-induced type (Nejm 1993;329:1406); weight-bearing exercise (Ann IM 1988;108:824); smoking cessation, exercise (Ann IM 1992;116:716); posture and balance exercise (fall prevention) walking (Jags 1996;44:756).
- Calcium replacement therapy (Med Lett 2000;42:29) w $CaCO_3$ 1.5 gm of elemental Ca++/d (milk has 300 mg Ca++/ cup; chewable Tums, 200-500 mg/tab; Os-Cal, 500 mg/tab) (Med Lett Drugs Ther 1989;31:101); first 800 mg qd as calcium citrate (Citracal), higher cost, but absorbed better, especially in achlorhydrics/elderly (Nejm 1985;313:70), then add $CaCO_3$ (Nejm 1990;323:878); substantial effect even without estrogen (Ann IM 1994;120:97), eg, 50% less loss/yr (Nejm 1993;328:460); calcium content in supplements and foods (Med Lett Drugs Ther 1996;38:108; Med Lett 2000; 42:29); incr protein in diet may exert calciuretic effect (Am J Clin Nutr 1988;48:880); no association of decreased fracture w incr dietary calcium (Am J Pub Hlth 1997;87:992).
- Vit D 400-800 IU qd; 400 IU in most multivitamins; 400 IU qd × 2 yr preserves femoral neck bone density in women > 70 yr (Jama 2001;285:785); 800 IU vit D prevents non-vertebral fx (Jama 2005;293:2267) sunscreen prevents vit D absorption–difficult trade-off w rising skin cancer rates.
- Estrogen risks greater than benefits.

- Mg increases BMD (Jags 2005;11:1875)
- Testosterone in men, especially if hypogonadism–watch for prostate cancer.
- Bisphosphonates should be stopped 1st 5 yr (Nejm 2004; 350:1189; Jama 2006;296:2927).
  - Alendronate (Fosamax) (Med Lett 1996;38:1; Nejm 1995;33:1437; Med Lett Drugs Ther 1996;38:965; Am Fam Phys 1996;54:2053), 10 mg po qd clearly helps prevent progression over 3 yr; prevents nonvertebral fx over 3 yrs (Jama 1997;277:1159; Lancet 1996;348:1535), also available for rx at 70 mg q wk; alendronate 5-10 mg qd for prevention in high risk women, eg, on steroids (J Bone Miner Res 2000; 15:993); long-term alendronate maintains BMD (Nejm 2004;350:1189); give when life expectancy at least 2-3 yr and pt is walking; analgesic effect (Bone Miner 1991; 15:237). Poor compliance a concern (Jags 2006;54:1015). Adverse effects: various gi sx, eg, esophagitis, diarrhea (Nejm 1996;335:1216); give w caution in pts w renal insufficiency; for men too (Nejm 2000;343:604); high cost; osteonecrosis of the jaw associated w bisphosphonates (J Oral Maxillofac Surg 2003;61:9; 2004;62:527; J Natl Cancer Inst 2007;99:1016).
  - Risedronate (Actonel) (Jama 1999;282:1344) 5 mg po qd (Med Lett 2000;7:26) reduces vertebral and hip fracture (Med Lett 2000;42:100); 35 mg weekly; etidronate disodium (Didronel) 400 mg po qd × 14 d, then 13 wk off in cycles (Nejm 1997;337:382) to avoid osteomalacia (Ger Rv Syllabus, 5th ed, 2002;186).
  - Pamidronate (Aredia) 150 mg po qd (Med Lett Drugs Ther 1992;34:1); 2 hr infusion 40-80 mg iv q 4 mo (Ann IM 2000;132:734; Am Fam Phys 2000;61:2732); fever in 20 of pts; monitor Cr prior to each dose.
  - Ibandronate 150 mg monthly po (Ann Rheum Dis 2006; 65:654).

- For all bisphosphonates, question long-term value, when to stop, micro fractures after 5 yr therapy (Cummings 2000; Jama 2006;296:2927).
- Zoledronic acid q yr (Nejm 2002;346:653).

- Calcitonin interferes w osteoclasts and inhibits bone resorption; 100 IU salmon calcitonin sc qd, may also relieve acute fx pain, possibly via opiate effect (J Fam Pract 1992;35:93); 200 IU qd alternating nostrils (Med Lett Drugs Ther 1996;38:965; Am J Med 1995;98:452); nausea from calcitonin self-limited and < 10% of pts discontinue med; other se include flushing, diarrhea, and pain at injection site; human calcitonin has more se than salmon calcitonin; recrudescence when therapy discontinued, even after 1 yr of therapy; PROOF trial supporting calcitonin flawed because ½ pts lost to f/u (Am J Med 2000; 109:330); alendronate maintains bone density more effectively than intranasal calcitonin (J Clin Endocrinol Metab 2000; 85:1783), calcitonin affects trabecular bone not cortical therefore vertebral, not hip fx (Am J Med Sci 1997;313:13).
- Thiazides may help bone density and fx rate (Ann IM 1993;118:657,666; 1996;129:187; Nejm 1990;322:286; Jags 2003;51:340); others report incr fracture rate (Nejm 1991; 325:1).
- Vertebraoplasty reinforces collapsing vertebrae w polymethylmethacrylate alleviating pain and increasing mobility; best for inpatients w 1-2 new fractures (Am J Neuroradiol 1997; 18:1897; J Neurosurg 2003;98:36; Clin Ger 2004;12:32).
- Kyphoplasty: sustained benefit after 2 yrs (Spine 2006;31:57).
- Teriparatide (Forteo) recombinant human parathyroid (Med Lett 2003;45:9; Jama 2004;5:382; Jags 2005;53:1658; 2006; 54:782,853).
- Use of β-blocker reduces risk via osteoblastic proliferation (Jama 2004;292:1326).

10.2 Hip Fracture

Nejm 1966;334:1519; Am Fam Phys 2003;67:537

Cause: Falls and osteoporosis.

Epidem: 90% pts > 50 yr old; rates lower in blacks; incr w low BMI (body mass index), maternal h/o hip fracture, alcohol use, CVA hx (Nejm 1994;330:1555), smoking (Nejm 1987;316:404), hyperthyroidism, increased homocysteine (Nejm 2004; 350:2089), visual impairment (Nejm 1991;324:1326), and drugs like long-acting benzodiazepines, tricyclics, SSRIs (Lancet 1998; 351:1303), and phenothiazines (Nejm 1987;316:363), as well as other psychoactive drugs, especially in NHs (Nejm 1992; 327:168). Paradoxically also may be increased by restraints (Ann IM 1992;116:369); associated w being on feet < 4 hr/d, higher resting pulse rate (Nejm 1995;332:767).

Pathophys: Falls and fxs occur in the elderly because:

- Slow gait results in more sideways and backward falls on hips, rather than on other body parts.
- Diminished protective responses; less fat and muscle protection.
- Diminished strength (J Gerontol 1989;44:M107).

Subcapital fracture (45%) disrupts blood supply to femoral head; higher incidence nonunion and necrosis of femoral head.

Intertrochanteric fx (10%) and subtrochanteric fx (45%) leaves blood supply to femoral head intact.

Sx: H/o fall; hip pain (may be vague in the elderly), may radiate to groin or knee.

Si: External rotation of the leg w shortening; pain w motion; persistent immobility in demented; occult hip fracture pain with internal rotation.

Crs: 20% of fall-induced hip fractures associated w death within 6 mo; 50% have subsequent functional dependence; 50% of pts are walking independently 1 yr after fracture (Am J Med 1997;103:205); pre-fracture mental status and physical functional level are best predictors of eventual outcome (Jags 1992;40:861).

Cmplc: R/o fx acetabulum or pubic ramus; after fx, frequently develop confusion (49%), UTI (33%), arrhythmia (26%), pneumonia (19%), depression (15%), CHF (7%), DVT; femoral neck fxs: avascular necrosis in 20%, nonunion 30%; intertrochanteric: failure of fixation devices (tremendous muscle forces on bone) (J Gen Intern Med 1987;2:78; Ger Rv Syllabus, 5th ed, 2002;90); fat emboli when there has been manipulation of intramedullary space as w prosthesis placement.

X-Ray: Fx, often subtle, especially if impacted. Best view: anteroposterior w internal rotation 15-20°; delayed repeat films may be necessary; after 72 hr, MRI if dx still in doubt (Am Fam Phys 2003;67:537).

Rx:

Prevention:

- Pos relationship between physical activity and lower risk of hip fx (Intern Med 1998;129:81).
- In elderly NH women, Ca 1200 mg + vit D 800 IU qd (Nejm 1992;327:1637) (see 10.1, Osteoporosis).
- Hip protectors in NH (Lancet 1993;341:11; Nejm 2000;343:1506).
- Statins (HMG-CoA reductase inhibitors) prevent hip fx (Jama 2000;283:3205,3211,3255; Lancet 2000;355:2185,2218).
- Avoid use of throw rugs in the home, and avoid restraints (Ann IM 1992;116:369).

Surgical:

- Subcapital fx: Austin-Moore prosthesis, early weight bearing; if nondisplaced: pin, wgt bearing in 12 wk.
- Intertrochanteric fx, subtrochanteric fx: screw w early ambulation.

Delay in surgery is associated w more post-op risk (J Bone Joint Surg Am 1995;77:1551); recombinant hirudin (desirudin) a specific inhibitor of thrombin administered 30 min before total hip replacement—more effective than enoxaparin in preventing DVT (Nejm 1997;337:1329).

After surgery, consider heparin and/or coumadin DVT prophylaxis if pt not able to get up quickly or at least compression stockings (Arch IM 1994;154:67); low molecular wt heparin q 12 hr for 1 mo post-op (Nejm 1996;335:696).

- Austin-Moore prosthesis: wt-bearing in 1-2 d.
- Compression screw internal fixation: wt-bearing in 2-3 d.
- Total hip replacement, limited in extremes of rotation.

Loosening of prosthesis: groin pain w acetabular component and upper thigh pain w femoral component.

Selected pts (eg, advanced Alzheimer's, Parkinson's, CHF, CVA, near terminal illness) for no repair if high surgical risk or nearing end of ambulatory life; pain management often no worse or prolonged than w post-op course.

Early rehab (Jama 1998;279:847) as good in NH as in rehabilitation unit (Jama 1997;277:396).

- Extended rehab and restorative training × 6 mo = improved outcome (Jama 2004;292:837).
- Anterior approach hip repair: rehab limited to flexion, adduction, internal rotation.
- Posterior approach should have less than 90° in relation to sitting surface and no internal rotation.
- Walker use s/p hip fracture (advance 20-30 cm, then move weak leg first).
- Cane use s/p hip fracture only if ipsilateral upper extremity and contralateral lower extremity are strong; < 25% of pt's wt should be placed on cane; when going up or down stairs, keep good leg up higher, ie, "up with good, down with bad"; although ipsilateral cane use can reduce the force acting on the hip, placing the cane in the contralateral hand is useful in relieving hip pain; watch for development of new shoulder prob-

lem with added stress (Jags 1996;44:434); cane height should allow 30° of flexion at the pt's elbow w top of cane parallel to greater trochanter.

Rx osteoporosis in walking NH patients (Jama 2000; 284:972).

10.3 Osteoarthritis

Kippel J, Dieppe P. Practical Rheumatology. St. Louis: Mosby 1995; Jama 1996;276:486; Kippel J. Primer on the Rheumatic Diseases, 12th ed, Atlanta: Arthritis Foundation, 2001. AGS Panel on Persistent Pain in Older Persons; The Management of Persistent Pain in Older Persons; J Am Ger Soc 2002;50:S205-S224; Ann IM 2000;133:635

Cause: Aging—decreased proteoglycan aggregation, decreased resistance of cartilage to procollagen (Lancet 1989;1:924); obesity; postural defects (genu valgum/varum); excessive repetitive stress; previous joint injuries, certain sport activities (marathon running, soccer, football), certain occupations (farmer—hip OA; jackhammer operator—elbow OA; miner—knee and spine OA; cotton mill worker—hand OA); crystalline deposit disease; previous inflammatory joint disease; hemochromatosis; Wilson's disease; acromegaly; in familial may be anka gene (Science 2000;289:265,289); heritability of hand OA is 65% (BMJ 1996;312:940); OA is a multigenic trait (Arthritis Rheum 1999;42:397); osteonecrosis, Paget's disease, Wilson's disease, acromegaly, hyperlaxity syndromes.

Epidem: Uncommon < 35 yr old, more common > 65 yr old (30-40% population > 65 having sx); men and women are affected equally, but women have symptoms that appear earlier and appear to be more severe (Arthritis Rheum 1998;41:778).

Pathophys: Injury to articular cartilage leads to destruction of proteoglycan matrix, which in turn leads to cellular proliferation in attempted repair, release of enzymes with increased destruction of all cartilage elements and proliferation of subchondral bone. OA is believed to be initiated by multiple factors, including genetic, developmental, metabolic, and traumatic.

Sx: Pain; aching worse with activity; relieved by rest; morning stiffness; hip arthritis begins in groin and radiates to thigh, getting up from chair. Knee OA may present with instability or buckling, particularly when descending stairs or stepping off curbs. Hand OA may present with problems with manual dexterity. Pts may notice sx are affected by the weather; may have increased pain during damp, cool, and rainy weather.

Older persons report their pain less frequently, and often have an atypical presentation of pain. May present with behavior changes, including restlessness or confusion (J Am Ger Soc 1990;38:409).

Common Pain Behaviors in Cognitively-Impaired Elderly Persons:

- Facial expressions: slight frown; verbalizations, vocalizations.
- Body movements: rigid, tense, fidgeting; changes in interpersonal interactions: aggressive, decreased social intractions; changes in activity patterns or routines like refusing food.
- Mental status changes.

Si: Affected joints: knee > hip > spine; elbows and wrists usually spared; first carpometacarpal joint commonly affected: joint crepitus; decreased range of motion, minimal soft tissue swelling + bony enlargement, minimal warmth or erythema; rare effusions; distal and proximal interphalangeal joint deformities (Heberden's and Bouchard's nodes).

Crs: Insidious onset; slowly progressive. Initially, pain is worsened with use of the affected joints, and relieved with rest and simple analgesics. With disease progression, pain may become persistent and require more substantial analgesics. Pain at rest or during the night is a feature of severe disease.

Cmplc: Joint pain and instability; contractures, tendonitis, bursitis; r/o osteoporosis, malignancy, Paget's, osteomyelitis, neuropathy, parkinsonism, avascular necrosis of hip, trochanteric bursitis (lateral bone pain instead of groin/hip pain seen w arthritis, also still have range of motion and no radicular signs), reflex sympathetic dystrophy (RSD; precipitated by trauma, stroke, MI, skin of hand hyperesthetic, warm vasodilation proceeding to cold vasoconstriction w edema on dorsum of fingers; after 6 mo skin becomes atrophied, proceeding in 6 mo to diffuse osteopenia; 3-phase bone scan to make dx early in disease, rx w steroids, stellate ganglion block), r/o polymyalgia rheumatica (OA of axial skeleton with muscle aches in neck, shoulder girdle, low back, and pelvic girdle with prolonged am stiffness, markedly elevated ESR, and normochromic, normocytic anemia; may coexist with temporal arteritis), r/o calcium pyrophosphate dehydrate deposition disease or hemochromatosis in patients with OA of atypical joints (metacarpophalangeal joints of hands, wrists, elbows, shoulders, or ankles.

- Of hand: r/o hypertrophic pulmonary osteoarthropathy (clubbing fingers, swollen wrists); de Quervain's (pain in base of thumb elicited by gripping thumb under fingers and flexing wrist in ulnar direction, rx w splinting and steroid injection, surgery); Dupuytren's contracture (fibrous contraction of palmar fascia causing flexion of fingers, rx'd w stretching, steroid injection and surgery).
- Of knee: r/o anserine bursitis (medial aspect of knee), Baker's cyst (rx w steroid injection into joint helps because of direct communication w joint and cyst); hip DJD, trochanteric bursitis (lateral tenderness), iliotibial band tightening, joint tumor (nocturnal or continuous pain), meniscal tear (knee locking, + McMurray's, + MRI), anterior cruciate ligament tear (+ Lachmans, + MRI).

Presence of pain in older people has been associated w depression, anxiety, decreased socialization, sleep disturbances, impaired ambulation, and increased healthcare utilization and costs. (J Am Ger Soc 1998;46:635).

Lab: ESR, CRP nl; synovial fluid wbc < 200/dL, protein < 4 gm/dL, glucose < serum glucose.

X-ray:

Early: slight loss of cartilage thickness with narrowing of joint space.

Middle: marginal osteophyte formation.

Late: loss of joint space, sclerosis of subchondral bone, subchondral cysts, loose bodies, subluxation deformity.

Hip films correlate w sx more than hand, knee films. MRI better to visualize cartilage directly, but plain radiography is preferred for diagnosis because of its availability and low cost.

Rx: Goals: relieving symptoms, maintaining and/or improving function, limiting physical disability, avoiding drug toxicity. Combine pharmacologic and nonpharmacologic rxs for best results and less toxicity.

Therapeutic:

Oral Medications: First choice is nonopioid analgesics (ie, acetaminophen), then NSAIDs, but caution in elderly; then opioids are the last drugs of choice; acetaminophen (Tylenol) is the initial drug of choice because of lower toxicity, but may not be as effective in some pts. NSAIDs may be more effective short term, but long-term chronic use may result in serious side effects (BMJ 2004;329:1317) (See Table 10.2.)

Oral corticosteroids with powerful anti-inflammatory properties do not significantly improve OA symptoms.

Opioids: Incidence of addictive behavior is low among pts taking prescription opioid drugs for medical indications (Am Pain Soc Bull 1991;1:1) and (Am Pain Soc Bull 2002;12:1); medical use of opioid analgesics to treat pain does not appear to contribute to increases in health consequences of opioid analgesic abuse (Jama 2000;283:1710). In chronic nonmalignant pain conditions, narcotic meds generally should be considered as a last resort and avoided if other effective therapy is available.

Adjuvant drugs are used alone or in combination with analgesics to treat persistent pain, especially neuropathic pain. Traditional antidepressants like amitriptyline, nortriptyline, and desipramine have effects on both pain and depression, but unwelcome se in elderly pts. SSRIs have a better se profile, but have not demonstrated effectiveness for pain. Gabapentin or other new anticonvulsant drugs may be better choice than older tricyclic antidepressants because of relatively low side-effect profiles (Jags 2002;50:586).

- Glucosamine sulfate 500 mg tid (Med Lett 1997;39:91), most se gi; must be taken for at least 1 mo before sx improve (Jama 2000;283:1469).
- Chondroitin sulfate demonstrated efficacy in improving the sx of OA after one mo (Jama 2000;283:1469). Well tolerated, may have slower onset of action, but work longer than NSAIDs (J Rheum 1996;23:1385) 400 mg tid.

Other agents being investigated: insulin-like growth factor 1, degradative enzyme inhibitors (Jags 1997;45:850).

- Vitamin D: Low levels of dietary intake or serum levels of vit D are associated with incr rates of OA progression (Ann IM 1996;125:353).

Topical treatments:

- US deep heat increases tolerance, not cost-effective (Ann IM 1994;121:133); TENS for knee pain.
- Lidocaine patch 5% significantly reduces pain intensity in pts w moderate-to-severe OA of the knee (Curr Med Res Opin 2004;20:13).

Invasive techniques:

- Joint injections:
- Corticosteroids: intra-articular knee injections significantly reduces pain for up to 4 wks (Arthritis Rheum 1999;42:475).

- Hylauronic acid: hylan G-F (Synvisc®) intra-articular injection over 4 wks works for 6-12 mo (Am Rheum Dis 1966;55:424; Jama 2003;290:3115).
- Epidural corticosteroid injections help approximately 60-70% of pts w low back pain and lumbosacral radiculopathy (Pain 1986;24:277; Anesthesiology 1999;91:1937).
- Acupuncture: Although advocated as a rx for OA, reviews of literature and clinical trials are controversial (Arthritis Rheum 2001;44:819). 1997 NIH Consensus Statement on acupuncture listed OA as one of the disorders "for which the research evidence is less convincing but for which there are some positive clinical trials" (Acupuncture. NIH Consensus Statement 1997;15:1). ↓ pain (Ann IM 2006;145:12).
- Cartilage repair and transplantation attempts generally not successful (Arthritis Rheum 1998;41:1331).
- Joint irrigation through arthroscope shown to significantly relieve pain for up to 24 wks (Arthritis Rheum 1999;42:475).
- Joint replacement good option in elderly without other med problems; consider when major instability in weight-bearing joint, loose bodies in joint, intractable pain.

Team Management/Nonpharmacologic Therapy: F/u frequently inadequate in clinical practice.

- Exercise improves function (Jama 1997;277:1863), preserves ROM and increases muscle strength and stability of joint; may reduce med requirements (Ann IM 1992;116:529); water exercises. Assist knee and quad strength with appropriately fitted chairs and toilets, wall support handles. Quadriceps weakness associated w instability and is responsive to isometric strengthening (Ann IM 2003;138:613). High impact activities may accelerate disease in a joint affected by OA and should be avoided.
- Emotional, social support; early education for long duration of disease. Older adults w good coping strategies have signifi-

cantly lower pain and psychologic disability (J Consult Clin Psychol 1987;55:208).

- Occupational therapy to evaluate pt's ability to perform ADLs, provide assistive devices, teach joint protection techniques and energy conservation skills. Interventions may include: splints to stabilize and reduce pain and inflammation (ie, thumb brace). Braces, canes, walkers, or other ambulatory aids (including insoles), patella taping, and other assistive devices including support proximal tarsal joint with lacing corset footwear; hallux valgus rocker shoe helps reduce stress on joint; cervical pillow; assistive devices, eg, jar holder, key holders.
- Decrease weight (Ann IM 1992;116:535) and prevent wgt gain. An increase from a normal wgt to overweight is associated with a higher risk of knee OA requiring arthroplasty than constant overweight (Ann Rheum Dis 2004;63:1434).
- NSAID use and interactions:
    1. Antacids make NSAIDs more tolerable, but decrease absorption; gi toxicity reduced by misoprostol 100 μg qid (limited by diarrhea), assessment and possible rx of *Helicobacter pylori* infection before commencing long-term course NSAIDs in pts w h/o recurrent PUD.
    2. With anticoagulation interactions, gi bleed risk; decrease anticoagulant to achieve same PT or PTT; ibuprofen (Motrin), tolmetin (Tolectin), sulindac (Clinoril, Vioxx, Celebrex) have least gi adverse effects.
    3. Antirheumatic agents: watch wbc, platelets.
    4. Diuretics: adjustment may be necessary to maintain antihypertensive effects.
    5. Lithium: decreased clearance so monitor level 7 d after beginning NSAID, indomethacin (Indocin), piroxicam (Feldene) in particular.
    6. Methotrexate: displacement from protein-binding site increases its toxicity.

7. Oral hypoglycemics: displacement from binding leads to sulfonylurea toxicity, particularly with fenoprofen (Nalfon), naproxen (Naprosyn), naproxen sodium (Anaprox).
8. Phenytoin: naproxen and fenoprofen (Nalfon) will displace, leading to phenytoin toxicity.
9. Probenecid: increases plasma levels of most NSAIDs—can reduce levels of some NSAIDs (ketoprofen, meclofenamate (Meclomen), indomethacin (Indocin).
10. Renal insufficiency relative contraindication; ASA alternative and can monitor w drug levels.

Table 10.2 Duration and Adverse Effects of NSAIDs

	Half-life		
	Short	**Intermediate**	**Long**
Least side effects	*Ibuprofen up to 3200 mg divided QID *Etoblac (Iodine) 200-400 divided TID	Sulindac (Clinoril) renal impairment? *Oxapiezin (Daypro) 1200 mg per day	*Nabumetone 500-1000 as BID (Relafen) *Diclofenal 500-1000 BID (Arthvotec 50)
Mild	Fenoprofen (Nalfon) Indomethacin (Indocin) GI, CNS Adv effects	*Naproxin 200-500 mg as TID (Naprosyn) *Ketoprofen 50-75 mg as TID (Orudis) Tolmetin (Tolectin)	Piroxicam (Feldene) CNS Adv. effects
Most side effects	Meclofenamate (Meclomen) diarrhea		

Adapted from BMJ 1996;312:1563.

10.4 Rheumatoid Arthritis

Jags 1991;39:284; Geriatrics 2000;55:30; Brit J Rheum 1996;35:453; Arthritis Rheum 1996;39:713; Clinics in Ger Med 2005;21:649

Cause: Humoral immune response (rheumatoid factor, IgM, IgG, or IgA complexed w antigens producing immune complexes w fixed complement) resulting in an inflammatory process; cellular immunity involving lymphocytes and macrophages; viral.

Epidem: 20% new onset after age 60 yr—elderly-onset RA (EORA).

Sx: Pain; inflammation small joints accompanied by constitutional sx such as malaise, anorexia, wgt loss; prolonged morning stiffness lasting > 1 hr.

Si: Criteria for dx (at least 4 of which must be present for 6 mo): morning stiffness; arthritis of 3 or more joint areas; hand-joint arthritis (symmetric involvement); rheumatoid nodules; rheumatoid factor; radiologic features.

Extra-articular manifestations of RA occur more in young-onset RA (YORA): anemia, thrombocytosis, eosinophilia, Felty's syndrome, splenomegaly, neutropenia, diffuse lymphadenopathy, osteoporosis, vasculitis, pericarditis w effusion, conduction abnormalities, valvular incompetence, Raynaud's phenomenon, pleuritis w effusion, interstitial fibrosis, bronchiolitis, entrapment syndromes (eg, carpal tunnel), atlanto-axial subluxation, monoarthritis multiplex, distal sensory abnormalities, autonomic changes, disuse atrophy, keratoconjunctivitis, scleritis, corneal ulceration, xerostomia, amyloidosis, cryoglobulinemia, hyperviscosity.

Crs: Possibilities include:

- Few months of sx followed by complete remission.
- Intermittent periods of active disease alternate w relative or complete remission.
- Unrelenting progressive disease.

Indicators of good px: monoarticular, unilateral, proximal, more abrupt onset, brief duration of initial sx, male sex, absence of IgM and rheumatoid factor, absence of high ESR or CRP, no extra-articular involvement, no erosions on x-ray; milder course has 50% chance remission vs 30% for YORA; only 6% w EORA have subcutaneous nodules vs 20% with YORA.

Cmplc: Late articular complications: deformities of knees and hips result in decreased ambulation; subluxation of cervical vertebrae may lead to neurologic deficits; septic arthritis of knees, elbows, wrists (staphylococcus most common)—19% mortality if not treated early.

R/o:

- OA: improves after rest and worsens w activity; weight-bearing joints; distal interphalangeal (Heberden's nodes); proximal interphalangeal.
- PMR (see 10.5).
- Gout (see 10.6).
- Pseudogout: common in knees, but may also be seen in the wrists, carpal joints; calcium pyrophosphate crystals in joint fluid.
- Primary Sjögren's syndrome in elderly: milder; less positive ANA, fewer antibodies to SS-A, SS-B (more in RA).
- Fibromyalgia: multiple tender points; disturbed sleep; no synovitis.
- Scleroderma: may present w diffuse swelling of digits, but will also see skin changes and anti-Sci-70 antibodies; Raynaud's phenomenon.
- SLE: 15% of pts present after 50 y/o; less female predominance in the elderly; milder course w fewer renal changes and more serositis and joint manifestations; rheumatoid factor occurs more frequently while hypocomplementemia and anti-double-stranded DNA antibodies occur less frequently in elderly SLE

pts; r/o rx-induced SLE with ∝ mitochondrial and ∝ histone antibodies.

- Polymyositis/dermatomyositis: Carcinomatous polyarthritis—direct invasion of bones or joints by lung or breast malignancy; asymmetric; spares small joints; mild inflammatory joint fluid; x-rays nl.

Lab: Rheumatoid factor pos in 70% of pts; ESR > 40 mm/hr (elderly run high); mild normochromic, normocytic anemia.

X-ray: Periarticular osteopenia; periarticular soft tissue swelling; symmetric joint involvement; loss of cartilage; deformities (usually in late disease).

Rx:

Therapeutic (Nejm 1994;330:1368):

- ASA 650-1000 mg qid (elderly more susceptible to salicylism and possible development of pulmonary edema and high risk for gi irritation and bleeding); ASA + NSAIDs may decrease institutionalization rate (Jags 1996;44:216).
- Gold 3 mg bid (toxic in elderly, causes diarrhea, rash, ulcers, nephropathy, marrow depression, colitis, so check CBC, UA, q 2 wk then q mo).
- D-penicillamine toxic in elderly; skin rash and taste abnormalities more common in elderly.
- Hydroxychloroquine—maculopathy more frequent in elderly.
- Azathioprine—beneficial effects within 2-6 mo, monitor CBC frequently.
- Methotrexate weekly (oral ulcers, liver abnormalities, marrow suppression, pneumonitis)—more early use recommended; monitor CBC, BUN, Cr, LFTs; supplement w folic acid.
- Sulfasalazine—nausea and vomiting more common in the elderly; monitor BP, lytes, glucose, CBC, LFTs, fecal occult blood test.

Steroid injections no more frequently than q 3 mo; use systemic steroids for short courses in conjunction w other agents; steroid se in 2-4 wk; low dose steroids 15 mg prednisone well tolerated during first 2 yr (BMJ 1998;316:811); > 7.5 mg/d glucocorticoid (prednisone) × 6 mo results in rapid loss of trabecular bone in hip, spine, forearm, therefore measure BMD and begin preventive measures w calcium, vit D, wgt-bearing exercise; if deterioration BMD give thiazide, sodium restriction, bisphosphonate, or calcitonin (Arthritis Rheum 1996;39:179); caution with > 3-5 steroid injections in joint pending replacement.

Early intervention w disease-modifying antirheumatic drugs (DMARDS) to control disease activity, alleviate pain, maintain function, and slow progression of joint damage:

- Hydroxychloroquine is recommended for pts w mild arthritis, f/u for retinal disease q 6 mo; methotrexate for moderate to severe disease, works in 3-6 wks, weekly dose; folic acid 1 mg/d to reduce toxicity; sulfasalazine an alternative to either drug (Med Lett 2000;42:57).
- Etanercept (Enbrel) inhibits tumor necrosis factor (TNF, a proinflammatory cytokine produced by synovial cells); can be used in combination w methotrexate, glucocorticoids, ASA, NSAIDs, or analgesics; response in 1-2 wks; lose effect after 1 mo discontinuation; 25 mg twice weekly sc; se (risk of sepsis, frequent infections); long-term effects unknown.
- Leflunomide (Arava) inhibits clonal expansion of T cells by inhibiting cell cycle progression; inhibits cytochrome P450; effect evident by 1 mo; 100 mg tab for 3 d then 20 mg qd; se include diarrhea, elevated ALT/AST, alopecia, rash; potential for immunosuppression; risk of sepsis, frequent infections; watch for renal insufficiency.
- Infliximab (Remicade) a monoclonal antibody that blocks TNF; (Lancet 1999;354:1932) can give w methotrexate; 3 mg/kg iv q 8 wks; watch immunosuppression; risk of sepsis, frequent infections.

Statins decrease inflammation RA (Lancet 2004;363:2015):

- Opioids have definite role in treating pain (Arthritis Rheum 1998;41:1603).
- Obtain neck films of pts w long-standing RA and limited ROM of neck to detect subluxation.

Team Management:

- Physical and occupational therapy.
- Acute episodes: avoid pillows under knees, prevents contractures.
- Knee, ankle, wrist splints part of the day to stabilize painful joint, while still allowing function.
- Isometric maximal contraction of muscle groups in mid-joint range.
- Raised soft heel protector for Achilles tendonitis.
- Molded insoles to maintain longitudinal arch of shoe.
- Hot soaks 20 min tid.
- If other associated joints functioning, can consider joint replacement.
- Walking (Jama 1997;277:25).
- Swimming, water exercise, if available.
- Establish long-term relationships w occupational, physical therapists.

10.5 Polymyalgia Rheumatica and Temporal Arteritis

Jags 1992;40:515; Am Fam Phys 2000;61:2061

Cause: HLA-D4 genetic susceptibility; inappropriate immune response.

Epidem: 0.1-1.0% of people over 70 yr; F/M = 2:1, white-black = 6:1.

Pathophys: Medium and large arteries segmentally; smaller arteries may also be involved, eg, lung.

Sx: May be sudden onset:

- Most w muscle pain which is relieved w activity.
- Fever.
- Jaw claudication.
- Transient blindness or blurred vision (occlusion of ciliary artery causing infarction of optic nerve head or, more commonly, central retinal artery causing normal-appearing disk with the remainder of the retina pale w segmented vessels).
- Diplopia.
- Headache, usually unilateral.
- Thickening of temporal artery.

Also slower onset:

- Malaise.
- Anorexia.
- Weight loss.
- Anemia.

Less common sx:

- Leg/arm claudication.
- CHF.
- Aortic arch syndrome.
- Facial swelling.
- Delirium/dementia.
- Peripheral neuropathy.

Si: Criteria for dx of PMR: pain and stiffness in two of the following areas: shoulders and upper arms, or pelvic girdle (hip and thighs), or neck and torso; morning stiffness > 1-hr duration; duration at least 4 wk; no muscle weakness on exam; no other collagen-vascular disease; elevated ESR (> 40 mm/hr); relief of symptoms within a few d of starting low-dose steroids (Clin Ger Med 1998;14:455).

Criteria for dx of Giant Cell Arteritis (3 of the following 5): > 50 yr old, new onset of localized headache, temporal artery tenderness or decreased temporal artery pulse, ESR > 50 mm/hr, abnormal temporal artery bx.

Crs: Average duration 3 yr.

Cmplc: Most PMR resolves uneventfully; 5% have synovitis in sternoclavicular joints; occasionally death from giant cell arteritis (cerebrovascular infarct, MI, aortic aneurysm) (Clin Ger Med 1998;14:455).

R/o: RA, which responds to NSAIDs whereas PMR does not.

Other causes of polymyalgia: SLE; dermatomyositis; periarteritis nodosa; neoplastic diseases, eg, carcinoma, multiple myeloma; Waldenström's macroglobulinemia; sarcoidosis; infective endocarditis; osteomalacia; HMG-CoA reductase inhibitors; weakness r/o myasthenia gravis (Jama 2002;3:322).

Lab: ESR > 30 mm/hr (80-95%), often > 100 mm/hr; elevated plasma viscosity and CRP (80-95%); normochromic, normocytic anemia (50-80%); elevated globulin fraction in serum electrophoresis (50%); elevated alkaline phosphatase (50%); neg rheumatoid factor (85%); neg ANA (85%).

Color duplex US for dx temporal arteritis (Nejm 1997; 337:1336).

Invasive: Temporal artery bx: not necessary in PMR without objective si of temporal arteritis because clinical outcomes for giant cell arteritis same as pts who only have PMR (Jags 1992;40:515; Drugs Aging 1998;13:109); excise 3-5 cm because shorter segment may miss involved segment; if bx neg, still a 5-10% chance that dx has been missed; bx rarely causes scalp necrosis, but more likely when both arteries are removed; 2 wks of steroid will not change characteristic pathological findings on temporal artery bx.

Rx:

Therapeutic: PMR: Prednisone 10-20 mg/d until ESR nl, asx; ↓ 1mg/d q 4 wk; monitor ESR q 4 wk × 3 mo, then q 2-3 mo until 1 yr, then q yr (Am Fam Phys 2000;61:2000).

Temporal arteritis pts need higher doses of steroids during infections, surgeries, increased physiologic stress; calcium, vit D supplementation and bisphosphonates; lose 20% BMD within 1 mo on high dose chronic steroids; alternate-day steroid therapy not recommended; after corticosteroids discontinued, monitor pt for at least 6 mo, checking ESR.

Prednisone 40-60 mg/d until ESR nl; ↓ 10% q 2 wk to 10 mg/d, then ↓ 1 mg/d q 4 wk; monitor ESR q 4 wk × 3 mo then q 2-3 mo until 1-1½ yr after cessation rx (Am Fam Phys 2000;61:2000).

10.6 Hyperuricemia and Gout

Ann IM 1979;90:812

Cause: Hyperuricemia defined as plasma urate > 420 mol/L (7.0 mg/dL); consequence of increased total body urate due to overproduction and/or under excretion of uric acid; plasma and extracellular fluid saturation with urate leads to crystal formation and deposition; uric acid is the final breakdown product of purine metabolism; 66-75% excreted in kidney, and the rest is excreted in the small intestine.

Epidem: More common in women.

Pathophys: Gout characterized by:

1. Hyperuricemia
2. Attacks of acute, monoarticular inflammatory arthritis.
3. Tophaceous deposition of urate crystals in and around joints (Calculi).
4. Interstitial deposition of urate crystals in the renal parenchyma.

Si: Extraordinarily painful joint, exquisitely sensitive to touch/pressure; pts do not tolerate any but gentle exam; may be subacute or chronic pain; tophi likely to occur in and around Heberden's nodes.

Cmplc: R/o pseudogout calcium pyrophosphate deposition (more common in elderly, in larger joints, often following trauma, surgery, or ischemic heart disease); gout associated w hyperthyroidism; pos birefringent rhomboid crystals under polarized light; x-ray reveals chondrocalcinosis in wrists, knees, pubis symphysis.

Crs: Attacks less frequent in the elderly.

Lab:

- Evaluation of hyperuricemia: > 800 mg/24 hr in urine indicates overproduction.
- Aspiration of involved joint or tissue key to dx with demonstration of intracellular mono urate crystals in synovial fluid, PMNLs or tophaceous aggregates; needle-shaped crystals show strong neg birefringence.

Rx:

Preventive: Most individuals who are hyperuricemic never develop gout; therefore, routine screening for asx hyperuricemia is not indicated; for diet, avoid high-purine foods (shellfish, wild game, organ meats); alcohol, dehydration can precipitate attack; if pt has diseases w incr cell breakdown, watch for incr production.

Therapeutic: Asx hyperuricemia: rx is not beneficial or cost-effective, except for chemotherapy pts (over-production) who are at risk for acute uric acid nephropathy.

Acute Gouty Arthritis

NSAIDs: Better tolerated than colchicine (former first-line rx); indomethacin-most widely used in younger age groups but more toxicity in elderly so use limited to < 7 d; continue rx 3-4 d after all si of inflammation have disappeared; use with caution in pts w PUD, heart failure, HT because of problems with salt retention; may precipitate hyperkalemia and renal insufficiency; anemia, check CBC early and during use.

Colchicine: Can be useful if NSAIDs not tolerated; incr toxicity in the elderly; inhibits the release of leukocyte-derived crystal-induced chemotactic factor; oral doses of 0.6 mg tid; cannot be tolerated in up to 80% pts because of abdominal pain, diarrhea, and nausea; increased toxicity when given w other drugs that are P-450 enzyme inhibitors, eg, cimetidine, erythromycin, tolbutamide (Nejm 1996;334:445); can also be given iv, but generally not recommended due to significant bone marrow toxicity risk; in pts with renal insufficiency, colchicine may produce a reversible neuromuscular toxicity that leads to a subacute myopathy, axonal neuropathy, and incr serum creatinine kinase; avoid iv if hepatic or renal disease, or if recently on oral colchicine.

Intra-Articular Injection of Corticosteroids: Use when pt cannot take po and when colchicine and NSAIDs are contraindicated or ineffective; po steroids (60-80 mg w quick taper), im steroids (methyl prednisone acetate [Depo-Medrol] 50 mg); im ACTH can also be effective (but unavailable at most pharmacies).

Chronic Gout (Pts with Recurrent Attacks, Chronic Sx, Evidence of Tophi, Gouty Arthritis, or Nephrolithiasis):

Biggest issue in elderly is toxicity of long-term med use for chronic gout; all use worth evaluating periodically; stop drugs if possible.

Before starting a urate-lowering agent, pt should be free of inflammation and have started colchicine for prophylaxis; rx goal is urate concentration < 300 μmol/L (< 5.0 mg/dl); diet modification plays a helpful role but pharmacotherapy is also effective; roles of hyperlipidemia, obesity, DM, HT, and ETOH abuse should be addressed.

Colchicine: at 0.6 mg/d for long-term suppression, if only sx is joint pain, monitor CBC.

Allopurinol (for Overproducers Only): potent competitive inhibitor of xanthine oxidase; absorbed from the gi tract; half-life = 3 hr; for pts with evidence of urate overproduction, nephrolithiasis, renal insufficiency (creatinine clearance < 80 mL/min), tophaceous deposits, pts at risk for acute uric acid nephropathy; maximum reduction in urate seen at 2 wk; initiation may induce gout attack so concomitant colchicine is usually prescribed; minor se: skin rash, gi, diarrhea, headache; serious se: alopecia, fever, lymphadenopathy, bone marrow suppression, hepatic toxicity, interstitial nephritis, renal failure, hypersensitivity vasculitis; death can occur in pts with renal insufficiency and pts taking diuretics; reduce dose in renal/hepatic impairment, monitor CBC.

Drug Interactions: Allopurinol prolongs the half-life of 6-mercaptopurine, cyclophosphamide, and azathioprine—all of which are degraded by xanthine oxidase; pts taking ampicillin or amoxicillin have a 3-fold increase in skin rashes; more toxic in the elderly, therefore reduce doses to 100 mg qod.

Uricosuric Agents (For Under Excretion, Most Common Cause): Decrease serum urate by inhibition of proximal tubule reabsorption; use carefully w renal monitoring in pts > 60 yr old, creatinine clearance < 80; most commonly used agents:

1. Probenecid 250 mg po bid up to 1.5 gm/d in 2-3 divided doses.
2. Sulfinpyrazone 50-100 mg qid, inhibits platelet function.

10.7 Cervical and Lumbar Stenosis (Spinal Stenosis)

Clin Ger Med 1994;10:557; Jama 1995;274:1949

Cause: Congenital size of spinal canal and progression of degenerative spinal disease (soft and bony tissue) lead to vascular compromise of nerve roots (claudication sx) caused by a 50% reduction in one segment relative to normal segments above and below as seen on CT.

Pathophys: Most common at L3/L4 or L4/L5 where there is disk degeneration leading to anterior, posterior disk height reduction and longitudinal ligament laxity and subluxation of facet joints; posterior ligamentum flavum hypertrophies in effort to keep segments from falling off each other, resulting in spinal stenosis.

Sx:

Cervical: upper extremity radiculopathy; loss bowel, bladder functions; lower extremity spasticity, Babinski, sensory changes. Cervical spondylotic myelopathy: neck stiffness, unilateral or bilateral deep aching neck, arm, shoulder pain; numbness, tingling hands; clumsiness while walking; weakness, stiffness in legs; electric shock down back w flexion (Lhermitte's sign); cervical spondylosis C5-6 no biceps reflex, but hyperreflexic triceps; Hoffmann's sign reflex contraction of the thumb and index finger after nipping the middle finger (Am Fam Phys 2000;62:1064).

Lumbar: calf, leg, quad, hip pain after walking a discrete distance; back pain less common; lumbar spinal canal increases in size w flexion and decreases w extension; therefore standing, walking on flat surface, or downhill, which extends the spine, increase pain.

Si: Neurologic exam usually neg w earliest sx but can progress to asymmetric ankle jerk, knee jerk; decreased quad, anterior tibial, extensor hallucis longus strength (check heel and toe walking, hip abduction); bicycle test (can bike further than can walk, for in sitting position lumbar spine is flexed, which opens up spinal canal and the foramen at each level); straight-leg raising neg; repeating exam after pt walks downhill may bring out subtle neurologic signs (Jama 1995;274:1949).

Cmplc:

R/o:

- Acute and chronic disk pain incr by sitting forward; pts often roll to one side and sit up sideways; plantar flexion = L4, dorsiflexion and hip adductors = L5; clearer dermatome pain distribution; chronic disk herniation pain may closely mimic spinal stenosis pain.
- Acute central disk: saddle anesthesia; sphincter tone loss (can be common finding in elderly); crossover leg pain (Bull Rheum Dis 1983;33:1).
- Peripheral vascular claudication: pulses absent.
- Tumor or infection: rapidly increasing pain or dysfunction, night pain.

X-ray: LS spine film helpful; MRI.

Rx:

Preventive: General conditioning, particularly walking.

Therapeutic:

- Conservative: bicycling program, follow pt over long enough time to get careful reading on trend of sx before costly therapy; walker, wheelchair for exercise (NH pts).
- Acupuncture, acupressure, stress reduction, pain rx programs (Semin Spine Surg 1994;6:156).
- Spinal manipulation not recommended (BMJ 1995;311:349; Ann IM 1992;117:590).
- Epidural steroids (Anesthesiology 1994;81:923).
- Surgical: posterior decompression helps calf pain (2-8 wk to normal activities); fusion (4-6 mo return to normal activities); 85% of pts helped, 12% of pts no better, 3% of pts worse (J Neurosurg 1994;81:699; Spine 1992;17:1); surg better than nonsurg rx early (Jags 2005;53:785); rapid increase in surgical intervention w high regional variation suggests need for more research on pt selection (Wennberg J. Dartmouth Atlas of

Health Care in the United States. Chicago: American Hospital Publishing, 1996).

10.8 Paget's Disease of the Bone

Clin Ger Med 1994;10:719

Cause: Autosomal dominant characteristics; 7 × greater risk if 1st-degree relative afflicted; may result from viral infection.

Epidem: Second most common bone disease (after osteoporosis) affecting older population; although severe disease much less common.

Pathophys: Localized incr rate of bone turnover and blood flow; pelvis, axial skeleton, skull and wgt-bearing bones affected most frequently; large increase in number and size of osteoclasts and increase in number of nucleoli; irregular resorption of bone produces "mosaic pattern"; reactive osteoblasts produce less organized "woven" bone.

Sx: 5% experience pain, especially at night in warm bed secondary to vasodilation in vascular bone; fractures, hip arthritis; 1% develop osteosarcoma which presents w excruciating pain unrelieved by analgesics; when pt's skull affected, may become apathetic and lethargic (South Med J 1993;10:1097); mental status changes could result from shunting of blood from internal to external carotid system through anastomotic channels; bone compression of CNs II, V, VII, VIII produces monocular visual loss, atypical trigeminal neuralgia, facial paresis or paralysis, hearing loss; middle ear ossicles may be affected, as well.

Si:

- Deformities: anterior tibial bowing along lines of least resistance; anterolateral femoral bowing; wgt of skull causes it to sink into spine, producing short neck and compression of CNs at the base of the skull, spinal neuropathy, hydrocephalus from distortion of the sylvian aqueduct and obstruction of CSF.

- Vertebrae: kyphosis, nerve entrapment, spinal stenosis, vascular steal syndrome which may be mistaken for direct cord compression (Aus NZ J Surg 1992;62:24).

Crs: Variable.

Cmplc: Osteosarcomatous changes (Clin Orthop 1991;265:306); high-output CHF; heart block due to bundle calcifications; renal stones, especially w immobilization; r/o viral, traumatic causes of bone pain.

Lab:

- Alkaline phosphatase reflects activity of the osteoblasts (Horm Metab Res 1991;23:559); be aware of commonness of minor alkaline phosphatase elevations in normal elderly; need elevations 1.5-2 × normal to pursue dx.
- Urinary hydroxyproline levels reflect activity of osteoclasts and bone resorption; both lab values used to monitor active disease and response to rx; free pyridinoline crosslinks, N-telopeptides-specific (Jags 1998;46:1025).
- Urine and serum calcium nl, unless suddenly immobilized; secondary hyperparathyroidism not uncommon.

X-ray: Trabecular and cortical bone irregularly thickened; sclerosis and deformity of periarticular bone; fissure fxs perpendicular to long axis of bone; inner and outer table of skull bones indistinguishable; thus entire thickness consists of spongiosa, producing "cotton wool" appearance; w osteosarcomas (most commonly in pelvis, femur, humerus) technetium uptake reduced and gallium uptake increased.

Rx

Therapeutic:

- Once r/o 2nd causes of alkaline phosphatase > 2-3× mL (liver disease, renal disease, hyperparathyroidism, malabsorption, rectal, prostate, breast cancer), treat asx Paget's disease of the skull or vertebrae; otherwise only rx disability, pain (not relieved by analgesics), incr bone deformity, frequent fractures, vertebral compression, rapid decline in hearing, high-output CHF.

- Early intervention w CN decompression results in better px.
- Biphosphonates: etidronate 200-300 mg/d in frail elderly for 6 mo; alendronate (Fosamax): reduces the rate of bone turnover and decreases bone blood flow; newly formed bone is lamellar; effects long lasting and persist after rx is stopped and more effective than etidronate and calcitonin (Nejm 1997; 336:558); tiludronate (Sarnoff) 200 mg might be tolerated better than other bisphosphonates (Med Lett 1997;39:65); Risedronate, Zoledronate—3rd generation.
- Calcitonin: 50-100 U sq/im qd or 3 × per wk (se, see Osteoporosis, 10.1).
- Plicamycin: cytotoxic antibiotic reserved for nerve compression; 15-20 μg/kg over 5-10 d period; give w calcium and vit D.

Surgical: Surgical hip replacement (J Bone Joint Surg Am 1987; 69:760); total knee replacement (J Bone Joint Surg Am 1991; 73:739).

F/u 6 mo and if no remission sx or alkaline phosphatase still abnormal, then considered rx failure (Jags 1998;46:1010).

10.9 Low Back Pain

Jags 1993;41:167

Cause: Major and minor soft tissue trauma and overuse injuries; UTI; cancer; spontaneous vertebral compression fractures (osteoporosis).

Epidem: Very common in elderly; frequently chronic or recurrent.

Sx: Nonspecific limb sx (pseudoclaudication), loss of continence.

Si: Decreased lower extremity muscle strength; decreased lower extremity muscle circumference; altered lower extremity reflexes; altered lower extremity sensory exam; pos straight-leg raising; check sitting knee extension; palpate for lower abdominal masses; pelvic and rectal exam, if pain severe or long-standing.

Palpate point and general tenderness—spinous processes of lumbar vertebrae, iliolumbar ligaments, lumbar paravertebral muscles, sacroiliac joints, gluteal muscles; evaluate landmark asymmetries—leg length discrepancies, tibial tuberosities, iliac crest heights; pelvic compression—osteopathic maneuver to detect sacroiliac joint instability; pelvic roll—osteopathic maneuver to detect mobility of LS spine; standing and seated flexion; sacral motion.

Cmplc: R/o fracture, spinal stenosis, infection, tumor, cauda equina syndrome.

Lab: CBC, alkaline phosphatase, Ca, ESR, UA, serum immunoelectrophoresis later if suspect multiple myeloma.

X-ray: LS plain films can be useful if suspect fx or neoplasm; prior film(s) always helpful for comparison; bone scan if suspect malignancy or osteomyelitis.

Rx: Brief bed rest periods only (if at all); encourage frequent brief walks; discourage sitting (particularly in auto) for any length of time; maintain regular f/u (frequency depends on pain); firm bed, lumbar pillow, abdominal muscle-strengthening exercises (after acute phase).

Osteopathic: Principles of treatment: use shorter, less frequent rx; avoid thrust techniques in people with severe osteoporosis or osteoarthritis; re-establish motion as quickly as possible; use steady, gentle techniques.

Specific manipulative treatments:

- Muscle and fascial stretching.
- Muscle energy technique: improve muscle-resting length by having pt actively engage the muscle group and then passively stretch it during relaxation.
- Counterstrain: reduction of inappropriate neuromuscular reflexes by placing joint into a position of comfort for 90 sec.
- Soft tissue release: massage of muscle to improve fluid mobilization.

Team Management: Establish physical therapy or osteopathic relationship early, if musculoskeletal origin of pain.

10.10 Adhesive Capsulitis of Shoulder

(BURSITIS, TENDONITIS)

Ger Rv Syllabus 1996;237; Jags 1998;46:1144

Cause: Primary capsulitis resulting from disuse secondary to rotator cuff pathology, fxs, cervical radiculitis, avascular necrosis and osteoarthritis, impingement syndromes, and systemic organic disease such as DM, tbc, RA, MI, chronic lung disease and lung cancer, scleroderma, thyroid disease, autoimmune disease.

Epidem: Most common in the 4th-6th decades of life; affects 2-3% of population, and in 15% is bilateral; F > M.

Pathophys: Adhesive capsulitis: contraction glenohumeral capsule.

Sx: Three phases:

1. Painful stage and increasing stiffness:
   Decreased ability to reach behind the back fastening garment or removing a wallet from the pocket, limited reaching overhead. Unable to scratch the back (Apley's test and NFL"Touchdown" test).

   Generalized pain with no clear pinpoint to exact location. Pain aggravated by movements, alleviated by rest. Sleep may be affected if pt rolls on the affected shoulder; condition progresses to stiffness, muscle spasm, diffuse tenderness about glenohumeral joint.

2. Adhesive stage: increasing stiffness and diminishing pain.
3. Recovery stage: Minimal pain with gradual and spontaneous increase in ROM.

Long head biceps tendonitis: arm motions w fixed flexed elbow, eg, screwing caps on jars; working overhead forcefully turns plantar surface of hand upward against resistance with elbow fixed; tennis serve motion.

Si:

- Adhesive capsulitis: decreased movement of the shoulder.
- Long head biceps tendonitis: tender bicipital groove, pain on resisted supination forearm w elbow adjacent to side and flexed 90°.
- Rotator cuff tendonitis (> 45 yr old): 60-120° extension with painful arc; pain at anterolateral aspect shoulder at greater tuberosity of humerus may lead to complication of subdeltoid bursitis, giving pain at tip acromion and over humeral head; supraspinatus: pain on resistance in abduction. Infraspinatus: pain on resistance in external rotation; no pain on resisted movement w subacromial bursitis. Rotator cuff tears: weakness w elevation of arm in abduction and external rotation. Impingement sign: putting hand behind head cannot hold hand in 90° position, infra- and supraspinatus atrophy (Jags 2000;48:1633); tendinitis of rotator cuff is most common cause of shoulder pain that manifests with pain on passive and active abduction; pain is greater with internal rotation than with external rotation.
- Subacromial bursitis: swelling, warm, tender; subacromial and subdeltoid bursitis-pain when pt lies on his/her shoulder; tenderness with palpation of the space on the lateral aspect of the shoulder just inferior to the acromion along deltoid.

- Acromiclavicular (AC) arthritis-tenderness at joint; aggravates by abduction 100°.

Crs:

- Adhesive capsulitis:
  - Painful stage lasts 3-8 mo, with active and passive motion in all planes lost. Early scapular thoracic rotation when abduction of arm attempted, distinguishes it from other pathologies.
  - Adhesive stage lasts 4-6 mo, and full recovery might take up to 3 yr.
  - External rotation improves first, followed by abduction and internal rotation.
  - 7-30% of the pts permanently lose ROM.
- R/o tumor from kidney, breast, lung, prostate when general exam is normal but pain severe.
- R/o cervical spine disease: pain w cervical extension, C5 weakness of shoulder adduction (deltoid, supraspinatus), C6 weak extension carpus radialis, C7 weak elbow extension (triceps); neck extension and lateral bending toward affected side closes neural foramina.

Cmplc: Stage III after 40 yr old: inflammation, permanent scarring, rotator cuff tendonitis tear, bone alterations, ruptured biceps.

X-ray: Mostly clinical dx. X-ray, limited use but can give information about secondary causes of adhesive capsulitis, such as osteoarthritis, fx, avascular necrosis, calcific tendonitis, and neoplasm; MRI changes are specific and sensitive, but decrease in joint volume not evaluated on MRI; arthrography, used to document decrease in joint volume; unaffected joint will accommodate 20-30 mL, whereas affected joint will be able to hold 5-10 mL. Most specific but invasive.

Subacromial bursitis: calcific deposits on x-ray.

Rx:

Therapeutic:

- Adhesive capsulitis: "If you don't use it, you lose it"; treat the underlying process and try to restore normal ROM; most cases respond to conservative therapy; 10% of pts will have long-term problems that require more aggressive surgical therapy.
- Acute period: limit overhead motion and lifting; NSAIDs may be used to relieve pain and inflammation, but caution in the elderly; nortryptiline may also be used.
- Exercise is the rx of choice during the acute phase, but vigorous and forceful exercises are contraindicated.
- Heat before, ice after more strenuous exercise (when ready) may preserve ROM.
- Long head biceps tendonitis: rx bid w exercise; should improve in 3 wk; if not better in 6 mo, consider surgery.
- Rotator cuff tendonitis exercises: pendulum, walk fingers up wall, exercises w arms close to body to avoid impingement, long stretches help to regain motor function; arthroscopic surgery for decompression impingement.
- Subacromial bursitis: improve with steroid injections, 1 cc depot steroid mixed w 1% lidocaine.
- Calcific tendonitis: may need closed lavage w lidocaine or surgical removal; regional anesthesia w interscalene block.
- Corticosteroid injections: subacromial injection may be indicated in pts with frozen shoulder who have concurrent rotator cuff or bicipital tenditinitis; addition of physical therapy may result in more rapid improvement than injections alone.
- Intraarticular dilation: hydroplasty.
- Glenohumeral injection with saline dilation is indication for pt with > 50% of loss ROM; requires fluoroscopy; usually total vol of contrast not to exceed 15 mL;

- Manipulation under anesthesia; capsular fibrosis is manually ruptured while pts are under general anesthesia or have had an interscalene brachial plexus block.
- Surgery not first line because the condition is self-limited; should be reserved for when physical therapy and corticosteroid injection fail.

Chapter 11

Gastrointestinal Disorders

Esophageal Disorders and Peptic Ulcer Disease

See Table 11.1.

11.1 Peptic Ulcer Disease

Surg Clin N Am 1994;74:93,113; Sci Am 1995;4:1; Jama 1996;275:622; Clin Ger Med 1999;15:439,457; J Fla Med Assoc 1997;84:101

Cause: Smoking, ASA, NSAIDs (greatest risk within first 3 mo), 15-35% PUD result of NSAIDs or ASA (Mayo Clin Proc 2004;79:129); *Helicobacter pylori* (50% seropositive by age 60) grows in mucus overlying antral gastric mucosa cells in 95% of pts w duodenal ulcers and 60-75% of pts w gastric ulcers; first degree relative = 3 × risk.

Epidem: Mortality duodenal ulcer 2-5:100,000 elderly/yr; 29-60% mortality from PUD in pts > 65 yr old; relapse 90% in 10 yr, quiescent after 10-15 yr; incidence increased in COPD, RA, cirrhosis, hyperparathyroidism.

Pathophys: Gastric acid secretion not decreased w aging in healthy individuals (GE 1996;110:1043); mucosal prostaglandin decreased, gastric bicarbonate decreased, and integrity of gastric mucosa decreased because of gastric blood flow; gastritis may be completely explained by *H. pylori* (Clin Ger Med 1999;15(3):439); gastric ulcers more often proximal in elderly.

Table 11.1 Dysphagia

	OROPHARYNGEAL (Can't initiate swallowing or transfer food bolus from mouth to upper esophageal sphincter)	ESOPHAGEAL (Can't transfer from esophagus to stomach) ACHALASIA-failure to relax lower esophageal sphincter
Cause	Neurological-brainstem, anterior cortical strike ALS, Parkinson's neoplasm, Alzheimer's Muscular-Myasthenia, Gravis, Eaton-Lambert, dermatomyositis, polymyositis Anatomic-neoplasm, Zenker's diverticula, cervical spurs, strictures, pemphigoid Iatrogenic-antipsychotics tardive dyskinesia, radiation	Achalasia, Esophageal Spasm, Scleroderma, Rings, Gerd
Epid		40s-50s 2nd peak in elderly
Sx		30-50% Retrosternal chest pain, gradual solid/liquid food dysphagia, 60-90% regurgitate undigested food ac If weight loss—15 lbs/1yr suspect malignancy
	Speech evil	R/o scleroderma, sarcoid
Course	Modified Ba swallow with fiberoptic endoscopic exam	
Tests		X-ray "bird beak" narrowing at gastroesophageal junction "sigmoid esoph"—very dilated Endoscopy to r/o malignancy
	Correct underlying disorder	
	Speech rx—turn head toward damaged side, strengthening tongue	Botulinum toxin injection into sphincter muscle lasts 24 mo—needs to be repeated
Rx		Pneumatic dilation (90% success rate), surgical myotomy laparoscopic (80-90% success)

Sx: Only 35% of elderly have pain; less pain w NSAID usage. Duodenal ulcer: deep epigastric pain relieved by food or antacids; hunger experienced 2 hr after meals; vomiting indicates ulcer within pyloric channel; melena from erosion at the base of the ulcer is an unusual complication; occasionally present w anemia, MI, CVA.

Crs: Gastric (bigger, bleed more in elderly) less common than duodenal.

Cmplc:

R/o:

1. Ischemic pain not relieved by food, but may respond to vasodilator.
2. Carcinoma: anorexia, nausea, weight loss.
3. Acute cholecystitis: lancinating pain, fever, weight loss.
4. Acute pancreatitis: nausea, emesis.
5. Acute appendicitis.
6. Other causes of upper gi bleeding (sources in order of decreasing prevalence): gastric ulcer, duodenal ulcer, gastric erosions, esophagitis, esophageal varices, neoplasm, Mallory-Weiss tears (Jags 1991;39:402).
7. GE reflux: rx w H2 antagonist; proton pump inhibitors effective, but more expensive.

Half of pts > 70 yr old have complications, higher mortality related to comorbidity, mortality rate 29-60%:

- Bleeding ulcers: mortality rate 10-15%; 10-20% have no sx; rebleed if hypotension or visible vessel or sentinel clot on endoscopy.
- Obstruction from edema or fibrosis in the region of the ulcer: distension or fullness before meal completed; > 300 mL gastric contents 4 hr after meal completed.
- Perforation (5-10% mortality): highest mortality/morbidity in the elderly; duodenal perforation 5 × more common than gastric perforation but gastric perforation mortality 5 × greater

(30-50%); severe progressive mid-epigastric pain, later localizing to right lower abdomen if gastric contents spill along surface of right colon; can get posterior ulcer penetrating into pancreas causing acute pancreatitis, which rarely becomes recurrent or chronic.

Lab:

- Endoscopy if gross upper gi bleed, no response to therapy, or multiple ulcers or gastric ulcer on previous exam.
- Basal and stimulated acid secretion when intractable to medical therapy; recurrent disease rapidly develops; gastric ulcer might be caused by carcinoma (33% of pts with ulcerated gastric carcinoma have achlorhydria after acid secretion stimulation whereas pts w benign disease have some acid secretion).
- Breath urea test for *H. pylori* or rapid serologic tests (Nejm 1996;333:984); antibody testing less specific than urease enzyme testing of bx specimen.

Rx:

Therapeutic:

- Diets not effective, although pts may prefer to avoid foods that have troubled them; avoid caffeine; refrain from eating at night.
- Avoid NSAIDs, especially indomethacin, try following alternatives for pain: tramadol, nonacetylated salicylates, intraarticular corticosteroids, possibly Cox-2 inhibitors (Mayo Clin Proc 2004;79:129), consider cardiovascular risk w Cox-2 inhibitors.
- Antacids 1 and 3 hr after meals and on retiring as good as H2-receptor antagonists (Drugs 1994;47:305); magnesium hydroxide-osmotic diarrhea; calcium carbonate-acid rebound; aluminum hypophosphatemia—good for renal failure; alternating magnesium, aluminum, and calcium antacids avoids side effects; avoid magnesium products in pts with renal dysfunction.

- H2 receptor antagonists: for less severe GERD and PUD prophylaxis (Am J Gastroenterol 1999;94:1430), rigorous separation of H2 receptors and antacids probably not necessary; cimetidine and ranitidine available generically, less expensive; se: cimetidine prolongs half-life of phenytoin, theophylline, coumadin, β-blockers, lidocaine, diazepam, chlordiazepoxide because interact w hepatic P-450 micro enzyme; ranitidine binds P-450 less, and famotidine, nizatidine do not bind P-450; cause mental confusion—concern in hospital, since extensively used postop; after 2-3 mo rx for gastric ulcer, re-evaluate (UGI or endoscopy) to identify 5% who progress to gastric cancer; if sx of duodenal ulcer improve, no further study needed.
- Sucralfate: 1 gm 1 hr ac 3 d and hs; works for multiple gastric erosions as well; affects aluminum absorption (use w caution in renal failure because of impaired excretion of aluminum); interferes w tetracycline absorption; constipation.
- Proton pump inhibitors (PPI): strongly inhibit hydrogen ion secretion by the gastric parietal cells; for resistant PUD, erosive gastritis esophagitis and GERD; better than ranitidine; misoprostol in ulcers associated w NSAIDs; healing in 4 wk; iv PPI in ICU, interference w drugs metabolized by P-450 system; decrease in the acid-induced metabolism of ingested digoxin (Ann IM 1991;115:540); acute hepatic toxicity (Am J Gastroenterol 1992;87:523).
- Misoprostol: 200 mg qid; synthetic prostaglandin E1 analogue for prevention of NSAID-induced gastric ulcers, also prevents duodenal ulcers; dose-related diarrhea 13-40%, abdominal pain 7-20% (Nejm 1992;327:1575).
- *H. pylori* treatment: 10-14 d course of amoxicillin 1 gm bid plus clarithromycin 500 bid w omeprazole 20 mg bid (Clin Ger Med 1999;15:467).

Surgery: Billroth I or II for recurrent ulcers produces dumping syndrome in 10% of pts.

11.2 Celiac Sprue

Sci Am 2000;11:3; Gastroenterology in Mansbach, CM. Malabsorption and Maldigestion; Nejm 1991;325:1709; GE 1998;114:424; Jags 2000;48:1690

Epidem: Short stature; 25% childhood or family hx; genetic predisposition (HLA) leads to intestinal reaction to x-gliadin fraction of gluten.

Pathophys: Saccharides degraded by luminal bacterial into 2- and 3-carbon fragments with increased osmotic effect leading to diarrhea; severe damage to villi; dietary CHO digested to monosaccharides by enzyme intestinal surface.

Sx: Profound fatigue by midday, cannot even do sedentary activity; stool change subtle, diarrhea intermittent for periods of 4-6 mo or less; anorexia after several mo/yr; glossitis; unexplained anemia (Minn Med 1995;78:29; Gut 1999;55:65); apathy, wasting, but not until severe.

Si: Anterior and lateral margins of tongue smooth; petechiae, ecchymosis, abdominal distention, ↑ BS, ↓ intestinal transit with advanced disease.

Crs:

Decreased vit A and vit K; decreased vit D leading to osteoporosis; decreased vit E may lead to spinal cerebellar degeneration; low B_{12} leading to ataxia—most common neurologic manifestation; low calcium and magnesium resulting in tetany, mental confusion (small percentage) (Arch IM 1997;15:1013); ulcer, colitis, or Crohn's may precede or follow sprue by months or years; 15-20% histiocytic lymphomas, adenocarcinomas.

Epilepsy in 3-5%; prolonged Q-T interval; tropical sprue: lymphocytic infiltration on bx, geographic location, severe megaloblastic anemia Hct = 20-25%; ischemic: bloody diarrhea and pain 15 min after eating; chronic radiation enteritis: may lead to stricture.

R/o dermatitis herpetiformis (pruritic red skin blisters on shoulder, buttocks, knees, elbows), diabetic autoimmune neuropathy, florid thyrotoxicosis.

Lab: Albumin < 2.5g/dL (protein loss through damaged surface membrane); megaloblastic anemia (50%); ↓ cholesterol; liver-abnormal AST, ALT resolve with rx (Clin Gastroenter 1995;20:90); ↑ antigliadin A, G, ↑ antiendomysial antibody titers corresponds to x-ray changes.

Rx: Diet excludes wheat, gluten, rye, barley, oats (Hosp Pract 1993;28:41); avoid milk—develop lactose intolerance; prednisone 20-40 mg if don't respond to gluten free diet; if becomes refractory to diet, look for tumors.

Table 11.2 Drug-induced Diarrhea

Drug-induced diarrhea (Clin Ger Med 2000;8:67)

Decreased gastric acid: leads to pathogens that cause diarrhea (*Shigella, Salmonella, Giardia lamblia,* and *Clostridium difficile*)
- Cimetidine (J Am Ger Soc 1993;41:940)
- PPI, H_2 blockers (Jama 2005;294:2989)

Decreased motility: gastric: leads to pathogens (Gastroenterol Clin N Am 1994;23:313)
- Metoclopramide
- Cisapride
- Erythromycin
- Diazepam

Small bowel: leads to pathogens
- Cholinomimetics, eg, tacrine (diarrhea rarely occurs w hypermotility of small bowel)

Secretory diarrhea: interferes w ATP pump
- Misoprostol
- 5-ASA
- Digoxin (second most common cause of drug-induced diarrhea)
- Colchicine

Osmotic diarrhea:
- Lactulose
- Acarbose

Mucosal damage:
- Antineoplastics
- Gold
- Penicillamine
- Methyldopa
- NSAIDs

11.3 Diverticular Disease: Diverticulitis and Diverticulosis

Surg Clin N Am 1994;74:293

Cause: Lack of dietary fiber.

Epidem: > 50% prevalence in persons over 70 yr old.

Pathophys: 90% in sigmoid colon because narrow caliber results in higher intraluminal pressure; found in R colon in the Asian population (Br J Surg 1971;58:902).

Sx: Pain 75% and hemorrhage 25%; abrupt, persistent L lower quadrant (sometimes R lower quadrant or suprapubic) colicky pain increasing in severity over time, exacerbated by meals, relieved by bowel movements; more often constipation than diarrhea or alternating; anorexia; vomiting; fever may be presenting complaint; peritonitis; elderly may not have pain or fever, therefore serial exams important.

Si: Distended abdomen, tympanic to percussion; bowel sounds diminished; localized tender mass; rebound tenderness locally; occult rectal bleeding.

Crs: 3-10 d; recurrence rate 25% in first 5 yr.

Cmplc: Perforation, fistula, abscess; urinary frequency, dysuria may suggest bladder involvement; most common cause of lower intestinal bleeding except angiodysplasia; w bleeding r/o colon cancer, ischemic bowel, angiodysplasia (R colon in 66% of pts, usually in the setting of previously undiagnosed asx disease, 70-80% resolve spontaneously, 3-5% require tfxs); B_{12} malabsorption → deficiency.

Lab: CBC: leukocytosis, anemia; white or red cells on UA, if ureteral inflammation.

X-ray:

- Saw-toothed pattern and thickening of muscular wall of colon considered prediverticular condition; adynamic ileus; mechanical obstruction.
- Perform sigmoidoscopy early without vigorous bowel preparation and minimal air insufflation; wait wks for full colonoscopy to r/o cancer proximal to rectosigmoid region.
- CT if suspect abscess.

- For continued bleeding: selective mesenteric arteriography to localize extravasation and distinguish from angiodysplasia; bleeding rate < 1 mL/min technetium-tagged rbc scan w diverticular bleeding.

Rx:

Therapeutic:

- Bowel rest w iv hydration.
- Surgical consultation early.
- Analgesics cautiously because they mask symptoms.
- Broad-spectrum antibiotics to cover gram-pos, anaerobic and aerobic gram-neg organisms; amoxicillin/clavulanate if no leukocytosis or fever.
- β-lactam antibiotic w activity against anaerobic and enteric Gram-neg organisms; if no improvement, CT to r/o intra-abdominal abscess (pain may be lacking, may not have increased wbc, anemia, increased alkaline phosphatase, ESR may be only clues), fistula formation; surgical mortality 20%, try percutaneous drainage first.
- Diet can be advanced over few days to normal diet.
- If severe, hemicolectomy indicated for spreading peritonitis; should be done in 2-stage procedure in the elderly, unless can attain preoperative percutaneous drainage of isolated diverticular abscess.
- For active bleeding, vasopressin for interarterial vasoconstriction, embolization; if pt exsanguinating, consider partial colectomy.
- In pts with early diverticulitis in NH or home w support, antibiotics and oral fluids w careful frequent evaluation appropriate.

Table 11.3 Diarrhea

	Crohn	Ulcerative Colitis	Diverticulitis	Mesenteric Ischemia	Villous Adenoma
Si/Sx/Lab	Blood/mucus/pus abdominal pain (postprandial)	Not as much bleeding as w younger pts	+/− Constipation, fever, leukocytosis, peritoneal sis; bleeding resolves spontaneously; be alert to presentation w few sx	L crampy postprandial pain; h/o decreased cardiac output, eg, afib; may lead to diarrhea, distension, and 50% bleed within 24 hr, and nausea and vomiting	Decreased K^+; chronic diarrhea presentation
Xray/endoscopy/complc	Ulcers on sigmoidoscopy; bx: transluminal granuloma; complc: obstruction, hemorrhage, perforation, fistula, malnutrition, weight loss large, arthritis, skin and oral lesions	Friable; avoid BE if fever; bleeding leads to toxic megacolon; 20% increase risk for colon cancer in 10 yr	Complc: obstruction, perforation, fistula, abscess, peritonitis from gram-neg and anaerobic organisms	BE thumbprinting blue submucosal hemorrhage adjacent to pallor; heal 2 wk or 15% stricture; 20% persistent; 10% gangrene (w 90% mortality)	Colonoscopy
Rx	See 11.4	See 11.5	Surgical resection > 2 episodes; early detection and rx w antibiotics important to prevent hospitalization	Rest bowel, parenteral fluids, NG tube, broad-spectrum antibiotics, surgery for gangrene or impending perforation, or if not resolved in 2-3 wk	Surgery

11.4 Inflammatory Bowel Disease: Crohn's

Epidem: Less common than ulcerative colitis; 16% of pts w Crohn's disease are > 65 yr old; bimodal population and involvement of different segments of the intestines (more distal) in later yr, suggests different disease entities (Med Clin N Am 1994;78:1303).

Pathophys: Transmural; more likely to be distal part of small bowel, narrowing ileal lumen.

Sx: Usually indolent; diarrhea persistent w large-bowel disease; less bleeding than w ulcerative colitis; mucus, pus, and abdominal pain (postprandial) may resemble small-bowel obstruction if terminal ileum involved (Am Fam Phys 1995;198:19).

Si: Aphthous ulcer in rectum; tender mass RLQ usually inflamed bowel, mesenteric lymph nodes, sometimes abscess (small sealed-off perforations); gross blood in stool unusual.

Crs: High (85%) postop recurrence (Med Clin N Am 1990;74;183). R/o other causes of diarrhea (see Tables 11.2 and 11.3).

Table 11.4 Inflammatory Bowel Disease in the Elderly

Ulcerative Colitis	Crohn
Slight male predominance	Female predominance
Severe initial attacks	Delays in dx
High mortality w severe attack	Mortality not increased
More frequent proctosigmoid	More colonic, less ileum involved
Lower relapse rate	Low postop recurrence rates
Good long-term prognosis	Good response med rx

Cmplc: Obstruction, perforation, fistula; malnutrition, 25 lb weight loss; arthritis; skin lesions; anal lesions; renal stones from calcium oxalate, if terminal ileum involved.

R/o:

- Cholelithiasis, cholecystitis.
- PUD.
- Mesenteric vascular insufficiency: pain disproportionate to belly tenderness; usually followed by bloody diarrhea within hours; treat w resection or re-establishment of arterial flow to involved bowel; chronic mesenteric ischemia presents w triad of postprandial pain, fear of eating, wgt loss.
- Tumors.
- Amoebic colitis: associated w inanition, fatigue.
- *Clostridium difficile*.
- Irritable bowel: recurrent crampy pain, bloating, flatulence, diarrhea and constipation; pain associated w stress, relieved by passage of flatus or stool. Bloating = bacterial overgrowth (Jama 2004;292:852).
- Diverticulitis: 3-6 cm of bowel, while Crohn's 10 cm segment w transverse fissures.
- Bowel obstruction: periumbilical pain waxes and wanes q 10 min in lower bowel.
- NSAID-induced enteropathy (Gut 1992;33:887): occult blood pos, anemia, Rx w misoprostol.

Lab: Anemia secondary to iron deficiency, ↓ vit B_{12} metabolized in terminal ileum; folate deficiency from sulfasalazine inhibition of its absorption; mild leukocytosis > 10 000/dL.

X-ray: Sigmoid ulceration on BE.

Rx:

- Sulfasalazine supplemented w folic acid, azathioprine, 6-mecaptopurine, methotrexate (Am Med J GE 1997;92:7703).
- Infliximab (tumor necrosis factor) (Br J Surg 1997;84:1051).
- Budesonide associated w reduced systemic se (Nejm 1998; 339:370).

- Poor candidates for ileoanal anastomoses because of disease and recurrences.
- Colonoscopic bx q 8-10 yr.

Team Management: In contrast to results in pts w ulcerative colitis, elemental diets, and TPN w bowel rest improve symptoms; inflammatory sequelae and nutritional status in pts w Crohn's (Nejm 1996;334:841).

11.5 Inflammatory Bowel Disease: Ulcerative Colitis

Sci Am 2001;4:4

Cause: Alteration in mucosal immune system.

Epidem: 12% of pts are > 60 yr old; 3 × more common than Crohn's disease; M > W (Gastroenterol Clin N Am 1990;19:361).

Sx: Tenesmus; presents more w diarrhea than bleeding in the elderly.

Crs:

Mild (60%), distal colon and rectum; even when disease remains quiescent, mucosa has abnormal dull flat or granular appearance.

Moderately severe (25%), > 5 stools/d gross blood, cramping pain, intermittent temperature to 100.4°F, intermittent fatigue, increased sleep requirement.

Severe (15%), extreme fatigue, weakness, prostration; distended abdomen, tympany, bowel sounds often absent; increased risk for colon cancer 20%/10-yr duration; cancer risk independent of disease activity.

Cmplc: Toxic megacolon 3%, perforation 3%, stricture 10%, severe hemorrhage 4%, cancer 3% (as high as 40% in pts who acquired the disease before 15 yr old) (Nejm 1990;323:1228); erythema nodosum 3%, aphthous mouth ulcers 10%, iritis 5%, arthritic large joints 5%, fatty liver 40%, pericholangitis 5%, cirrhosis 3%, sclerosing cholangitis 2.5%, pyoderma gangrenosum, uveitis, spondylitis (HLA-B27).

- R/o bacterial gastroenteritis, ischemic colitis, diverticulitis, amebiasis, Crohn's, irritable bowel.

Lab: CBC, lytes, liver profile, blood cultures; can also see granulomas on bx in ulcerative colitis.

X-ray: Avoid BE if fever or tachycardia or increased rectal bleeding, since may cause toxic megacolon; friable sigmoid and rectum (grades 1-4 ranging from friability after swabbing to unprovoked bleeding before swabbing); small bowel follow-through; pseudopolyps (nodules of regenerative mucosa); aphthous ulcer rectum.

Table 11.5 Findings on BE

Ulcerative Colitis	Crohn
Loss of haustra; multiple 1-mm diameter "collar button" ulcers	"Rose thorn" ulcers w deep tracts; ileum involvement w skip lesions; "thumbprinting"; transmural involvement; fistulas

Rx:

Preventive: Serial colonoscopies q yr w bxs q 10 cm for 8 yr after onset.

Therapeutic: Antidiarrhea agents: diphenoxylate, loperamide, tincture of opium.

- Sulfasalazine and 5-aminosalicylates (5-ASA) derivatives (mesalamine) for remissions or mild sx.
- Olsalazine (Gut 1994;35:1282), mesalamine for mild flares (Med Lett 2007;49:25); corticosteroid enemas for mild to moderately active.
- Azathioprine for several mo; when bone marrow depression occurs, 3 d off drug will allow parameters to return to nl; qd for moderate to severe sx.

- Add cyclosporine iv for fulminant colitis or toxic megacolon; response in 4 d.
- Diet: watch for lactose intolerance; Fe po.
- Erythropoietin (Nejm 1996;334:619), tfx for anemia.
- Indications for proctocolectomy:
  1. Failure of intensive drug therapy after 2-4 wk.
  2. Failure of toxic megacolon to improve after 4 d of intensive therapy.
  3. Cannot distinguish stricture from cancer.
  4. Severe extracolonic manifestations, ileal-rectal anastomosis or ileoanal pouch (Am J Gastroenterol 1998;93:166).
- Antibiotics of no help (Am J Gastroenterol 1994;89:43).

11.6 Ischemic Bowel

Med Clin N Am 1994;78:1303; Clin Ger Med 1999;15:527

Table 11.6 Mesenteric Ischemia

	Epidem	Sx	Rx
Acute			
Arterial			
Superior mesenteric artery (SMA) embolus	*77 yr, 40-50%, cardiac origin, SMA not occluded explaining why proximal small bowel spared	Severe abd pn out of proportion to exam, gut emptying, severe cardiac disease, progresses to peritoneal irritation	Rx < 12 hr, heparin, antibx, resect necrotic bowel, 2nd look operation 24-48 hr or thrombolytics? (Ann Vasc Surg 1998;12:187)
SMA thrombus	*77 yr, 18-25%, diffuse ASVD	Same as CMI, distention in 12-24 hr, bloody stool, electrolyte abn late, irreversible, occlusion at origin SMA, collateral formation limits ischemic injury	Revasc to achieve SMA patency, no percutaneous transluminal angioplasty because increased risk of thrombus
Nonocclusive mesenteric ischemia	*63 yr, 20%	Low flow states superimposed on ASVD, patchy diffuse involvement, colicky, periumb pn	Vasodilators, eg, papaverine × 24 hr

continues

Table 11.6 continued

	Epidem	Sx	Rx
Venous			
Mesenteric venous thrombosis	*66 yr, 5%	Mild distention, pn weeks, abd trauma, sepsis, portal HT, hypercoagulability, OCPs, protein def	Revasc
Chronic			
Arterial			
Chronic mesenteric ischemia (CMI)	Younger women	Postprandial pn 4 hr, weight loss (food fear), visceral angina, ASVD of mesenteric circ usually 2 ves occluded SMA, celiac, IMA less common	
Venous			
Chronic mesenteric venous thrombosis	*74 yr		

*Average.
Source: Med Clin N Am 1994;78:1303; Clin Ger Med 1999;15:527.

Cause: Associated w artificial mitral valve, Afib, surgical bypass.

Epidem: Most common cause of noninfectious colitis in the elderly; 1% of all admissions for acute abdomen.

Pathophys: Mucosal, then serosal involvement; L colon (splenic flexure); "watershed" area prone to ischemia because of poor circulation.

Sx: Abdominal pain (left-sided cramps in 75%), bleeding (50% within 24 hr), distension, diarrhea, nausea, vomiting.

Si: Decreased cardiac output.

Crs: Bloody diarrhea, wgt loss, decreased albumin; generally complete healing in 2 wk.

Cmplc: Pseudo-obstruction, 15% strictures, 20% persistent ischemic colitis, 10% gangrene; 90% mortality.

X-ray:

- Supine abdomen: gas in portal vein-poor px; done primarily to exclude other causes.
- BE: thumbprinting; sigmoidoscopy: focal hemorrhagic lesions, ischemic ulcerations (dark blue submucosal ulcerations adjacent to areas of pallor); C-T, MRI: nonspecific edema; duplex US: to dx chronic mesenteric ischemia early by arterial narrowing, decreased blood flow.

Rx:

Therapeutic: Bowel rest, parenteral fluids, NG tube; broad-spectrum antibiotics; surgery, if suspect gangrene or perforation impending or not resolved within couple of wks; pseudo-obstruction: colonic decompression if cecal diameter > 9 cm.

11.7 GI Bleeding (Angiodysplasia)

Clin Ger Med 1994;10:1; 1999;15:511

Cause: NSAIDs and ASA cause gastritis, gastric and duodenal ulcers (epigastric pain); Malory-Weiss tear (usually h/o vomiting);

ETOH; potassium, vit C, quinidine, tetracycline, alendronate cause esophagitis or ulcer; aortoenteric fistula (h/o AAA repair or bypass); varices (portal HT, gastropathy liver disease); Rendu-Osler-Weber (h/o epistaxis).

Epidem:

- Mortality in old-old correlates w severe bleeding, ulcer > 2 cm, bilirubin > 2.0; early endoscopy w heater probe decreases mortality (Br J Surg 1998;85:121); *H. pylori* rx decreases risk of gi bleed.
- Angiodysplasia: one of the most common etiologies of gi bleeding in the elderly; 25% associated w aortic stenosis (Am J Surg 1979;137:57).

Pathophys: Increased intraluminal pressure in the R colon leads to decreased mucosal blood flow and mesenteric ischemia leading to AV shunting in the submucosal layer of the bowel (Am Fam Phys 1985;32:93).

Sx:

Melena = UGI, or small bowel or proximal colon bleed.
Hematochezia = LGI bleed or brisk UGI bleed.

Si: Stigmata of liver disease commonly seen; bleeding from diverticular lesions (arterial source) more severe than from ectasias (venous source).

Crs:

- Gi bleed; mortality related to smoking; in 80 yr old mortality is 35% related to underlying DM, HT, CAD, meds.
- Angiodysplasias: usually stop spontaneously.

Cmplc: Resting tachycardia = 10% blood loss; pulse increased 20 bpm or sys BP decreased 20 pts = 20-30% blood loss.

Lab: BUN/Cr ratio 20:1 suggests UGI bleed (absorption in proximal small bowel of Hb); also a sign of prerenal azotemia.

X-ray:

- Avoid BE; gastrografin, if contrast agent necessary.
- Colonoscopic findings: telangiectasias, surface erosions < 5 mm cecum and ascending colon, tortuous veins.

Rx:

Therapeutic: Vit K, fresh frozen plasma if on coumadin; O_2; angiodysplasia: vasopressin, chemical embolization, electrocoagulation, laser, segmental resection, hemicolectomy; hormonal therapy controversial.

11.8 Pancreatitis/Cholecystitis

Surg Clin N Am 1994;74:317; Clin Ger Med 1999;15:571,579

Cause:

- Pancreatitis: ETOH > 12-15 yr, gallstones (most common, 75% of cases of acute pancreatitis in pts > 80 yr old), meds (ethacrynic acid, corticosteroids, metronidazole, thiazide, estrogen), metabolic (hypercalcemia, hypertriglyceridemia, uremia), surgery, ERCP, sphincter of Oddi dysfunction, tumors, ischemia, perhaps periampullary diverticula, hereditary (trypsinogen, cystic fibrosis).

Epidem:

- Biliary disease leading indication for acute abdominal surgery in elderly.
- Pancreatitis: acute mortality rate 20% (Am J Surg 1986; 152:638).

Pathophys: *E. coli* and Klebsiella most common organisms in cholecystitis; anaerobic infections also; larger common bile duct in elderly; change in biliary metabolism (cholesterol saturation of bile is increased); predispose pts to cholecystitis.

Sx:

- Cholecystitis: peritoneal signs are seen in < 50% of pts and some pts have no abdominal tenderness; frequently low grade temp elevations, but may be toxic-appearing w pt disoriented and showing no abdominal signs; 40% of acutely ill pts have empyema, perforation, gangrene; 15% have subphrenic abscess or liver abscess; acalculous cholecystitis similar to acute calculous cholecystitis in presentation, but most prevalent after surgery, trauma, repeated transfusions, burns, prolonged parenteral nutrition, cancer.
- Pancreatitis: altered mental status may be only presenting sx; epigastric pain radiating to back, pt sits forward; tachycardia, nausea, vomiting, fever, ileus, shock; chronic pancreatitis presents w pain; nutritional deficiency w protein and fat malabsorption; glucose intolerance more common than in young people.

Cmplc:

- Choledocholithiasis 10-20% of time: 75% present w pain and jaundice, 18% w pain, 6% w jaundice; endoscopic sphincterotomy if unfit for surgery; mortality rates for operative common duct exploration are 6-12%, usually cardiac cause.
- Gallbladder perforation due to decreased vascularity of fundus of gallbladder w aging.
- Pancreatitis: left-sided effusions, localized parenchymal infiltrates (pancreatic effects on pulmonary surfactant) (Gastrointest Endosc Clin N Am 1990;19:433); renal failure and ARDS early, infection late.
- Severe if one of the following (Jama 2004;291:2805):
  1. Organ failure (one or more of the following: systolic BP < 90, PaO_2 < 60, Cr > 2.0, bleeding > 500 cc/24 hr
  2. One of the following complications: pseudocyst, abscess, necrosis
  3. At least 3 Ranson criteria.
  4. At least 4 APACHE II.

- Underlying adenocarcinoma of the gallbladder: especially in women in 6th and 7th decades w gallstones.
- R/o appendicitis.
- R/o pancreatic cancer w CA 19-9 marker (Clin Ger Med 1999;15:579).
- R/o perforated PUD, bowel obstruction, bowel perforation, mesenteric ischemia.

Lab:

- Cholecystitis: leukocytosis in 66% of pts, sometimes only elevated alkaline phosphatase (Ger Rv Syllabus 2004;5:330).
- Pancreatitis: elevation of enzymes not correlated w px or severity of disease, CRP > 150 measurement severe, Hct < 39 female, 43 male neg predictor.

X-ray: If dx uncertain, obtain CT w contrast; ensure adequate renal function prior to contrast, MRI better for seeing necrosis or pseudocyst.

Rx:

- 9.8% mortality from surgery for acute cholecystitis because of delayed dx and comorbidities; laparoscopic cholecystectomy preferred (Ann Surg 1991;213:665).
- Pancreatitis: ERCP, sphincterotomy for gallstone pancreatitis (Lancet 1988;2:979); npo; NSAIDs for pain; ICU if severe to monitor cardiac, fluid, and electrolyte status and start enteral or parenteral feeding; abx if not better 5 d or ascites or pseudocyst or pancreatic necrosis; imipenem, consider adding fluconazole; platelet activation factor receptor antagonist decreases mortality in severe acute pancreatitis (GE 1997;112:A453); pancreatin, 8 tabs w meal for malabsorption.
- Pancreatitis: APACHE II better predictor of px than Ranson criteria (see table on p. 586 in Clin Ger Med 1999;15:579).

11.9 Liver Disease

Table 11.7 Liver Disease in the Elderly

	Hep B/C	Pyogenic Liver Abscess	Autoimmune Liver Disease	Hepatic Ischemia	PBC	Neoplasm
Cause		Direct extension from biliary tract, pancreatitis hematogenous from portal v. (divertic, appendicitis, Crohns), hematogenous from hepatic artery (endocarditis, prosthesis) malignancy		Results from hypertension and shock, ASCVD		Mets from colorectal CA most common. 25% of colorectal CA pts have Mets on presentation. Abdomen, brain, lung, neuroendocrine mets to liver
Epid	Prevalence Hep B $\uparrow$ 3$\times$ in pts 64-74, 43% Hep C compared to younger group 7%	Primarily affects elderly	22% of pts with AH > 65 yr, less severe (aminotransferase levels not as high) (Age Aging 1997;26:441)	6th, 7th decades	As many as 38% of new cases > 65 yr (Gut 1997;41:430)	Pts > 60 yr lower survival rates; however, tumor size most important prognostic factor
Sx	Mild, subclinical in Hep B & C			Critically ill or anorexic, fatigue	Extrahepatic disorders: hypothyroid, sicca syndrome, cutaneous xanthoma	

Si	5% Hep B lead to chronic hepatitis lead to HCC: the longer the infection exposure, the more the chance of HCC. Hep C ↑ mortality rate in elderly		Pts with AST > 10× or Gamma globular > 5× have 3-yr mortality rate of 50% (Med Clin N Am 1996;80:973)		Once 5× of pruritus jaundice, hepatosplenomegaly and complications of cirrhosis develop advage poor px (> 90% die of liver disease)	
Lab		US, MRI not accurate, needle bx liver	Liver bx or might miss dx	Serum transaminase 25-250× nl during acute insult return to nl in 7-10 days, bili, alk phos 3-4× nl, PT nl		Difficult detect tumor Less than 1 cm radiologically and may not be assoc with alpha FP. Screen pts with Hep C with US and alpha FP of 6 mo

Source: Clin Geriatr Med 1999;15:559.

11.10 Enteral Feeding

Nejm 1997;226:41; Crit Care Clin 1997;13:669

Indications: Pts with a functional gi tract who are unable to sustain adequate caloric intake by mouth; significant muscle wasting occurs after npo 7-10 d; discussion of alternative feeds, if no hope for resuming po; no increase in lean body mass (LBM), but attenuation in the rate of loss of LBM (especially muscle) (Nutr 1999; 15:158).

- Neurologic disorders: trauma, CVA, and disease.
- Malignancy: especially head and neck.
- Burns.
- Chemotherapy and radiation therapy.
- Gi disorder, eg, IBD, enterocutaneous fistula.

Caloric Requirements:

- Adult: 25-35 kcal/d
- Elderly: 15-20 kcal/d
- Resting energy expenditure (REE): M REE = $(789 \times \text{BSA}) + 137$, F REE = $(544 \times \text{BSA}) + 414$.
- Hospitalized pts need 20% in excess of REE; burn pts need 100% in excess of REE.
- Use LR as first fluid in hospital: 28 mEq/L lactate combats muscle wasting; D5 provides 50 g dextrose (min caloric supply).

Types of Tubes:

- NG tube: 8-10 Fr with mercury-weighted tip, pliable.
- Gastro/jejunostomy tube: percutaneous endoscopic placement with conscious sedation at bedside by gi or intra-operative placement by surgeon; 1% major complication rate; wait 2-3 d after placement for use; clean dressing changes qd; secure tube to prevent dislodgement.

Types of Formulas:

- Polymeric: nutrients intact, nl gi function required; varieties containing lactose, lactose free, with fiber.
- Monomeric or elemental formulas for compromised digestion/absorption, highly osmolar, impalatable: protein hydrolysates or amino acids, glucose, oligosaccharides, medium chain triglycerides; require min digestion; use in pancreatitis, ulcerative colitis, gi fistula; 1 kcal/mL.
  - *Vivamax* and *Vivamax HN* (high nitrogen).
  - *Vital:* good for fluid restricted pts.
- Specialty formulas designed for specific disease:
  - Intact protein isolates, starches and long-chain fatty acids; fed to stomach or small bowel; pt must have normal proteolytic and lipolytic functions; minimally hyperosmolar, 1 kcal/mL, come premixed.
    1. *Osmolite*
    2. *Osmolite HN* (high nitrogen) better for smaller people
    3. *Jevity:* equivalent to *osmolite HN* with fiber added; good for diarrhea and constipation; tolerated well
    4. *Magna cal:* 2 cal/mL (double that of standard formulas); good for fluid restricted pts.
    5. *Criticare:* formulated for pts under stress.
  - Immunoenhanced: specific nutrients including glutamine, arginine, omega-3 fatty acids and nucleotides improve infection rate and hospital length of stay; no effect on mortality (Crit Care Med 1999;27:2799).
    1. *IMPACT*
    2. Lipid emulsions: concentrated source of energy (FFA).
    3. *Immun-Aid:* adds glutamine for improved 6 mo survival in critically ill pts (Nutr 1997;13:752); branched-chain amino acids.
- Modular feedings provide supplemental single nutrient source: elements individually mixed by pharmacy to specific pt needs; most expensive.

Administration:

- Aspiration precautions: head up at 30°, CXR for tube placement prior to use, ongoing clinical vigilance for continuing bowel function.
- Begin with 1/4th strength at 20 mL/hr to prevent hypernatremia; for gastric feeding, increase concentration first, then vol; for small bowel feeding, increase vol first vs starting at full strength (Ger Rv Syllabus 2002;5:197) and bolusing several times per d over 20-30 min to avoid infusion pumps.
- May need TPN w enteral nutrition while building to adequate caloric and protein requirement.
- Check residuals every two hrs for first 48 hr of feeding.
- Decrease rate (hold feeds for 2 hr) for residuals > 100 mL.
- Continuous infusion (gravity or pump) during sleeping hours for small bowel feeding; start 30 mL/hr and increase by 30-50 mL q 8-12 hr; bolus of 200-400 mL q 4 hr for gastric feeding.
- Flush tube with 25-100 mL water after each continuous feed or bolus.
- Limit bacterial overgrowth by refrigerating tube feeds; no more than 4 hr at room temperature.

Complications: (See Table 11.8)

- Gastrointestinal: cramping, bloating, diarrhea; may rx by changing formula, concentrations of feeds or adding bulk agent; for poor gastric emptying may need metoclopramide or erythromycin.
- Mechanical: tube obstruction, dislodgement; gi obstruction and peritoneal leakage, necrosis gastric wall.
- Fluid, electrolyte abnormalities: hyperglycemia, hypernatremia, azotemia, hyperosmolar, non-ketonic coma, hypomagnesemia; daily electrolyte and glucose monitoring for first 48 hr; may add insulin to feeds to combat hyperglycemia; start with sliding scale; add approximate 24-hr sliding scale requirement to feeds.
- Aspiration: common, may be lethal (see above) a major cause of ARDS.

Table 11.8 Complications of Tube Feeding

Complication	Intervention
Aspiration pneumonia	Check tube placement before commencing feeding Elevate head properly while feeding Adjust feeding rate to minimize gastric distention
Diarrhea	Switch to different formula or dilution Administer kaolin-pectin suspension, paregoric, diphenoxylate, or codeine
Hyponatremia	Decrease water flushes Add sodium chloride to the formula Switch to a nutrient-dense formula
Skin irritation around tube site	Use cleansing mechanical barriers Use H2-blockers to decrease gastric acidity
Refeeding (decrease K, decrease PO4, decrease Mg)	Cautious advance over several days monitoring electrolytes

Adapted from Annals of Long-Term Care 1998;6(10):329.

GASTROINTESTINAL DISORDERS

11.11 Hyponatremia

Nejm 2000;342:1581

Table 11.9 Hyponatremia (< 135 mEq/L; < 120 mEq/L = seizures)

Decreased Serum Osm (< 275)			NI Osm	Increased Osm
Increased ECF	**NI ECF**	**Decreased ECF**	**Hyperlipidemia**	**Hyperglycemia**
Urine Na < 20 mEq/L CHF Cirrhosis	SIADH (CNS, lung, stress) Dilutional hyponatremia Urine Na > 20 mEq/L Urine Osm > 200 Morphine, tricyclics, nicotine, NSAIDs, sulfonylureas, hyponatremia, adrenal insufficiency	Urine Na > 20 mEq/L Renal Diuretic Addison's Dehydration	Hyperproteinemia	—
Rx: fluid restrict + furosemide; ?captopril	Water restrict; 0.9 or 3% saline + furosemide (increase Na 20 mEq/L/48 h)	Replace fluid; rx underlying disorder	—	—

ECF = extracellular fluid.

Reproduced with permission from Annals of Long-Term Care 98;6(supplement):4.

$$\text{Fractional excretion of } Na^+ = \frac{\text{Urine } Na^+/\text{Plasma } Na^+}{\text{Urine Cr/Plasma Cr}} \times 100$$

- Prerenal < 1%
- Renal (ATN) > 1%

Chapter 12

Dermatology

12.1 Skin Problems (Benign and Malignant Lesions)

Am J Med 1995;98:99S; J Am Acad Derm 1992;26:521; Nejm 1991;325:171; Am Fam Phys 1995;193; Geriatrics 1993;48:30; UCLA Ger Rv 9/2002. Skin Problems

Epidem: The incidence of skin cancers increases exponentially with age and is thought to be related to UVB irradiation cumulated over a life span; worse in geographical areas of decreased ozone.

Pathophys: Changes of aging skin.

Epidermis:

- Flattening of dermal-epidermal junction leads to incr propensity to blister and erode w shear force.
- Decreased moisture content of the stratum corneum; decreased secretion from sweat glands; xerosis.
- Decreased epidermal turnover: slowed wound healing; increased secondary infection following minor trauma; hyperproliferative disorders, such as psoriasis, tend to improve with age.
- Melanocytes decrease by about 10% every decade after 30 yr old, leading to depigmentation; melanin normally functions to absorb carcinogenic UV light.
- Cell-mediated immune response decreased (Langerhans' cells or macrophages in the epidermis); more susceptibility to cutaneous tumors, but less potential for allergic contact sensitization.

Dermis:

- The dermis decreases in density; relatively acellular, avascular, leading to poor insulation, pale skin, and hypo/hyperthermia; regression of subepidermal elastic fibers causes skin wrinkling; dermal clearance of foreign material decreased, prolonging contact dermatitis duration.

Skin Appendages:

- Sweat glands decreased causing dry skin, less body odor.
- Pacinian and Meissner's corpuscles decrease by approximately ⅔, predisposing elderly to trauma, burns and decreased ability to perform fine hand maneuvers.
- Subcutaneous tissue volume decreased within wt-bearing surfaces, such as feet, causing calluses, corns, ulcerations, and chronic pain.
- Wrinkles.

Rx: Topical Tretinoin inhibits irradiation-induced matrix metalloproteinase (Nejm 1997;337:1419); for non-sun-exposed (J Am Acad Derm 1993;29:25).

Prevention: Sunblock (15-30 SPF) applied q morning.

Photodermatitis

Appearance: Vesicles, papules, pustules; patches sun-exposed and lightly clothed areas.

Cause: Long wave UV light, drug induced (thiazides, furosemide, sulfonamides, NSAIDs floroquinolones amiodarone).

Eczema

Appearance: Dry skin, fine fissuring, pruritic; lower legs; worsening in the wintertime.

Rx: Of highest importance, increase hydration by applying emollients and bath oils, particularly after bathing; avoid excess exposure to water; increase use of room humidifiers; use steroid preparations only if severe or chronic.

- Topical steroids: low potency (triamcinolone 0.025%-0.1% cream); mid-potency (triamcinolone 0.1% lotion or ointment); high potency (triamcinolone 0.5% cream; high potency (fluocinonide 0.05% cream); super high potency (betamethasone dipropionate 0.05% ointment).
- Lotion or gel for acute lesion (oozing, crusting, vesicles) to help drying; cream for subacute lesions (scales, patches); ointment for chronic lesions (dry skin, plaques, lichenification).

Atopic Dermatitis

Rx: Although less common in elderly, best rx'd w lowest potency topical steroid, 2nd generation H1-antihistamines for sx relief. Calcineurin inhibitor (pimerolimus Elidel, tacrolimus Protopic), no skin atrophy, no adrenal suppression, no adverse ocular SE, expensive (Treat Guide L Med Lett 2007;5:79).

Seborrheic Dermatitis

Appearance: Greasy yellow scale w or w/o erythematous base on nasolabial folds, eyebrows, hairline, sideburns, posterior auricular, mid chest.

Rx: Hydrocortisone 1% × 2 wks, selenium sulfide.

Rosacea (Nejm 2005;352:793)

Appearance: Transient flushing, non-transient erythema, papules, pustules, telangectasia.

Cause: Facial mite (possibly), ETOH, spicy foods, hot drinks, sun-exposure, stress, exercise.

Rx: Metronidazole 0.75% cream or gel bid for 6-9 wk; rx pustules w doxycycline 100 mg po, telangiectasias w electrodesiccation, rhinophyma w plastic surgery.

Psoriasis

Appearance: (J Am Acad Derm 2002;46:1) Scaly, erythematous plaques on scalp, extensor surfaces; small pustules palms and soles.

Cause: T lymphocyte immune response systemic disorder.

Rx: Avoid drugs that adversely affect: β-blockers, lithium, ACE inhibitors, anti-malarials, systemic steroids, bupropion, radiologic contrast dye; mild limited, rx w topical corticosteroids; anthralin, tar 1-4% messy and irritating; recalcitrant cases w UV light, PUVA, topical vit D (calcipotriene) in limited doses for non-facial area, because irritating; yrs of rx w UV light, methotrexate, cyclosporine, strong topical steroids may predispose pts to other health problems.

Seborrheic Keratosis

Appearance: Disseminated, pigmented, waxy, "stuck on"; may be very large or thickened.

Crs: Benign.

Rx: Electrocautery, particularly for large lesions; liquid nitrogen may work.

Look-alikes: Bowen's disease, superficial spreading melanoma.

Actinic Keratosis

Appearance/Location: Multiple, red/brown, flat/raised, with adherent scale, "sandpaper" feel.

Crs: Most common precancerous lesion in whites, but frequency of overall conversion debated.

Rx: Liquid nitrogen, light 20-sec freeze; 5-fluorouracil 2-5% qd × 2-3 wk, may react w sun; warn pts of duration of sx of rx.

Bowen's Dermatosis

Appearance: 66% solitary, 33% multiple, sharply demarcated, scaly, flat or raised.

Crs: Not sun-induced; good prognosis.

Rx: Curettage; electrodesiccation; deep excision if hair follicle; topical fluorouracil bid several weeks to larger lesions; Moh's surgery (serial layers excised until no microscopic evidence of Ca remains) and laser therapy also are options.

Look Alikes: Eczema (palpable, thickened, red/brown w deepened skin lines), tinea, superficial basal cell carcinoma, irritated seborrheic keratosis.

Keratoacanthoma

Appearance: Common in elderly men, dome-shaped, flesh-colored smooth nodule with depressed center filled with keratin plug; sun-exposed areas; backs of hands, arms, central face.

Crs: Rapid growth 2 wk, stationary, involution.

Rx: Hard to distinguish from squamous cell cancer, so excision, or curettage; fulguration for lesions < 2 cm.

Squamous Cell Ca

Cause: Sun, coal tar, creosote oil, paraffin oil exposures.

Appearance/Location: Head, forearm, neck, back; firm erythematous nodule with indistinct margins.

Crs: Metastasize unpredictably to lymph nodes; most convert to malignant from actinic keratosis; ulcer indicates aggressive.

Rx: Electrosurgery; chemotherapy; Moh's surgery; surgery—wide excision or Moh's dependent on location; radiation.

Leukoplakia

Appearance: White plaque mucous membranes; hypertrophic.

Crs: Precancerous; 10-17% develop into squamous cell carcinoma (floor of mouth, ventral surface of tongue) 1-20 yr after initial onset.

Rx: Excisional bx, electrodesiccation, liquid nitrogen, topical fluorouracil, laser.

Look Alikes: Candidiasis, secondary syphilis, vulvar atrophy; lichen sclerosis et atrophicus (extends beyond mucous membrane to skin; if doesn't respond to topical estrogen or corticosteroid, should bx, although potential for malignancy is small).

Scabies (Arch Derm 2002;136:387)

Appearance: Itching erythematous, papular eruption; excoriation, secondary infection; axillary, waist, inner thigh, back, arm, leg; burrows between fingers.

Crs: Persists for decades untreated.

Rx: Scrape skin parallel to surface of burrow deep enough to cause pinpoint bleeding, use mineral oil and coverslip on slide to identify mite, egg or fecal material; lindane (Kwell) 1% or crotamiton (Eurax) 10% or permethrin cream (Elimite) 5% 12 hr, reapply in 1 wk, itches for 2 wk; vacuum rugs, hot water wash, then heat-dry clothes; treat close contacts; in NH: ivermectin 200 μgm/kg po × 1 dose.

Look Alikes: Other bites (not in web spaces).

Herpes Zoster

Appearance: Usually unilateral tingling or pain 4-5 d; erythematous grouped vesicles/crust; occasionally nodules, papules; may affect eye (corneal ulceration); any dermatomes may be involved.

Eye Findings:

1. Simplex: dendritic ulcers of cornea.
2. Zoster: periphery of cornea with vascularization, ulceration, dendrites can happen—uncommon.

Crs: Often extended course of many wks to several mo w "postherpetic" pain; some communicability and best to avoid unnecessary exposure; NH staff require gloves if vesicles, crusting.

Rx: If early, valacyclovir 1 gm tid × 7 d or famciclovir 500 mg tid × 7 d or acyclovir 800 mg 5 d 7-10 d; if established for > 3 d, antivirals not helpful (and are expensive); if no contraindication to corticosteroids (DM, HT, glaucoma) prednisone 60 mg tapered over 21 d may decrease risk of post-herpetic neuralgia (Nejm 1996;335:32); uveitis: topical corticosteroids w ophthalmologic consult, atropine to dilate pupils; pain management often a longer problem, since may require codeine or other opioids; for extended courses, long-term lower-dose anti-virals can be helpful; cover acute lesions to decrease communicability.

Pemphigus Vulgaris

Jags 1998;46:92

Appearance: Oral mucosa and skin; IgG, C3 deposits stratum malpighii; increased pemphigus antibody corresponds to severity of disease; Px favorable for older people; 50% Jewish.

Rx: Triamcinolone acetonide.

Bullous Pemphigoid

Nejm 1995;333:1475

Appearance: Sudden-onset urticarial plaques or intact tense blisters; flexural blisters, rapid spread; immuno-fluorescent studies: C3 along basement membrane.

Rx: Untreated lesions may become extensive and highly symptomatic, resulting in death; early administration of prednisone 40-60 mg/d gives best response and begin tapering when no new lesions appearing; 2nd rx: azathioprine, cyclophosphamide, cyclosporine, methotrexate, tetracycline, dapsone, sulfapyridine, gold; pulsed corticosteroids, plasmapheresis, high-dose immune globulin.

Look-Alikes: Pemphigus vulgaris: no urticarial plaques; immunofluorescent studies: antibodies against intercellular cement.

Onychogryphosis

Appearance: Nails patchy distal yellow discoloration; raised edge; fragile; later thickening and curvature of nails due to chronic trauma; more common in pts w atherosclerosis, fungi, or chronic paronychial infection (usually secondary to candidal infection).

Crs: Chronic; rx expensive and of limited value in elderly w few long-term cures.

Rx: Acetic acid (VoSol) or rubbing alcohol to affected nail fold results in evaporation of water in 10 min; if pseudomonas present, use gentamicin ointment; treat surrounding skin infections aggressively to improve comfort; nail cutting, grinding to reduce mass of nail important for foot comfort and injury prevention; onychomycosis—oral fluconazole 150 mg po/wk × 6 mo; oral terbinafine (lamisil) 250 mg/d × 3-4 mo, 60% cure rate, hepatic risk (3%) check liver function, may inhibit metabolism of antidepressants; Itraconozole pulse rx 200 bid × 7 d q mo × 3-4 mo.

Melanoma

Appearance: Worrisome if asymmetric, irregular borders, > 0.6 cm, multiple colors white, red, blue, black, evolving size, shape sx (itching, tender) surface (bleeding) shades of color (Jama 2004;296:2771).

Lab: Pathology of bx specimen. Clark levels:
I: limited to epidermis, no invasion
II: into but not filling papillary dermis, 95% 5-yr survival
III: filling papillary dermis
IV: reticular dermis
V: subcuticular fat, 5-yr survival 40%

Rx: Full excision primary lesion.

Oral Cancer

Epidem: Squamous 95%; risk factors: age, male, previous oral malignancy, tobacco, alcohol, exposure to sunlight (lip).

Crs: Prognosis without lymph node involvement: 50% 5-yr survival rate for tongue; 95% 5-yr survival rate for lip.

Rx:

Preventive: Quit smoking.

Therapeutic: High morbidity from surgical resection, irradiation, cytotoxic chemotherapy: disfigurement, speech impediment, salivary gland hypofunction, osteomyelitis.

12.2 Pressure Ulcers

J Am Ger Soc 1995;43:919; Geriatric Review Course September 2002, Assessment Pressure sores, Barbara Bates-Jensen; Jama 2003;289:223

Epidem: 50-70% in pts > 70 yr old in NH (J Am Ger Soc 1988;36:807); hospital prevalence 3-11%, with highest in coronary care unit; on admission to NH 11-35%.

Pathophys: When pressure exceeds 32 mmHg, capillary blood flow is halted; prolonged hypoperfusion leads to hypoxia, acidosis, hemorrhage into the interstitium (nonblanchable erythema), toxic cellular wastes, cell death, and tissue necrosis (Med Clin N Am 1989;73:1511); pressure against the epidermis results in highest pressure nearest the bone, because pressure is more easily dissipated w deformation of the more superficial tissues.

- Pressure, friction, shear, chronic exposure to water (Ped Derm 1994;11:18); deficiencies in ascorbic acid, zinc, Fe (J Am Ger Soc 1993;41:357).

Si: (See Table 12.1) Check collateral circulation with ankle brachial index; deep tissue injury w purple black discoloration of tissue; size (length, width) exudates amount, tissue type predict healing

Table 12.1	Staging of Pressure Sores
Stage I	Nonblanchable erythema of intact skin; early pressure sore may appear postoperatively as bruising
Stage II	Abrasion, opened blister, partial thickness involving epidermis and/or dermis
Stage III	Necrosis, undermining; full-thickness loss into the subcutaneous tissue
Stage IV	Sinus tracts, extension into the fascia, muscle, bone

Note: Most commonly scapula, iliac crest, sacrum, ischium, trochanter, lateral malleolus, heel, lateral edge of foot.

of ulcer, use PUSH (Pressure Ulcer Healing Graph) tool (http://www.npuap.org/push3-0.html).

Cmplc: Offending organisms in sepsis: *Proteus mirabilis*, *E. coli*, *Pseudomonas aeruginosa*, *Klebsiella*, *Bacteroides* fragilis; recurrence of pressure ulcer within 2 yr of surgical primary wound closure (Adv Wound Care 1994;7:40).

Lab:

- ESR to r/o osteomyelitis; serum albumin; CBC; serum glucose.
- Suspect osteomyelitis w elevated wbc, fever, and poor wound healing.

Rx:

Preventive:

- Braden scale predictive value 64-77% (Decubitus 1989;2:44); Norton scale predictive value 0-37%; other similar scales (Am Fam Phys 1996;54:1519).
- Address risk factors for pressure sores in all pts: lymphopenia, immobility, dry skin, decreased body weight (Jama 1995; 273:865).

Nonblanchable erythema is very important early sign (address immediately); turn sequentially from back to left to right side q 2 hr; avoid direct pressure on the greater trochanter and lateral malleolus by positioning back at a 30° angle to the bed w pillows between knees and lower legs and along back and arms to maintain optimal positioning (AHCPR Public No. 92-0047, 1992); reposition pts in chairs q 1 hr; use trapezes, draw sheets; sitting on doughnut-type padding may cause ischemia (Ann IM 1986;105:337); education of multidisciplinary team decreased incidence of pressure sores by 63% (Arch IM 1988;148:2241).

Therapeutic: (See Table 12.2)

J Palliative Care Med 2007;10:1161

1. Relieve pressure: mattresses and beds (list-J Am Ger Soc 1995;43:919); low-air-loss mattress cost-effective (Jama 1993;269:494; J Gerontol 1995;141:6); air-fluidized beds for stages III-IV on two of the following areas: left hip, right hip, sacrum; or w recalcitrant wounds (J Am Ger Soc 1989; 37:235); 4-layer compression bandage more cost effective in persistent venous ulcers (BMJ 1998;316:1487). In hosp: alternative pressure mattress better results (BMJ 2006;332:1416).
2. Remove necrotic debris: autolytic, enzymatic, or sharp debridement.
3. Control local infection: avoid systemic antibiotics unless there is an abscess or expanding cellulitis, then use clindamycin and fluoroquinolones; avoid topical antiseptics such as hydrogen peroxide, potassium hypochlorite (Dakin's solution), acetic acid, povidone-iodine (Betadine), may inhibit fibroblast growth (Clin Ger Med 1992;8:835; J Trauma 1993;35:8); MRSA-infected wound: topical mupirocin (Bactroban); malodorous pressure sores: metronidazole gel (Am Fam Phys 1996;54:1519) or crushed metronidazole tablets less expensive.
4. Protect healthy tissue: stages II and III w little exudate; use foam island or hydrocolloid, change q 3 d.
5. Promote granulation: moist environment hastens healing w increased migration of fibroblasts and growth factor; hydrocolloid dressing q 3-5 d for stages III and IV, better than wet to dry, watch for infection; deep wound packing w space-occupying (eg, calcium alginates) or salt-impregnated dressings (Mesalt) for stages III and IV (J Am Ger Soc 1995;43:919).

Table 12.2 Categories of Products and Devices Commonly Used in Wound Care

Category	Description	Characteristics	Concerns	Applications
Gauze, dry or wet	• Woven natural cotton fibers; non-woven rayon and polyester blends • Available in pads and rolls, sterile and non-sterile	• May be dampened with saline or water • Inexpensive • Facilitates wet-to-dry debridement • Non-adherent when used as wet-to-moist dressing • Minimally to moderately absorbent	• Wet-to-dry debridement painful, may damage healthy tissue • Woven variety is abrasive • May dehydrate wound • Requires frequent changes • Packing may harden, causing further pressure injury	*As primary dressing:* • Deep wounds; can be packed into undermined or tunneling areas *As secondary dressing:* • Can maintain a moist environment if kept moist, or under an occlusive secondary dressing • Can be used in large, necrotic wounds or presence of soft tissue infection
Impregnated gauze pads	• Woven or non-woven materials in which substances such as saline, water, iodinated agents, petrolatum, zinc compounds, sodium chloride, chlorhexadine gluconate, bismuth tribromophenate, or other materials have been incorporated	• Inexpensive • Non-adherent with specific product formulations	• Some impregnated materials may be toxic to living tissue	• See above

Pressure Ulcer Therapy Companion Clinical Practice Guideline, Columbia, MD 1999;21-22. "Copyright © 1998 American Medical Directors Association, All Rights Reserved"

6. General condition: high-protein diet (24% protein) enhances wound healing (J Am Ger Soc 1993;41:357); ascorbic acid 500 mg bid (J Gen Intern Med 1991;6:81); zinc 200-600 mg qd (Ann IM 1986;105:342; Adv Wound Care 1996;9:8); nitro paste 2% for vasodilation (Jags 1997;45:895).
   - Other rx options: fibroblast growth factor (J Clin Invest 1993;92:2841), hyperbaric oxygen (Jama 1990; 263:2216; Nejm 1996;334:1642); silver dressings to reduce infection, wound warming therapy, becaplermin (Regranex) for diabetic ulcers, recombinant human platelet derived growth factor for full thickness neuropathic ulcer-not if infected.
   - Expected rate of healing: stage I : 1 d-1 wk, stage II: 5 d-3 mo, stage III: 1-6 mo; stage IV: 6 mo-1 yr).

Chapter 13

Ethics

Clin Ger Med 1994;10:403; Arch IM 1995;155:502; Nejm 2007;357:1834

13.1 Competency (Decision-Making Capacity)

Legal standards for competency (Jags 2000;48:913); capacity is medical assessment, while competency is legal assessment.

"Informed consent" depends on competency, a legal definition; pt must demonstrate: (See Table 13.2)

1. Ability to evidence a choice about treatment.
2. Capacity to have factual understanding of the information that the average pt would consider material to making the health care decision in question.
3. The ability to rationally manipulate information.
4. The capacity to appreciate the nature of the specific situation (Am J Psych 1977;134:3).

Mini-Mental State Exam (MMSE) not good for predicting competency; scores < 7 incompetent; score $> 27 =$ competent; scores 7-27 not helpful; decision-making capacity in elderly does not compare well to MMSE, and should be assessed by direct methods (J Am Ger Soc 1990;38:1097; Am J Psych 1977;134:3); autonomy assumes that persons possess the capacity to decide, to carry out decisions, and to manage and be accountable for the consequences of their decisions (J Am Ger Soc 1995;43:1437). 50% elderly inpatients lack capacity (Lancet 2004;354:1421).

Table 13.1 Competency Profile

Name:	SS#:	Date:	
Decision to be made:			
Criterion	**Independent**	**With Assistance**	**Unable**
1. Receives information			
2. Recognizes relevant information as information			
3. Remembers information			
4. Relates situation to oneself, values, and circumstances			
5. Reasons about alternatives			
6. Ranks alternatives in order of preference			
7. Resolves situations (dilemmas)			
8. Resigns self to the decision			
9. Recounts one's decision-making process			
10. Organizes effort to implement the decision			

Adapted from Nursing Home Medicine 1996;4(8):49A.

Advance Directives (Jama 1997;277:1854)

Pts, families, and providers need to consider the following rx decisions:

1. Cardiac arrest
2. Acute, reversible, life-threatening event
3. Acute, non-reversible, life-threatening event
4. Nutrition
5. Routine blood work (J Am Ger Soc 1991;39:396,1221)
6. Artificial hydration
7. Antibiotics at end of life

Directives completed at higher rates w physician-directed intervention (Arch IM 1994;154:2321); pre-hospital code status

Table 13.2 Mnemonic for Evaluating Competency

"C"—consistent	Consistent on serial Mini Mental State Exam (MMSE); consistent decision on serial questioning; and consistent w life values
"O"—other alternatives to therapy	Understands other care alternatives, which, in turn, requires ability to understand factual material and manipulate information rationally
"M"—malleable	Physician must remain malleable; pts and families change their minds about end-of-life decisions in different settings and decisions should be reviewed w a change of setting
"P"—particulars	Pt must be able to appreciate the nature of the particular situation; physician must be particular about what pt is competent to do, eg, can decide health care but not run a household; degree of competence (supramaximal, full, limited) may differ depending on the domain (civil, personal, financial, health care) (Nurs Home Med 1996;4:81); least restrictive guardianship is the goal (partial capacity)

can be effectively made in the NH setting; have no effect on the short term but decrease use of hospital in the last months of life (J Am Ger Soc 1995;43:113).

Pts overemphasize benefit of CPR (J Gen Intern Med 1993; 8:295), but prognostic information influences decisions and most elderly do not want CPR (Nejm 1994;4:330,545); 14% of elderly will change opinion based on more information (Jama 1995; 274:1775); doctors inaccurate in predicting survival of most terminally ill pts, perhaps why continued low rate of hospice referrals (BMJ 2000;320:469).

Medical futility: physiologic intervention no plausible effect on disease (Clinics in Ger Med 2005;21:211). Quantitative: extremely unlikely to have effect on disease. Qualitative: not improved, possibly diminished quality of life.

APACHE (Acute Physiology and Chronic Health Evaluation) predictors of mortality depend on severity of illness and not age; age alone does not predict survival (J Am Ger Soc 1995;43: 520,1131; Am J Emerg Med 1995;13:389; Jama 1990;264:2109); decreased survival in hospitalized pts > 70 yr old probably due to underlying med problems; predictors of poor outcome following CPR: hct < 35, creatinine > 1.5, BUN > 65, albumin < 2.7 gm/dL (Ann IM 1989;7:199; J Am Ger Soc 1990;38:1057); success rate of CPR in elderly > 70 yr old so low may not be worthwhile (Ann IM 1989;111:193,199; Arch IM 1993;153:1293); poor outcome in NH facilities (J Am Ger Soc 1993;41:163,384).

Life values and resuscitation preferences are related; therefore important to discuss together (J Am Ger Soc 1996;44:958).

Nutrition:

- Basic human need vs extraordinary medical intervention (Clin Ger Med 1994;10:475); survey of NG tube feeds in elderly pts in a community hospital found that 53% of the time restraints were needed, and 24 of 29 pts were judged to be incompetent (Clin Ger Med 1994;10:475; Arch IM 1989;149:1937).
- States have various statutes regarding when tube feeding can be stopped or not started (Clin Ger Med 1994;10:475).
- Complete starvation associated with euphoria and analgesia (J Gen Intern Med 1993;8:220; Clin Ger Med 1994;10:475).
- Hypernatremia, hypercalciuria, hyperosmolarity, azotemia all produce sedation during dying process (P. Rousseau *Hospice: Ethical issues in End-of-life care* Mar 1998 San Antonio, Texas-American Medical Directors Association Annual Conference).
- Feeding tubes do not prevent aspiration; pts w dementia who are fed by tube vs by hand have same survival rates; long-term rates of complications from tube feeding 32-70% including restraining pt; pts cannot enjoy eating w feeding tube; most pts change their mind about tube feeding when told they might have to be restrained (Nejm 2000;342:206), not helpful for terminally ill (Am J Hosp Palliat Care 2006;23:369).

Substituted Judgment

- Competent pt can leave advance directives (a living will, or durable power of attorney for health care); cannot infer CPR decision on basis of pt having a "living will" (Arch IM 1995;155:171).
- Majority directives to carry out CPR are made by pts; the majority of DNR orders are made by families (Arch IM 1992; 152:561; Jama 1985;253:2236); physicians and families are not good at predicting pt preferences (Arch Fam Med 1994;3:1057).
- Long-term care residents at NH do not have long-term survival from CPR (J Am Ger Med 1993;41:163).
- Poor survival in NH patients w unwitnessed arrest or asystole, electrical mechanical dissociation (J Am Ger Soc 1995; 43:520); NH medical directors are more likely to support withholding rx in terminally ill pts, but are generally not in favor of mandatory DNR orders (J Am Ger Med 1995;43:1131; J Am Board Fam Pract 1993;6:91; Ann EM 1994;23:997).
- If no appropriate surrogate can be found, then group of individuals who care for the pt may determine treatment (multidisciplinary health care team) according to AGS ethics committee position 3 (J Am Ger Soc 1996;44:986).
- Terminal pts request aggressive rx when physicians have not given them realistic assessment of their px (Jama 1998; 279:1709); families more likely to be accurate when have spoken w pt about end-of-life decisions, when pt has private insurance, when either have high school diploma; less accurate when surrogate has personal experience w life-sustaining therapy, attended religious services or when pt anticipated living > 10 y/o (Ann IM 1998;128:621).
- Prior competent choice may be superceded by best interest standards if pt's subjective experience at time of therapy clearly indicates change in preference (Jags 1998;46:922).

Refusal of Treatment

Competent Patients: Have the right to refuse rx; rx against pt's wishes can be construed as assault and battery and has been prosecuted as such (Clin Ger Med 1994;10:475).

Incapacitated Patients: Rigid criteria such as permanent unconsciousness or poorly defined categories such as terminal condition inadequate alone to determine whether surrogate should have authority to refuse life-sustaining rx for pt because often substantial uncertainty about px and most pt preferences are based on projected quality, not quantity, of life (AGS ethics committee position 8-J Am Ger Soc 1996;44:986).

Physician-Assisted Suicide (Euthanasia):

- More ethical solution might be rx of pain, especially in dying pts, and compassionate care; pts unduly influenced by physical suffering, impairment, abandonment, financial bankruptcy (J Am Ger Soc 1995;43:553); rx of mild-to-moderate depression does not necessarily result in increased desire for life-sustaining measures (J Gerontol 1994;49:M15; Nejm 1997; 337:1234; Palliat Med 1998;12:255).
- Assess cognitive status; assess how support people and family feel about suicide plan; explore unresolved religious, spiritual concerns (Ann IM 2000;132:209).

Principle of Double Effect: If primary intent of treatment is to do good, but may be accompanied by harm, then ethically acceptable to administer treatment.

Withdrawing of Therapy: Not obligated to continue a therapy that is not accomplishing any of the predefined goals of therapy, if the following conditions apply:

1. Pt has irreversible loss of cognitive function.
2. No goal other than sustaining organic life is accomplished by therapy.
3. No other goals of therapy can be achieved.

4. Pt has not previously expressed preference for being sustained on support (Clin Ger Med 1994;10:475); position supported by AMA council on ethical and judicial affairs.

Withholding rx vs withdrawing rx may or not be morally equivalent (J Am Ger Soc 1995;43:716; President's Commission for the Study of Ethical Problems in Biomedical and Behavioral Research, City U.S. Government Printing Office 1983); distinction exists between withholding and withdrawing very low-burden interventions in chronically ill patients, eg, pacemaker: changing timing of death, not killing (Jama 2000;283:1061)

Truth Telling (eg, Alzheimer's):

When pt's decision-making capacity and ability to cope w med information is impaired enough to warrant withholding information vs withholding information that deprives pt of opportunity to act on important medical and non-med (financial planning) life decisions.

Index

INDEX

C

D

E

F

G

H

I

J

K

L

M

N

O

P

Q

R

S

T

U

V

W

Y

Z